Personalized Immunosuppression in Transplantation

Personalized Immunosuppression in Transplantation
Role of Biomarker Monitoring and Therapeutic Drug Monitoring

Edited by

Michael Oellerich, MD

Lower Saxony Distinguished Professor of Clinical Chemistry,
George-August University, University Medicine Göttingen,
Göttingen, Germany

and

Amitava Dasgupta, PhD

Professor of Pathology and Laboratory Medicine,
University of Texas Medical School at Houston,
Houston, TX, USA

AMSTERDAM • BOSTON • HEIDELBERG • LONDON
NEW YORK • OXFORD • PARIS • SAN DIEGO
SAN FRANCISCO • SINGAPORE • SYDNEY • TOKYO

ELSEVIER

Elsevier
Radarweg 29, PO Box 211, 1000 AE Amsterdam, Netherlands
The Boulevard, Langford Lane, Kidlington, Oxford OX5 1GB, UK
225 Wyman Street, Waltham, MA 02451, USA

British Library Cataloguing-in-Publication Data
A catalogue record for this book is available from the British Library

Library of Congress Cataloging-in-Publication Data
A catalog record for this book is available from the Library of Congress

ISBN: 978-0-12-800885-0

For Information on all Elsevier books,
visit our website at http://store.elsevier.com/

Printed and bound in the United States of America

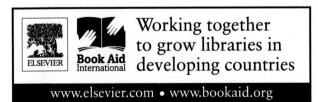

www.elsevier.com • www.bookaid.org

Publisher: Mica Haley
Acquisition Editor: Mara Conner
Editorial Project Manager: Jeffrey Rossetti
Production Project Manager: Melissa Read
Designer: Maria Ines Cruz

Contents

Preface

Approximately 30,000 patients per year in the United States receive a transplanted organ. There are another 100,000 on US waiting lists due to the shortage of donor organs, and currently approximately 200,000 living graft recipients live in the United States. In the European Union, approximately 64,000 patients were on the waiting list in 2012, of which approximately 6% died while waiting for an organ. The discrepancy between donor availability and patients waiting for organs mandates continuing attempts to both increase donor numbers and maximize transplantation outcomes. After transplantation, these patients receive lifelong therapy with various immunosuppressant drugs. Although therapeutic drug monitoring is useful in preventing toxicity of various immunosuppressants, unfortunately, even highly accurate therapeutic drug monitoring using chromatography combined with tandem mass spectrometry cannot precisely predict efficacy or the possibility of rejection. In addition, genetic variation in *CYP3A5* may affect the metabolism and disposition of certain immunosuppressants, so therapeutic drug monitoring is useful only as a phenotype approach to personalize immunosuppressant therapy in transplant patients. Direct pharmacogenomics testing prior to the administration of immunosuppressants may be a superior approach into managing immunosuppressant therapy compared to traditional therapeutic drug monitoring. Recently, biomarker monitoring such as interleukin-2 expression by CD8$^+$ T lymphocytes or graft-derived cell-free DNA among other markers is gaining importance as a complementary approach for personalized immunosuppression to guide therapeutic decision-making following organ transplantation. Conventional biomarkers such as creatinine are often increased only after 50% loss of kidney function, and reliable noninvasive markers for cardiac rejection are lacking. Very recently, monitoring graft-derived circulating cell-free DNA has shown promise in the early detection of transplant injury as a "liquid biopsy" and may enable earlier intervention.

This book is directed at professionals including pathologists, toxicologists, and transplant surgeons who are involved in the management of transplant patients. As such, this book provides in-depth coverage of the management of immunosuppressant therapy in transplant patients with a goal of personalized therapy so that each patient can obtain the maximum benefit of his or her drug therapy with minimal risk of experiencing drug toxicity. Practical guidelines are included for managing immunosuppressant therapy, including the therapeutic ranges of various immunosuppressants, the pitfalls of methodologies used for determination of these immunosuppressants in whole blood or plasma, appropriate pharmacogenomics testing for organ transplant recipients, and when biomarker monitoring could be helpful. To our knowledge, this is the first book to focus on the personalized management of immunosuppression therapy in individual transplant patients: how to provide a given patient with an optimal immunosuppression therapy to avoid acute organ rejection or irreversible chronic allograft dysfunction while at the same time avoid or minimize the toxicity of these agents.

There are 11 chapters. In the first four chapters, issues of therapeutic drug monitoring of various immunosuppressants are addressed, including methodological challenges and problems of interferences in therapeutic drug monitoring of immunosuppressants using immunoassays. Chapter 4 addresses the clinical utility of monitoring free (unbound) mycophenolic acid, whereas Chapter 5 addresses pharmacogenomics issues related to therapy with immunosuppressants. Chapter 6 provides an overview of biomarker monitoring during immunosuppressant therapy, and Chapters 7–11 address various biomarker monitoring strategies during immunosuppressant therapy with a goal of achieving personalized immunosuppression. Chapter 7 discusses recent discoveries of graft-derived circulating cell-free DNA as a marker of graft injury in organ transplantation. Chapter 8 focuses on biomarkers of tolerance in kidney transplantation. Chapter 9 addresses issues of intracellular concentrations of immunosuppressants. Chapter 10 focuses on markers of lymphocyte activation and proliferation. Finally, Chapter 11 is devoted to discussion of NFAT-regulated gene expression.

We are grateful to all contributors, who are internationally known experts in their respected fields. Without their dedicated efforts, we would not have been able to publish this book. We also thank our wives, Pushpa (Oellerich) and Alice (Dasgupta), for putting up with us during long evening and weekend hours we devoted to writing chapters and editing this book. Lastly, our readers will be the final judge of the quality of our book. If readers enjoy reading this book, the efforts of all contributors and editors will be duly rewarded.

Michael Oellerich
Göttingen, Germany

Amitava Dasgupta
Houston, TX, USA

List of Contributors

Daniel Baron
INSERM, Nantes, France, CHU de Nantes, ITUN, Nantes, France, and Université de Nantes, Faculté de Médecine, Nantes, France

Julia Beck
Chronix Biomedical GmbH, Göttingen, Germany

Stein Bergan
Department of Pharmacology, Oslo University Hospital, Oslo, Norway; School of Pharmacy, University of Oslo, Oslo, Norway

Heike Bittersohl
Institute of Clinical Chemistry and Pathobiochemistry, Klinikum rechts der Isar der TU München, Munich, Germany

Sara Bremer
Department of Medical Biochemistry, Oslo University Hospital, Oslo, Norway

Sophie Brouard
INSERM, Nantes, France, CHU de Nantes, ITUN, Nantes, France, and Université de Nantes, Faculté de Médecine, Nantes, France

Amitava Dasgupta
Department of Pathology and Laboratory Medicine, University of Texas–Houston Medical School, Houston, TX, USA

Magali Giral
INSERM, Nantes, France, CHU de Nantes, ITUN, Nantes, France, and Université de Nantes, Faculté de Médecine, Nantes, France

Kamisha L. Johnson-Davis
Department of Pathology, University of Utah Health Sciences Center, Salt Lake City, UT, USA, and ARUP Institute for Clinical and Experimental Pathology, Salt Lake City, UT, USA

Philipp Kanzow
Department of Clinical Pharmacology, University Medicine Göttingen, Göttingen, Germany; Department of Preventive Dentistry, Periodontology and Cardiology, University Medicine Göttingen, Göttingen, Germany

Otto Kollmar
Department of General Visceral and Paediatric Surgery, University Medicine Göttingen, Göttingen, Germany

Loralie Langman
Department of Laboratory Medicine and Pathology, Mayo Clinic College of Medicine, Rochester, MN, USA

Gwendolyn A. McMillin
Department of Pathology, University of Utah Health Sciences Center, Salt Lake City, UT, USA, and ARUP Institute for Clinical and Experimental Pathology, Salt Lake City, UT, USA

Michael C. Milone
Hospital of the University of Pennsylvania, Philadelphia, PA, USA

Michael Oellerich
Department of Clinical Pharmacology, University Medicine Göttingen, Göttingen, Germany

Jessica Schmitz
Department of Clinical Pharmacology, University Medicine Göttingen, Göttingen, Germany

Ekkehard Schütz
Chronix Biomedical GmbH, Göttingen, Germany

Maria Shipkova
Head Laboratory for Therapeutic Drug Monitoring and Clinical Toxicology, Central Institute for Clinical Chemistry and Laboratory Medicine, Klinikum Stuttgart, Germany

Werner Steimer
Institute of Clinical Chemistry and Pathobiochemistry, Klinikum rechts der Isar der TU München, Munich, Germany

Teun van Gelder
Departments of Internal Medicine and Hospital Pharmacy, Erasmus University Medical Center, Rotterdam, Netherlands

Ron H.N. van Schaik
European Specialist Laboratory Medicine, Department of Clinical Chemistry, Erasmus University Medical Center, Rotterdam, Netherlands

Nils Tore Vethe
Department of Pharmacology, Oslo University Hospital, Oslo, Norway

Philip D. Walson
Department of Clinical Pharmacology, University Medicine Göttingen, Göttingen, Germany

Eberhard Wieland
Central Institute for Clinical Chemistry and Laboratory Medicine, Klinikum Stuttgart, Stuttgart, Germany

Overview of the pharmacology and toxicology of immunosuppressant agents that require therapeutic drug monitoring

1

Michael C. Milone

Hospital of the University of Pennsylvania, Philadelphia, PA, USA

1.1 INTRODUCTION

More than 100,000 solid organ and 50,000 allogeneic bone marrow transplants are currently performed worldwide each year. Outcomes vary widely depending on the transplant type and underlying disease; however, solid organ allograft survival has improved significantly during the past quarter century coinciding with the introduction of new immunosuppressive drugs (ISDs). ISDs are critical to transplantation success due to the potent cellular and humoral immune mechanisms that restrict allogeneic transplantation. Whereas early ISDs consisted primarily of glucocorticoids and antimetabolite drugs to block lymphocyte proliferation, several ISDs with differing mechanisms of action have been introduced, including the recent introduction of the first biologic agent, belatacept (Nulojix, a CTLA4–Ig fusion protein), which interferes with a critical step in the initiation of T cell-mediated immunity. Although these agents have significantly improved outcomes, their benefits often come at a cost of increased risk of infection as well as toxicity. The use of ISDs to control allograft rejection and graft-versus-host disease is very difficult because errors can lead to serious and sometimes fatal consequences for the transplant recipient.

One of the greatest challenges to effectively using ISDs is their widely variable pharmacokinetic behavior across individuals. This pharmacokinetic variability makes it difficult to predict a priori an individual's response to a drug following administration of a particular dose. Applying knowledge of a drug's concentration and pharmacokinetic behavior within an individual to the clinical use of a drug, often termed therapeutic drug monitoring (TDM), has therefore become a standard approach to ISD therapy aimed at mitigating the risks associated with the use of these drugs. An important prerequisite to successful TDM is the ability to measure a drug of interest. Using modern technologies that are available within most analytical

M. Oellerich & A. Dasgupta (Eds): Personalized Immunosuppression in Transplantation.
DOI: http://dx.doi.org/10.1016/B978-0-12-800885-0.00001-1

chemistry laboratories, the measurement of drugs, including ISDs and their metabolites, is readily achieved as described in the following chapters of this book.

Unfortunately, having the plasma or whole blood concentration of a drug is not enough for proper patient management. Effective use of drug concentration data also requires a thorough understanding of the pharmacodynamics relationship between drug exposure and important clinical outcomes of toxicity or efficacy. Like pharmacokinetics, the pharmacodynamics of ISDs also vary greatly across individuals [1], but a measured drug concentration does not provide insight into this variability. Biomarkers of organ function, tissue injury, and immune function provide some insight into the pharmacodynamics of ISDs. In the broadest sense, TDM may be considered to encompass an array of testing modalities beyond traditional concentration monitoring, such as the use of serum creatinine to monitor the nephrotoxic effects of drugs such as the calcineurin inhibitors, tacrolimus, or cyclosporine. Several of the subsequent chapters are devoted to exploring these biomarker-based testing approaches. In this chapter, the ISDs currently approved for use in solid organ and bone marrow transplantation are discussed with a focus on their pharmacology and clinical use.

1.2 CALCINEURIN INHIBITORS

Currently, two calcineurin inhibitors (CNIs), cyclosporine and tacrolimus, are commonly used clinically as immunosuppressants. This section provides an overview of these two drugs.

1.2.1 CYCLOSPORINE A

Introduced in the 1980s, cyclosporine A (CsA) revolutionized the care of transplant patients through its potent inhibition of acute cellular transplant rejection. Although its use has gradually been replaced by tacrolimus, it is currently used in approximately 10% of transplants. It is typically used in combination with other immunosuppressive drugs such as mycophenolic acid, azathioprine, and glucocorticoids. Originally isolated in 1969 from the soil fungus *Tolypocladium inflatum* by Hans Peter Frey, a biologist working at Sandoz Pharmaceuticals, CsA is a lipophilic, cyclic endecapeptide composed of *N*-methylated amino acids, making it resistant to intestinal digestion as shown in Figure 1.1A. It is highly lipophilic and only slightly water-soluble. It derives its primary immunosuppressive activity by selectively binding to cyclophilin A, a peptidylprolyl isomerase present within the cytoplasm of cells. Once bound, the CsA/cyclophilin complex inhibits the enzymatic activity of the calcineurin (CN), a heterodimeric, calcium-dependent serine/threonine phosphatase composed of CNA and CNB subunits that is activated by the rapid rise in intracellular calcium following T cell receptor engagement. CN removes a critical regulatory phosphorylation on nuclear factor of activated T cells (NFATc) triggering its translocation to the nucleus of T cells, where it synergizes with other factors to mediate the transcription

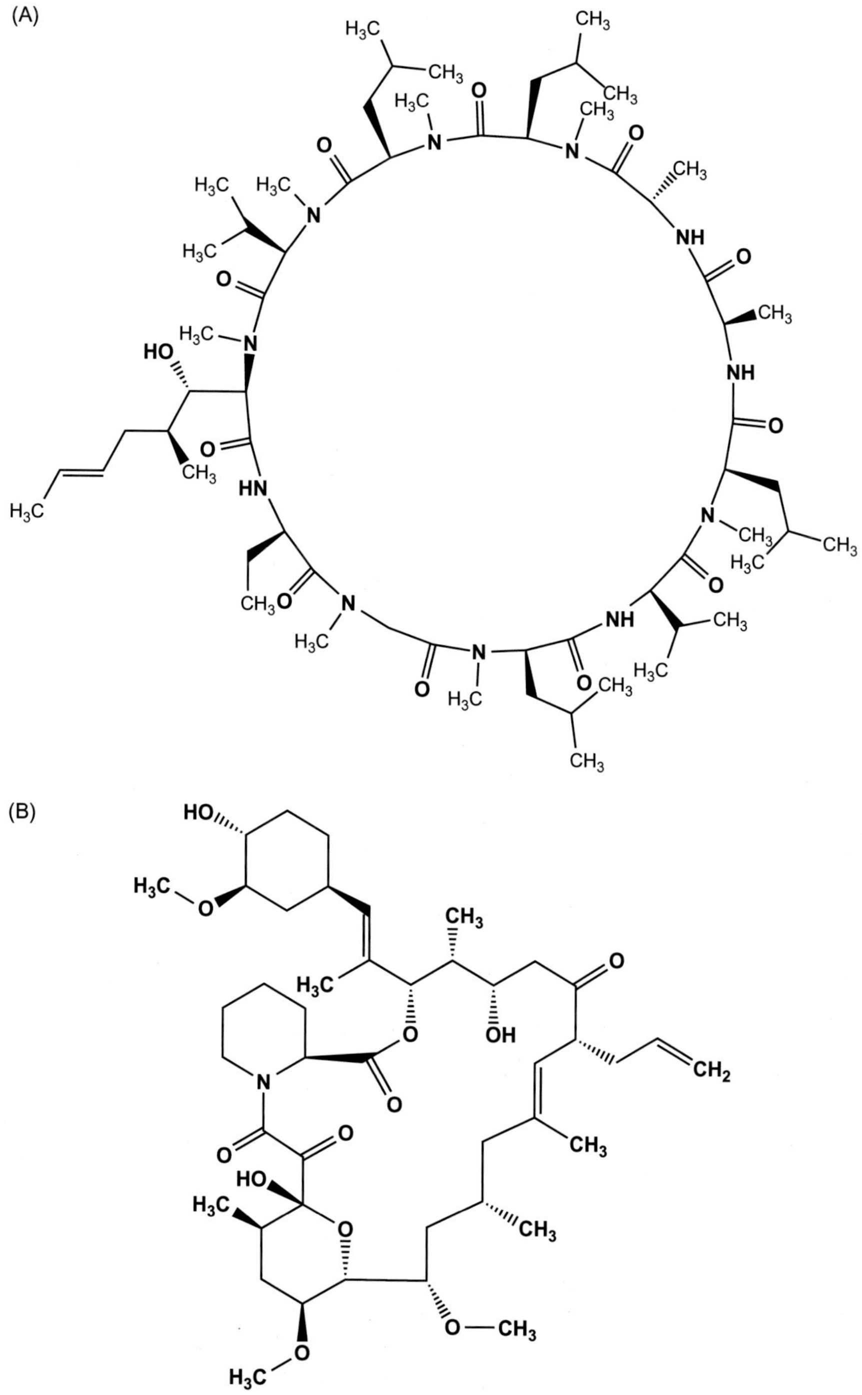

FIGURE 1.1 Calcineurin inhibitors and their mechanism of action.

(A) Structure of cyclosporine A; (B) structure of tacrolimus;

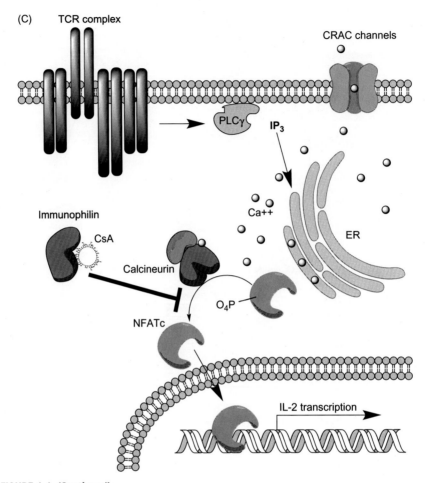

FIGURE 1.1 (Continued)

(C) schematic of calcineurin–NFATc signaling pathway in T cells that is inhibited by CsA and TRL. CRAC channel, calcium release activated channel (Orai1); PLCγ, phospholipase Cγ; IP_3, inositol triphosphate.

of a large number of genes, including interleukin-2 (IL-2), an important cytokine for T cell proliferation, and CD40 ligand (CD40L), an important costimulatory ligand for B cells, as schematically diagrammed in Figure 1.1B. Although the calcineurin–NFATc pathway is critical to T cell activation, this pathway plays a role in diverse cell types, including neurons [2,3], skeletal and cardiac myocytes [4,5], and endothelium [6]. These non-immune roles of calcineurin–NFATc signaling may contribute to the toxicity observed with the clinical use of cyclosporine, which includes nephrotoxicity, neurologic toxicity (e.g., tremors and headaches), and diabetes.

Due to the highly lipophilic nature of CsA, the original therapeutic formulation of CsA (Sandimmune) was an oral solution of the drug dissolved in oil. This solution was then mixed with a liquid such as juice prior to consumption. Early pharmacokinetic studies revealed that CsA absorption with this formulation was slow and erratic with poor bioavailability, leading to significant intra- and interindividual variability in CsA exposure. Studies of CsA given to healthy volunteers by intravenous (IV) and oral routes demonstrated a median oral bioavailability of 21.2% [7]. CsA is highly protein bound and exhibits a large volume of distribution at steady state that ranges from 3 to 5 L/kg due to the high affinity for cyclophilins within tissues including red blood cells (RBCs) [8]. As a result of the extensive binding to RBCs, whole blood concentrations of CsA are commonly used for most pharmacokinetic (PK) studies. In addition to highly variable bioavailability, CsA also displays significant variability in clearance that spans greater than an order of magnitude (0.63–23.9 ml/min/kg) in healthy individuals [7].

Due to the poor oral bioavailability observed with these early preparations of CsA, formulations based on an oil-based microemulsion (Neoral or Gengraf) were developed in an effort to improve absorption [9]. The oral bioavailability of the microemulsion formulations was significantly improved. Bioavailability is still lower in liver transplant recipients compared to kidney transplant recipients [8]. Biliary flow and the presence of bile is a major factor affecting intestinal absorption of CsA, as illustrated by the greater than fourfold increase in bioavailability observed in liver transplant patients following T-tube clamping [10]. The improved bioavailability of CsA microemulsion is paralleled by improvements in absorption kinetics leading to a more consistent time to peak concentration and superior dose linearity with exposure. Despite these improvements in formulation, significant pharmacokinetic variability remains, with the dose-adjusted area under the concentration curve (AUC) of microemulsion-formulated cyclosporine demonstrating a greater than 20% coefficient of variation (CV) across individuals [11].

In addition to the wide variability in absorption, the variability in CsA metabolism and elimination is also clinically important. CsA is extensively metabolized to more than 25 different metabolites primarily via the cytochrome P450 3A (CYP3A) system [8,12–14]. Excretion is mostly biliary, with greater than 90% of the parent drug eliminated by this route. Renal excretion in urine accounts for only approximately 6% of drug elimination, with the vast majority excreted as CsA metabolites. As a result, renal failure has minimal effect on the clearance of CsA compared with the dramatic alterations in CsA absorption and clearance in patients with liver failure. CsA is also highly bound to cyclophilins within tissues, including RBCs. Due to the high protein binding, little CsA is also removed by hemodialysis [15]. CsA is subject to numerous drug and food interactions. Grapefruit and red wine, as well as herbal medicines such as St. John's wort, exhibit significant interactions with CsA through their common metabolism by the CYP3A enzymatic system and membrane transport by P-glycoprotein (also known as MDR1). Commonly co-administered immunosuppressive drugs such as corticosteroids and sirolimus also show clinically relevant effects on CsA pharmacokinetics.

The relationship between CsA exposure and clinically relevant endpoints such as nephrotoxicity and organ rejection was investigated early during the use of CsA due to the highly variable pharmacokinetic behavior of the drug. In one of the earliest studies of CsA pharmacokinetics, Lindholm et al. reported on a population of 160 consecutive kidney transplant patients treated with once-daily IV or oral CsA [16]. Although transplant rejection (40%) and graft loss (23%) were significantly higher in this study compared with the incidence observed with current induction and maintenance immunosuppressive regimens, patients with higher CsA concentrations had significantly lower rates of graft rejection and higher rates of graft survival at 1 year. Subsequent studies have supported the pharmacodynamic relationship between CsA exposure and clinically relevant endpoints [17–22]. These studies have also confirmed the wide variability in pharmacokinetic behavior of this drug, particularly during the early part of the dose interval. Thus, concentration monitoring of CsA is generally considered a standard of care across transplant centers.

Although AUC_{0-12h} provides the best measure of drug exposure, the impracticality of making these AUC measurements, particularly in the outpatient setting, has led to the use of other surrogate measures of exposure. Because most of the variability in CsA pharmacokinetics occurs during the initial 4 h following dosing, AUC over this early post-dose period (e.g., AUC_{0-4h}) has been explored as a surrogate for the full-dose interval AUC_{0-12h}; however, even these abbreviated sampling approaches pose real challenges to collection in the clinic [22]. Pre-dose concentration (C0) represents the simplest measure of CsA exposure. Unfortunately, the correlation between C0 and AUC_{0-12} for CsA is relatively poor. Reported r^2 (r = correlation coefficient) values for the relationship between C0 and AUC_{0-12h} or AUC_{0-4h} generally fall within the 0.4–0.6 range. C0 also appears to be a poor predictor of CsA efficacy or toxicity [17–22]. In a prospective study by Grant et al. that compared the pharmacokinetics of Neoral and Sandimmune formulations of CsA, AUC_{0-6h} demonstrated a significant correlation with graft rejection, with patients in the lowest quartile of AUC exposure showing a more than twofold increased incidence of rejection compared to those in the highest exposure quartile. No significant relationship between C0 and efficacy or toxicity endpoints in either formulation group could be demonstrated [19].

Despite the limitations, C0 (trough or pre-dose concentration) remains a commonly used single, timed concentration for CsA monitoring. The typical target pre-dose concentrations vary significantly across transplant type, time post-transplant, and transplant center [23]. Selection of a target concentration should also take the method used for measurement into consideration. Early PK studies used immunoassays with limited specificity for CsA relative to metabolites. Differences between some analytical platforms were reported to be as large as 100% [24]. More recent versions of automated CsA immunoassays, such as the chemiluminescent microparticle immunoassay marketed by Abbott Laboratories or the Roche automated electrochemiluminescence immunoassay, appear to show improved agreement with liquid chromatography–mass spectrometry-based assays, with a mean positive bias of less than 10% for both methods [25,26].

Although no single, timed concentration is likely to provide as much information regarding CsA exposure as an AUC, 1- or 2-h post-dose concentration, close to the C_{max} for microemulsion-formulated CsA, has been proposed as a significantly better surrogate for the 12-h dose interval AUC compared with C0. Correlations between these early post-dose time points and AUC_{0-12} are reported with r^2 values generally greater than 0.8 [17–21,27–29]. Based on the improved correlation with AUC, the 2-h post-dose concentration (C2) has been advocated as a single concentration monitoring alternative to C0 in several transplant settings. Knight and Morris systematically reviewed the literature for studies directly comparing C2 and C0 monitoring in both de novo and stable kidney, liver, heart, and lung transplant recipients [30]. Although most retrospective studies demonstrate a relationship between C2 and clinically relevant endpoints such as rejection and nephrotoxicity, prospective studies of the benefits of C2 monitoring on clinically relevant endpoints are limited. Of the 10 randomized, controlled studies comparing C2 to C0 monitoring, only a single study demonstrated a significant improvement in rejection and nephrotoxicity with C2 monitoring; however, this study lacks many important details, such as the C0 target range used or the fraction of patients achieving the target concentration [31]. Thus, currently, there appears to be insufficient evidence to support C2 monitoring as superior to C0 despite the improved correlation with AUC.

1.2.2 TACROLIMUS

Tacrolimus, also known as FK506, was introduced into clinical practice in 1989 as an alternative to cyclosporine, and it achieved US Food and Drug Administration (FDA) approval for use in patients following liver transplantation in 1994. Tacrolimus has assumed a central role in the primary prophylaxis against organ rejection, with approval in most transplant settings. In 2012, approximately 90% of kidney and liver transplant recipients were treated with a tacrolimus-based immunosuppressive regimen [32]. Tacrolimus, like CsA, is typically used in combination with other immunosuppressive drugs.

Tacrolimus is a macrocyclic lactone (macrolide) compound that was originally isolated from *Streptomyces tsukubaensis* in 1984. It is very poorly soluble in water but highly soluble in alcohol. Due to the poor aqueous solubility, IV formulations such as Prograf contain tacrolimus solubilized in polyoxyl 60 hydrogenated castor oil (HCO-60) mixed with alcohol.

The mechanism of action for tacrolimus-induced immunosuppression is very similar to that for CsA. Tacrolimus demonstrates high-affinity binding to a distinct family of ubiquitously expressed peptidyl-prolyl isomerases termed FK506-binding proteins (FKBPs) or immunophilins. Although immunophilins share functional activity with the cyclophilins that bind CsA, they do not share amino acid similarity. The tacrolimus–FKBP complex that forms within the cytoplasm of T lymphocytes binds to the calcineurin complex blocking its phosphatase activity with similar inhibitory effects on NFATc translocation: T cell activation and T cell proliferation to those observed with cyclosporine (see Figure 1.1). Interestingly, tacrolimus shares structural similarity and binding to immunophilins with sirolimus and everolimus; however, these ISDs mediate their immunosuppressive effects by a very distinct mechanism from tacrolimus and CsA. As a result of the overlapping mechanism of action for tacrolimus and CsA, they share many of the same adverse effects, such as renal and neurologic toxicity.

The oral bioavailability of tacrolimus, like that of CsA, varies widely from as low as 5% to as high as 95% in some individuals [33,34]. In studies of liver transplant patients, tacrolimus exhibited a mean oral bioavailability of approximately 25%. Unlike CsA, little change in absorption was observed with T-tube closure, suggesting that bile does not play an important role in absorption [35]. Tacrolimus displays an apparent volume of distribution of 1.94 ± 0.053 L/kg in healthy individuals with extensive binding to FKBP in most tissues including RBCs. Like CsA, whole blood concentrations are the primary measurements for most PK studies.

In healthy individuals, clearance following IV administration is estimated at 0.040 ± 0.008 ml/min/kg; however, clearance varies substantially, with some studies showing as much as a 50% CV. Tacrolimus undergoes extensive metabolism by the liver and gastrointestinal cytochrome P450 (CYP) enzyme system, with less than 0.5% of the parent drug excreted unchanged in the feces and urine. Much of the variability in elimination as well as absorption may be explained by genetic differences among individuals in the cytochrome P450 enzymes and the P-glycoprotein drug transporter (see Chapter 5). At least 15 different metabolites of tacrolimus have also been described. Some of the metabolites of tacrolimus exhibit immunosuppressive activity; however, metabolites of tacrolimus with immunosuppressive activity generally represent only a small fraction of the total immunosuppressive activity of tacrolimus [36–38]. Tacrolimus pharmacokinetics is also affected by age, gender, several drug interactions, and especially liver function [39]. Significant diurnal variation has also been observed with lower clearance after the morning dose compared with the evening dose, resulting in an average 20% difference in exposure [40].

Although pharmacokinetics is variable, tacrolimus exposure appears to correlate with the important clinical endpoints of rejection and toxicity. Laskow et al. were the first to document a clear pharmacokinetic–pharmacodynamic relationship for tacrolimus in a prospective, concentration-controlled exposure escalation trial [41]. In this study, 120 kidney transplant recipients were prospectively randomized during the first 2-week period following transplant to three different levels of tacrolimus exposure with low (C0, 5–15 ng/mL), intermediate (C0, 16–25 ng/mL), or high (C0, 26–40 ng/mL) target blood trough concentrations adjusted over 42 days. Logistic regression analysis of trough concentrations in relation to both rejection and toxicity endpoints demonstrated a significant relationship, with more rejection events occurring in the low exposure group and more toxicity, including severe, life-threatening toxicity, observed in the high target exposure group. Serum creatinine and estimated glomerular filtration rate were not significantly different among the three target groups; however, the follow-up period in this study was short. Venkataramanan et al. conducted a prospective study of liver transplant recipients receiving tacrolimus with a longer 4-month follow-up period and demonstrated a strong concentration–response relationship between rejection as well as nephrotoxicity. Toxicity was observed even at the lowest exposures, with the lowest probability of toxicity (<10%) at tacrolimus trough concentrations less than 5 ng/mL rising to greater than 80% probability of nephrotoxicity at concentrations greater than 20 ng/mL [42]. These pharmacodynamics relationships were further supported by several subsequent studies that were thoroughly reviewed by Staatz and Tett [39].

Tacrolimus dosing is presumed to benefit from concentration-monitored therapy due to the narrow therapeutic index of this drug and the overall variable pharmacokinetic behavior. The package insert currently recommends concentration-monitored therapy, which is considered the standard of care in all centers using the drug. Although widely used, there are limited data from concentration-controlled studies to support its use. The study by Laskow et al. represents the only prospective trial that evaluated the ability of concentration-controlled therapy to achieve desired exposure levels [41]. Unfortunately, due to ethical concerns with study design, a control arm managed without TDM was not included for comparison to demonstrate a benefit to monitored therapy.

Monitoring of trough (pre-dose) tacrolimus concentration (C0) is by far the most commonly applied TDM approach supported by the published, pharmacodynamic relationships observed with trough measurements [41,42]. This is undoubtedly due to the ease of collecting this specimen over other timed specimens or the multiple samples required over a dose interval for AUC estimation. The strength of the correlation between C0 and exposure as assessed in a full-dose interval AUC has been the subject of some debate. The correlation between trough tacrolimus and AUC is variable, with r^2 values ranging from 0.97 to 0.34 in published studies [43–48]. The wide differences in the correlation between C0 and AUC across studies is unclear, but they may be related to differences in the study populations or analytical methods used for measurement. The introduction of new, extended-release formulations of tacrolimus with altered PK may necessitate a re-evaluation of monitoring methods; however, early PK data from studies of these formulations suggest that C0 and AUC correlations may be similar despite the altered PK [49,50].

Alternative single time point concentrations and limited sampling strategies (LSS) have been explored to enhance the accuracy of estimating the tacrolimus AUC while retaining a sample collection scheme that is reasonable to apply to the outpatient clinic setting. Ting et al. provides the most recent critical analysis of LSS for tacrolimus AUC estimation [51]. Of the seven published approaches available in 2006, all utilized multiple linear regression to derive relationships between either single or multiple timed tacrolimus concentrations within the initial 6-h period following tacrolimus dosing and tacrolimus AUC. Only a single published study by Dansirikul et al. used prospectively collected data and provided validation of the derived LSS equation in a separate group of patients [52]. A few additional studies have been published beyond those reviewed by Ting et al. with similar results and limitations as those of the previously published studies [53–58]. These approaches may provide some utility in the evaluation of challenging patients; however, the improvement over traditional C0 monitoring remains unknown. The transferability of LSS derived in one patient population to another, given the variability in transplant type, concomitant drug therapy, and genetic factors (e.g., *CYP3A5* genetic differences among racial groups) that influence tacrolimus pharmacokinetics presents an additional major challenge to using any LSS. Caution must therefore be exercised with their use.

Notwithstanding the lack of randomized controlled trial evidence to support the use of TDM to optimize tacrolimus therapy, the substantial evidence showing a correlation between whole blood tacrolimus concentrations and toxicity has led to monitoring as standard of care. C0 monitoring remains the primary approach even in light of the known limitations; however, AUC measurements should be considered for some patients, particularly those with clinical findings of rejection or toxicity that are inconsistent with the apparent level of immunosuppression.

1.3 ANTIMETABOLITE DRUG

Mycophenolic acid (MPA; formulated as the 1,4-morpholinoethyl ester of MPA prodrug (mycophenolic acid mofetil, CellCept)), an antimetabolite drug, was first FDA approved for prevention of kidney transplant rejection in 1995. It has since become the predominant antimetabolite ISD used in the transplant setting. MPA is a fungal metabolite originally described by Bartolomeo Gosio in 1893 as an antibiotic with activity toward *Bacillus anthracis*, making it the first antibiotic purified from a mold [59]. However, immunosuppressive activity of MPA was recognized by Planterose almost 80 years later [60]. Its first clinical use was in the treatment of psoriasis [61–63].

As an ISD, the primary mode of action of MPA is noncompetitive inhibition of the enzyme inosine 5′-monophosphate dehydrogenase (IMPDH; EC 1.1.1.205). Two isoforms of IMPDH have been identified, and both are sensitive to MPA, with the IMPDH-II isoform showing slightly more sensitivity to inhibition by MPA [64]. IMPDH plays an important role in the de novo synthesis of guanine nucleotides by catalyzing the conversion of IMP to the critical precursor xanthine 5′-monophosphate (XMP), as shown in Figure 1.2. Because lymphocytes rely heavily on de novo nucleotide synthesis for their proliferation and function [65], inhibition of IMPDH by MPA results in a significant block in cell-mediated adaptive immunity [66–68].

MPA is currently used clinically both as prodrug, mycophenolic acid mofetil (MMF), and an enteric-coated sodium salt (EC-mycophenolate sodium [EC-MPA], Myfortic). MMF is rapidly hydrolyzed, mostly in the upper gastrointestinal tract, to produce MPA and hydroxyethyl morpholine, an inactive metabolite that is rapidly metabolized and excreted in urine [69]. Peak concentrations are typically achieved within 1 or 2 h following oral dosing of MMF and 1.5–2.75 h for the sodium salt with a lag in absorption of 0.25 to 1.25 h, most likely due to the enteric coating. The bioavailability of MPA is relatively high, with MMF exhibiting oral bioavailability of 80–90% and comparable bioavailability for EC-MPA [70,71]. Once absorbed, MPA exhibits complex pharmacokinetics. Distribution within blood is primarily within the plasma compartment, with 97–99% bound to albumin [72,73]. The 12-h

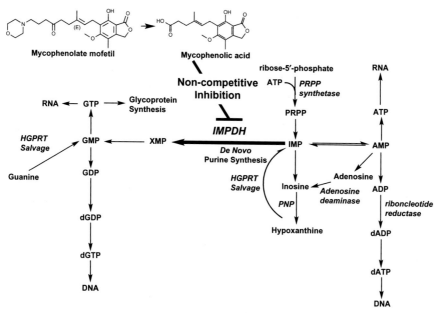

FIGURE 1.2 Schematic of guanine nucleotide synthesis showing mechanism of action for MPA.

HGPRT, hypoxanthine–guanine phosphoribosyl transferase; XMP, xanthosine-5′-monophosphate; IMP, inosine-5′-monophosphate; GMP, guanosine-5′-monophosphate; GDP, guanosine-5′-diphosphate; GTP, guanosine-5′- triphosphate; dGDP, deoxyguanosine-5′-diphosphate; dGTP, deoxyguanosine-5′-triphosphate; PRPP, phosphoribosyl pyrophosphate; AMP, adenosine-5′-monophosphate; ADP, adenosine-5′-diphosphate; ATP, adenosine-5′- triphosphate; dADP, deoxyadenosine-5′-diphosphate; dATP, deoxyadenosine-5′-triphosphate; PNP, purine nucleotide phosphorylase.

dose-interval MPA plasma concentration versus time profile is characterized by rapid absorption, reaching maximal concentration within 1 h followed by rapid distribution to tissues and falling plasma concentration, reaching a plateau within 3 or 4 h. A second peak concentration is often present within the latter half of the dosing interval. This latter peak is variable in both time and intensity, with complete absence in some patients. MPA is metabolized mostly via the UDP glucuronyl transferase (UGT) system within the liver [74]. The primary inactive metabolite is the phenolic glucuronide MPAG, which is transported from liver cells into bile most likely via the ATP binding cassette transporter, MDR1-related protein 2 (Mrp2) [75–78]. Following biliary excretion, MPAG can be converted back into MPA by glucuronidase produced presumably by intestinal bacteria, resulting in reabsorption of MPA. This enterohepatic cycle (EHC) of excretion followed by reabsorption is responsible for the secondary peak in concentration often observed with MPA, and EHC is estimated to contribute 10–60% of the overall AUC for MPA [79].

Despite the complex PK of MPA, exposure as assessed by AUC displays a relatively linear relationship with dose [71,80]. Clearance of MPA, however, varies considerably across individuals as well as within an individual [79,81]. Studies in healthy individuals show interindividual variability of 25–30% for AUC following a single 1-g dose of MMF. It is also clear from studies in transplant recipients that MPA PK changes over time following transplantation, with lower maximal concentration (C_{max}) and lower AUC during the early post-transplant period followed by a gradual rise during the first 3 or 4 months [79]. A lag in absorption is also noted in the early post-transplant where C_{max} is often not reached until 4 or 5 h compared with the typical achievement of C_{max} at approximately 1 h in the stable post-transplant period. Although drug absorption may contribute to some of the changes in PK, these changes are also observed with MPA administered intravenously. It is therefore likely that the change in PK is related, in part, to restrictive clearance mechanisms that likely result from the high protein binding of MPA [82]. The free (non-protein-bound) fraction of MPA, which is the fraction metabolized, is likely higher in the immediate post-transplant period due to lower albumin concentration or altered protein binding associated with displacement by drugs or endogenous compounds present in disease states such as renal and hepatic failure [72]. As albumin concentration normalizes in the post-transplant period, MPA clearance declines, presumably leading to the observed increase in AUC. These changes in MPA PK over time have been observed in most transplant settings, with the most pronounced change observed in the liver transplant setting.

Although monitoring is not currently recommended in the package insert for either MMF or EC-MPA, the variability in exposure to MPA across individuals taking a fixed dose of the drug has led to efforts to improve control of exposure by concentration monitoring of therapy. A relationship between MPA exposure and the clinically relevant pharmacodynamic endpoint of transplant rejection has also been demonstrated. The Randomized Concentration-Controlled Trial (RCCT) [83], designed to evaluate the impact of MPA TDM on outcome, randomized 154 adult patients following kidney transplant into three groups with different MPA AUC targets. All patients in this study were receiving concomitant CsA and prednisone therapy as maintenance immunosuppression. Although patients within the three groups achieved average AUC target levels that were higher than originally proposed, a pharmacokinetic–pharmacodynamic analysis of this study demonstrated that the median MPA AUC during the 6-month time course of the study was inversely related to incidence of acute rejection. No relationship was apparent between MPA dose and efficacy. Three studies more recently evaluated prospectively the utility of TDM using either (1) a Bayesian forecasting approach for AUC determination [84], (2) an abbreviated sampling AUC estimation approach [85], or (3) the C0 concentration [86] to adjust MMF dosing. Each of these three studies utilized a no TDM empiric dosing control group. The APOMYGRE study largely confirmed the previous findings in the RCCT study for renal transplant patients receiving concomitant CsA immunosuppression. However, the FDCC and Opticept studies (each included a majority of patients on tacrolimus therapy) did not demonstrate a significantly lower rate of rejection in concentration-controlled patients compared to empirically dosed patients [85,86] in a setting in which the rejection rates at 1 year were less than 10% across the study arms. Because the rejection incidence was substantially below the anticipated rate of rejection based on previous studies (~20%), these studies were largely underpowered. Interestingly, both Opticept and FDDC studies did demonstrate a statistically significant relationship between AUC and risk for rejection (FDCC) or trough concentration and risk for rejection (Opticept). The use of tacrolimus as the predominant concomitant ISD instead of CsA in these studies may have also contributed to the difference in outcomes. Studies in additional transplant groups other than kidney have shown similar pharmacodynamic relationships between MPA exposure and efficacy, as reviewed by Staatz and Tett [81]. The association between MPA AUC and adverse events such as suppression of hematopoiesis, gastrointestinal toxicity, or infectious complications is less clear. A few studies have supported a relationship between some of these endpoints and pharmacokinetic measures [87,88]; however, a significant association with toxicity could not be observed in any of the prospective, randomized concentration-controlled studies [84–86].

Although a relationship between MPA exposure and clinical outcome clearly exists, the clinical utility of concentration monitoring, particularly C0 monitoring, for MMF has been questioned due to the results of the prospective, concentration-controlled studies described previously. Although these studies were anticipated to fully clarify the utility of monitored MMF therapy, the outcomes from these studies are conflicting and have done little to settle the controversies surrounding this area of therapeutic drug monitoring. Based on the marked PK variability observed with MPA and the pharmacodynamic relationship of PK parameters to rejection outcome, several scientific societies and consensus conferences have advocated the use of concentration monitoring for patients undergoing treatment with MMF or EC-MPA [89]. C0 measurements or AUC estimations based on an LSS are the primary methods used for monitoring MMF therapy. When combined with CsA, the recommended target ranges for MPA are 1–3.5 mg/L and 30–60 mg∗/L for C0 and AUC, respectively. For the combination with tacrolimus, the target ranges of 1.9–4.0 mg/L and 30–60 mg∗h/L for C0 and AUC measurements, respectively, have been suggested [90].

1.4 MAMMALIAN TARGET OF RAPAMYCIN INHIBITORS

The mammalian target of rapamycin (m-TOR) inhibitors were developed as an alternative to calcineurin inhibitor-based immunosuppressive therapy in order to reduce side effects of calcineurin inhibitors, such as nephrotoxicity and viral infection. Currently, the m-TOR inhibitors sirolimus and everolimus are used in clinical practice.

1.4.1 SIROLIMUS (RAPAMYCIN)

Sirolimus was introduced in the United States in 1999 as an immunosuppressive drug that when administered together with CsA reduced the incidence of acute rejection in renal transplant recipients [91]. In 2003, sirolimus was approved by the FDA for a second indication, namely substitution for and reduction of the nephrotoxic burden of the calcineurin inhibitors CsA or tacrolimus. Approved use of sirolimus is restricted to renal transplant patients older than age 13 years [92]. An ester form of sirolimus, temsirolimus (CCl-779), also exists for intravenous administration. The formulation is rapidly hydrolyzed to sirolimus by plasma esterases, and it is currently FDA approved for use in renal cell carcinoma as an anticancer agent. It has not been studied as an immunosuppressive agent in humans, and it does not currently have approval for any transplant indications.

Sirolimus is a cyclic 31-membered ring macrolide antibiotic (shown in Figure 1.3A) with low aqueous solubility that was first isolated from *Streptomyces hygroscopicus*, a fungus isolated from soil samples collected at the Vai Atari region of Rapa Nui (Easter Island). Early studies of sirolimus demonstrated its potent immunosuppressive effects associated with the inhibition of IL-2-mediated T cell proliferation due to a block in cell cycle progression at the G_1 to S phase transition [93–97]. Sirolimus shows structural similarity to tacrolimus, and it binds the same immunophilins; however, sirolimus complexed to FKBP12 does not inhibit calcineurin. Instead, the sirolimus/FKBP12 complex acts as an allosteric inhibitor of mTOR [98] that is present within cells in two distinct, functional complexes. The first form, known as mTORC1, is composed of mTOR, mammalian lethal with additional proteins including sec-13 protein 8 (mLST8), and regulatory-associated protein of TOR (raptor). In mTORC2, raptor is replaced by rapamycin insensitive companion of mTOR (rictor) with addition of stress-activated protein kinase-interacting protein 1 (mSIN1). Of the two complexes of mTOR, mTORC1 is primarily sensitive to sirolimus, with mTORC2 activity decreasing only after prolonged exposure, presumably due to mTOR depletion. Activated by growth factor receptors, nutrients (e.g., amino acids), and cellular energy state (AMP:ATP ratio), mTORC1 controls a number or processes, including ribosomal biosynthesis, macromolecular biosynthesis in relation to nutrient availability, and regulation of energy metabolism as diagrammed in Figure 1.3C. mTORC1 therefore plays a central role within cells, controlling multiple cellular processes required for cell growth and proliferation [99,100]. In addition to the profound effects of sirolimus on T cell proliferation, mTOR inhibition also inhibits CD4[+] and CD8[+] T cell differentiation and promotes the differentiation of CD4[+]CD25[+]FOXP3[+] regulatory T cells (Tregs) that together may contribute to the immunosuppressive effects of sirolimus [101–103]. Likely related to ubiquitous expression of mTOR and its role in a wide array of biological processes, sirolimus causes pleiotropic adverse effects, including hyperlipidemia [104], bone marrow suppression [105], and defects in wound healing [106]. Significant proteinuria has also been observed with sirolimus immunosuppression, particularly in the setting of conversion from a calcineurin inhibitor-based regimen to a sirolimus-based regimen in patients with deteriorating renal function and existing proteinuria following kidney transplant [107–110]. The mechanism for increased proteinuria following conversion from calcineurin inhibitor to sirolimus has not been fully elucidated, but it may be related to direct toxic effects of mTOR inhibitors on kidney podocytes

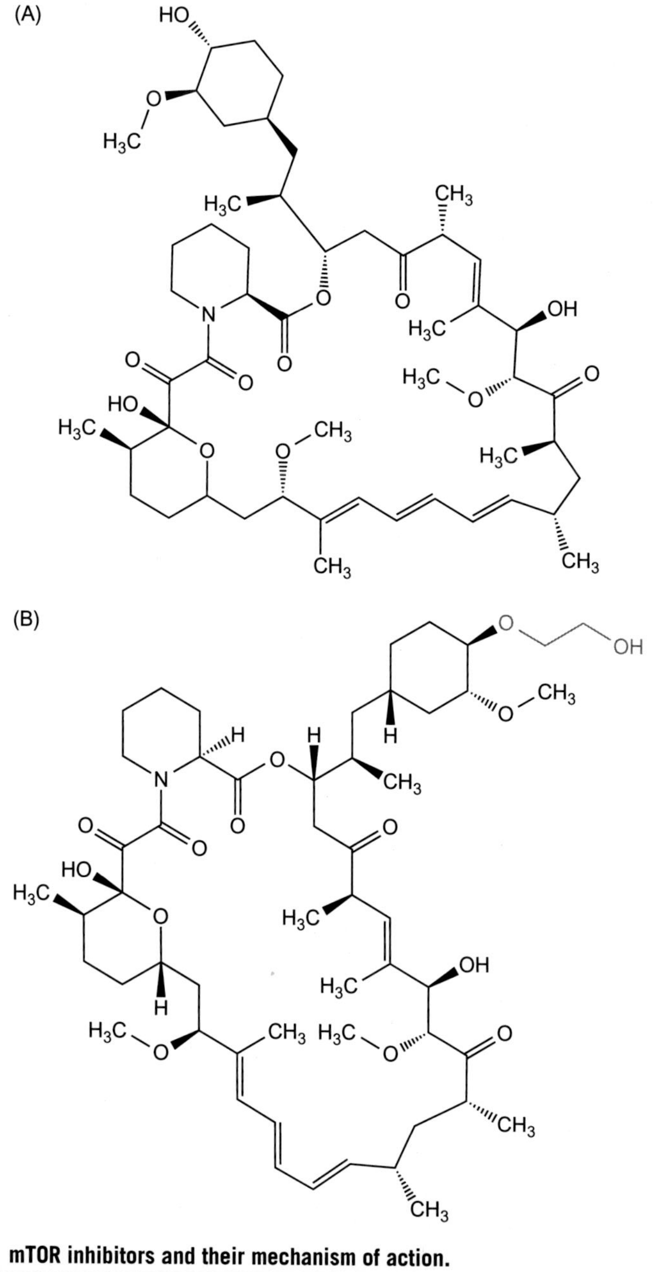

FIGURE 1.3 mTOR inhibitors and their mechanism of action.

(A) Structure of sirolimus; (B) structure of everolimus with C40 hydroxylethyl moiety highlighted in red;

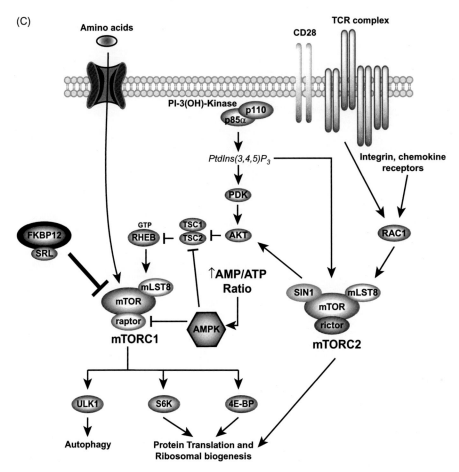

FIGURE 1.3 (Continued)

(C) schematic of mTOR signaling in T cells that is inhibited by the mTOR inhibitors sirolimus and everolimus. PDK, phosphoinositide-dependent kinase 1; AKT, serine/threonine kinase also known as protein kinase B (PKB); RHEB, ras homolog enriched in brain; TSC1, tuberous sclerosis 1 (hamartin); TSC2, tuberous sclerosis 2 (tuberin); ULK1, Unc51-like kinase 1; S6K, ribosomal protein S6 kinase; 4E-BP, eukaryotic translation initiation factor 4E-binding protein 1; RAC1, ras-related C3 botulinum toxin substrate 1.

or tubular cells or changing intrarenal physiology following CNI withdrawal in an already injured kidney [111].

Sirolimus absorption, metabolism, and clearance are highly variable and subject to clinically important drug–drug interactions. Oral bioavailability is low, with an average of 13.6% (10.3–16.9%, 95% confidence interval) using the solution formulation and slightly higher bioavailability with the tablet form. Like CsA and tacrolimus, sirolimus is highly protein bound in vivo, with rapid partitioning into cells and tissues. In whole blood, approximately 95% of sirolimus is found with RBCs. Sirolimus exhibits a high apparent volume of distribution with a mean of 12 ± 8 L/kg. Sirolimus displays a slow clearance with a terminal elimination half-life of 62 ± 16 hr (mean $\pm$ SD) [112]. Clearance varies considerably, with studies in kidney transplant recipients showing as much as an eightfold difference between individuals [113,114]. Biliary secretion appears to be the primary mode of sirolimus excretion, with greater than 90% eliminated in the feces [115]. Sirolimus trough concentrations and AUC over the 24-h dose interval are highly correlated ($r = 0.96$), supporting the use of C0 for sirolimus exposure measurement [116]. Trough concentrations vary widely within and among patients on sirolimus (%CV, 45% and 38%, respectively), likely due to the drug's highly variable clearance described previously [116]. Sirolimus is also subject to numerous drug–drug interactions, including with CsA, diltiazem, ketoconazole, erythromycin, verapamil [117,118]. Sirolimus is primarily metabolized via oxidative metabolism by multiple cytochrome P450 isoforms of the CYP3A family [119]. The P-glycoprotein countertransport system appears to be the major transport system governing gastrointestinal absorption and distribution into and out of tissues [120]. These two processes are the likely sites for drug–drug interactions via competition for binding sites between sirolimus and the interacting drugs.

The extensive variability of sirolimus clearance explains the unpredictability of blood concentration per unit of drug dose. Investigations of the relationship between steady-state trough sirolimus concentration and clinical effects (acute rejection and side effects) led to the recommendation of therapeutic drug monitoring for all patients taking sirolimus [92]. Close monitoring of blood sirolimus concentration is especially important at the initiation of therapy in conjunction with a loading dose, when there is a change in the dosage form of the drug, when there is significant change in liver function, or when concomitant CsA dosage is tapered or withdrawn. Kahan and colleagues provided the first retrospective analysis of sirolimus blood concentration versus clinical outcome data in a cohort of 150 renal transplant patients who received concomitant CsA [121]. Sirolimus was measured in whole blood samples using a well-validated high-performance liquid chromatography with ultraviolet methodology [122]. According to their analyses, there was a significant association between trough sirolimus concentrations less than 5 ng/mL and the incidence of acute rejection. Trough concentrations were reported to be significantly higher in subjects at the time when they were experiencing adverse effects, including thrombocytopenia ($<100,000$ mm^3), leukopenia (<4000 mm^3), and hypertriglyceridemia (>400 mg/dL), leading to a provisional recommendation of 15 ng/mL as the upper end of the therapeutic range. Statistical analyses of sirolimus concentration versus acute rejection in five clinical studies during the clinical development of the drug in renal transplant patients receiving concomitant CsA confirmed the significantly increased risk of acute rejection below 5 ng/mL [123]. The recommended target ranges for sirolimus when used in combination with CsA are listed in the package insert as "16 to 24 ng/mL for the first year following transplantation. Thereafter, the target sirolimus concentrations should be 12 to 20 ng/mL" [112]. No specific recommendations are given for use in other combinations. Although sirolimus TDM is considered a standard of practice for transplant patients prescribed this immunosuppressant, and is recommended by the manufacturer, there is only retrospective concentration versus clinical outcome data for the combination of sirolimus, CsA, and corticosteroid therapy. Due to the widespread use of immunoassays with varying metabolite bias, use of different regimens (e.g., sirolimus in combination with tacrolimus), and lack of prospective studies using therapeutic drug monitoring of sirolimus in contemporary practice, further investigation of sirolimus TDM is certainly warranted.

1.4.2 EVEROLIMUS (RAD001)

In 2010, everolimus was approved for use in the United States for calcineurin inhibitor-sparing immunosuppression regimens. This approval was extended in 2013 to liver transplant on a tacrolimus-sparing regimen.

Everolimus is very similar to sirolimus, with a 40-*O*-(2 hydroxyethyl) substitution on the sirolimus structure as shown in Figure 1.3B. Everolimus was designed to be more water-soluble and rapidly absorbed. Because the C40 modification on everolimus is located away from the region of the molecule involved with binding to FKBP12 and mTOR [124], everolimus mediates immunosuppression by the same mechanism of mTOR inhibition as sirolimus. Although less extensively studied as an ISD, everolimus also appears to show a similar toxicity profile to sirolimus, as reviewed in Zaza et al. [125].

Despite the improved aqueous solubility and reduced metabolism afforded by the C40 modification [126], everolimus still shows relatively low bioavailability that is comparable to sirolimus. The reasons for poor bioavailability are unknown, but studies in rats suggest that poor oral bioavailability of sirolimus and everolimus may occur by different mechanisms, with the latter showing greater intrinsic membrane permeability that is balanced by greater first-pass, intestinal metabolism [127,128]. The distribution of everolimus in humans is unknown, but it is likely similar to sirolimus due to the ubiquitous expression of mTOR. The apparent volume of distribution of everolimus is estimated at approximately 2.2 L/kg based on a population PK study in renal transplant recipients. In blood, greater than 75% of everolimus is found within RBCs, and greater than 75% of plasma everolimus is protein bound [129]. Studies in nonhuman primates demonstrate wide distribution of everolimus in tissues, with the highest concentrations in gall bladder, pancreas, lung, kidneys, cerebellum, and spleen [130].

Everolimus also shows wide variability in clearance, similar to CsA, tacrolimus, and sirolimus. The variation in clearance is likely governed by extensive CYP3A metabolism and P-glycoprotein transport that varies both genetically and due to concomitant drug interactions. The within- and between-patient variability of dose-interval AUC was 27% and 31%, respectively, in a study of 731 renal transplant patients studied during a 6-month period post-transplantation [131]. There was no detectable influence of sex, age (16–66 years), or weight (42–132 kg) on AUC, but everolimus exposure was significantly lower by an average of 20% in blacks. Everolimus shows a reasonably good correlation between trough concentration and AUC ($r^2 = 0.79$).

The package insert for everolimus recommends the use of C0 monitoring to guide therapy, with a recommended target range of 3–8 ng/mL [132]. These recommendations are based on early phase clinical data as well as the pooled analysis of three randomized, multicenter, clinical trials of everolimus in de novo kidney transplant [133]. A follow-up analysis of everolimus concentrations performed by the same group in a prospectively monitored de novo kidney transplant population confirmed the increased likelihood of acute rejection when C0 is less than 3 ng/mL [134]. Correlation between everolimus C0 and safety endpoints of thrombocytopenia, leukopenia, hypertriglyceridemia, or hypercholesterolemia have also been observed; however, defining the upper boundary of the target range has been more challenging [133–135]. Retrospective analysis of clinical trial data of everolimus in heart transplant suggests that the target range of 3–8 ng/mL may be transferable to this transplant population [136]. Pharmacodynamic data relating concentration data to outcomes in liver transplantation are currently sparse. However, in the pivotal study that led to everolimus approval for use in liver transplantation, everolimus concentrations were prospectively maintained within the 3–8 ng/mL range, documenting the efficacy and safety of this approach [137,138]. Unfortunately, there have been no prospective concentration-controlled trials to date to demonstrate the benefits of maintaining patients within the recommended target range.

1.5 CONCLUSIONS

Currently, cyclosporine, tacrolimus, mycophenolic acid, sirolimus, and everolimus are used as immunosuppressive agents in the management of organ transplant patients. Pharmacokinetics of all these agents is complex and variable. Moreover, therapeutic drug monitoring of these drugs is needed due to their narrow therapeutic ranges, significant variability in blood concentrations between individual patients, gender differences in drug metabolism, and drug–nutrient as well as drug–drug interactions. In this chapter, an overview of pharmacology and toxicology of these drugs was provided along with an in-depth discussion on various aspects of therapeutic drug monitoring of these agents.

REFERENCES

[1] Yatscoff RW, Aspeslet LJ, Gallant HL. Pharmacodynamic monitoring of immunosuppressive drugs. Clin Chem 1998;44(2):428–32.
[2] Malleret G, Haditsch U, Genoux D, Jones MW, et al. Inducible and reversible enhancement of learning, memory, and long-term potentiation by genetic inhibition of calcineurin. Cell 2001;104(5):675–86.
[3] Graef IA, Mermelstein PG, Stankunas K, Neilson JR, et al. L-type calcium channels and GSK-3 regulate the activity of NF-ATc4 in hippocampal neurons. Nature 1999;401(6754):703–8.

[4] Musaro A, McCullagh KJ, Naya FJ, Olson EN, et al. IGF-1 induces skeletal myocyte hypertrophy through calcineurin in association with GATA-2 and NF-ATc1. Nature 1999;400(6744):581–5.

[5] Wu H, Rothermel B, Kanatous S, Rosenberg P, et al. Activation of MEF2 by muscle activity is mediated through a calcineurin-dependent pathway. EMBO J 2001;20(22):6414–23.

[6] Hernandez GL, Volpert OV, Iniguez MA, Lorenzo E, et al. Selective inhibition of vascular endothelial growth factor-mediated angiogenesis by cyclosporin A: roles of the nuclear factor of activated T cells and cyclooxygenase 2. J Exp Med 2001;193(5):607–20.

[7] Ptachcinski RJ, Venkataramanan R, Burckart GJ, Gray JA, et al. Cyclosporine kinetics in healthy volunteers. J Clin Pharmacol 1987;27(3):243–8.

[8] Novartis. Neoral Package Insert. <https://http://www.pharma.us.novartis.com/product/pi/pdf/neoral.pdf>. Novartis; 2013.

[9] Dunn CJ, Wagstaff AJ, Perry CM, Plosker GL, et al. Cyclosporin: an updated review of the pharmacokinetic properties, clinical efficacy and tolerability of a microemulsion-based formulation (neoral)1 in organ transplantation. Drugs 2001;61(13):1957–2016.

[10] Andrews W, Iwatsuki S, Shaw Jr. BW, Starzl TE. Cyclosporine monitoring in liver transplant patients. Transplantation 1985;39(3):338.

[11] Keown P, Landsberg D, Halloran P, Shoker A, et al. A randomized, prospective multicenter pharmacoepidemiologic study of cyclosporine microemulsion in stable renal graft recipients. Report of the Canadian Neoral Renal Transplantation Study Group. Transplantation 1996;62(12):1744–52.

[12] Maurer G, Loosli HR, Schreier E, Keller B. Disposition of cyclosporine in several animal species and man. I. Structural elucidation of its metabolites. Drug Metab Dispos 1984;12(1):120–6.

[13] Combalbert J, Fabre I, Fabre G, Dalet I, et al. Metabolism of cyclosporin A. IV. Purification and identification of the rifampicin-inducible human liver cytochrome P-450 (cyclosporin A oxidase) as a product of P450IIIA gene subfamily. Drug Metab Dispos 1989;17(2):197–207.

[14] Christians U, Sewing KF. Cyclosporin metabolism in transplant patients. Pharmacol Ther 1993;57(2–3):291–345.

[15] Venkataramanan R, Ptachcinski RJ, Burckart GJ, Yang SL, et al. The clearance of cyclosporine by hemodialysis. J Clin Pharmacol 1984;24(11–12):528–31.

[16] Lindholm A, Kahan BD. Influence of cyclosporine pharmacokinetics, trough concentrations, and AUC monitoring on outcome after kidney transplantation. Clin Pharmacol Ther 1993;54(2):205–18.

[17] Clase CM, Mahalati K, Kiberd BA, Lawen JG, et al. Adequate early cyclosporin exposure is critical to prevent renal allograft rejection: patients monitored by absorption profiling. Am J Transplant 2002;2(8):789–95.

[18] Cantarovich M, Barkun JS, Tchervenkov JI, Besner JG, et al. Comparison of neoral dose monitoring with cyclosporine through levels versus 2-hr postdose levels in stable liver transplant patients. Transplantation 1998;66(12):1621–7.

[19] Grant D, Kneteman N, Tchervenkov J, Roy A, et al. Peak cyclosporine levels (Cmax) correlate with freedom from liver graft rejection: results of a prospective, randomized comparison of neoral and sandimmune for liver transplantation (NOF-8). Transplantation 1999;67(8):1133–7.

[20] Barakat O, Peaston R, Rai R, Talbot D, et al. Clinical benefit of monitoring cyclosporine C2 and C4 in long-term liver transplant recipients. Transplant Proc 2002;34(5):1535–7.

[21] International Neoral Renal Transplantation Study Group. Cyclosporine microemulsion (Neoral) absorption profiling and sparse-sample predictors during the first 3 months after renal transplantation. Am J Transplant 2002;2(2):148–56.

[22] Mahalati K, Belitsky P, West K, Kiberd B, et al. Approaching the therapeutic window for cyclosporine in kidney transplantation: a prospective study. J Am Soc Nephrol 2001;12(4):828–33.

[23] Proceedings of the international consensus conference on immunosuppressive drugs. Lake Louise, Alberta, Canada, May 5–7, 1995. Ther Drug Monit 1995;17(6):559–703.

[24] Burton ME. Applied pharmacokinetics & pharmacodynamics: principles of therapeutic drug monitoring, 4th ed. Philadelphia, PA: Lippincott Williams & Wilkins; 2006. xvii, 867 pp.

[25] Vogeser M, Shipkova M, Rigo-Bonnin R, Wallemacq P, et al. Multicenter analytical evaluation of the automated electrochemiluminescence immunoassay for cyclosporine. Ther Drug Monit 2014;36(5):640–50.

[26] Brate EM, Finley DM, Grote J, Holets-McCormack S, et al. Development of an Abbott ARCHITECT cyclosporine immunoassay without metabolite cross-reactivity. Clin Biochem 2010;43(13–14):1152–7.

[27] Cantarovich M, Barkun J, Besner JG, Metrakos P, et al. Cyclosporine peak levels provide a better correlation with the area-under-the-curve than trough levels in liver transplant patients treated with neoral. Transplant Proc 1998;30(4):1462–3.

[28] Cantarovich M, Besner JG, Barkun JS, Elstein E, et al. Two-hour cyclosporine level determination is the appropriate tool to monitor Neoral therapy. Clin Transplant 1998;12(3):243–9.

[29] Jaksch P, Kocher A, Neuhauser P, Sarahrudi K, et al. Monitoring C2 level predicts exposure in maintenance lung transplant patients receiving the microemulsion formulation of cyclosporine (Neoral). J Heart Lung Transplant 2005;24(8):1076–80.

[30] Knight SR, Morris PJ. The clinical benefits of cyclosporine C2-level monitoring: a systematic review. Transplantation 2007;83(12):1525–35.

[31] Wang X, Xu D, editors. Using neoral C2 monitoring as the predictor in de novo renal transplant patients: a prospective study. In: XIXth international congress of the transplantation society. Miami, FL. 2002 Aug 25–30.

[32] 2012 Annual data report: scientific registry of transplant recipients. Available at: <http://srtr.transplant.hrsa.gov/annual_reports/2012/pdf/2012_SRTR_ADR_updated_full_intro.pdf>; 2014 [29.12.14].

[33] Astellas. PROGRAF (tacrolimus) package Insert. <http://www.astellas.us/docs/prograf.pdf> Astellas; 2013.

[34] Wallemacq PE, Furlan V, Moller A, Schafer A, et al. Pharmacokinetics of tacrolimus (FK506) in paediatric liver transplant recipients. Eur J Drug Metab Pharmacokinet 1998;23(3):367–70.

[35] Venkataramanan R, Jain A, Warty VW, Abu-Elmagd K, et al. Pharmacokinetics of FK 506 following oral administration: a comparison of FK 506 and cyclosporine. Transplant Proc 1991;23(1 Pt 2):931–3.

[36] Iwasaki K, Shiraga T, Nagase K, Tozuka Z, et al. Isolation, identification, and biological activities of oxidative metabolites of FK506, a potent immunosuppressive macrolide lactone. Drug Metab Dispos 1993;21(6):971–7.

[37] Alak AM, Moy S. Biological activity of tacrolimus (FK506) and its metabolites from whole blood of kidney transplant patients. Transplant Proc 1997;29(5):2487–90.

[38] Gonschior AK, Christians U, Winkler M, Linck A, et al. Tacrolimus (FK506) metabolite patterns in blood from liver and kidney transplant patients. Clin Chem 1996;42(9):1426–32.

[39] Staatz CE, Tett SE. Clinical pharmacokinetics and pharmacodynamics of tacrolimus in solid organ transplantation. Clin Pharmacokinet 2004;43(10):623–53.

[40] Min DI, Chen HY, Fabrega A, Ukah FO, et al. Circadian variation of tacrolimus disposition in liver allograft recipients. Transplantation 1996;62(8):1190–2.

[41] Laskow DA, Vincenti F, Neylan JF, Mendez R, et al. An open-label, concentration-ranging trial of FK506 in primary kidney transplantation: a report of the United States Multicenter FK506 Kidney Transplant Group. Transplantation 1996;62(7):900–5.

[42] Venkataramanan R, Shaw LM, Sarkozi L, Mullins R, et al. Clinical utility of monitoring tacrolimus blood concentrations in liver transplant patients. J Clin Pharmacol 2001;41(5):542–51.

[43] Jorgensen K, Povlsen J, Madsen S, Madsen M, et al. C2 (2-h) levels are not superior to trough levels as estimates of the area under the curve in tacrolimus-treated renal-transplant patients. Nephrol Dial Transplant 2002;17(8):1487–90.

[44] Jorgensen KA, Povlsen JV, Poulsen JH. Optimal time for determination of blood tacrolimus level. Transplant Proc 2001;33(7–8):3164–5.

[45] Braun F, Peters B, Schutz E, Lorf T, et al. Therapeutic drug monitoring of tacrolimus early after liver transplantation. Transplant Proc 2002;34(5):1538–9.

[46] Wong KM, Shek CC, Chau KF, Li CS. Abbreviated tacrolimus area-under-the-curve monitoring for renal transplant recipients. Am J Kidney Dis 2000;35(4):660–6.

[47] Cantarovich M, Fridell J, Barkun J, Metrakos P, et al. Optimal time points for the prediction of the area-under-the-curve in liver transplant patients receiving tacrolimus. Transplant Proc 1998;30(4):1460–1.

[48] Ku YM, Min DI. An abbreviated area-under-the-curve monitoring for tacrolimus in patients with liver transplants. Ther Drug Monit 1998;20(2):219–23.

[49] Alloway RR, Eckhoff DE, Washburn WK, Teperman LW. Conversion from twice daily tacrolimus capsules to once daily extended-release tacrolimus (LCP-Tacro): phase 2 trial of stable liver transplant recipients. Liver Transpl 2014;20(5):564–75.

[50] Gaber AO, Alloway RR, Bodziak K, Kaplan B, et al. Conversion from twice-daily tacrolimus capsules to once-daily extended-release tacrolimus (LCPT): a phase 2 trial of stable renal transplant recipients. Transplantation 2013;96(2):191–7.

[51] Ting L, Villeneuve E, Ensom M. Beyond Cyclosporine: a systematic review of limited sampling strategies for other immunosuppressants. Ther Drug Monit 2006;28(3).

[52] Dansirikul C, Staatz CE, Duffull SB, Taylor PJ, et al. Sampling times for monitoring tacrolimus in stable adult liver transplant recipients. Ther Drug Monit 2004;26(6):593–9.

[53] Armendariz Y, Pou L, Cantarell C, Lopez R, et al. Evaluation of a limited sampling strategy to estimate area under the curve of tacrolimus in adult renal transplant patient. Ther Drug Monit 2005;27(4):431–4.

[54] Delaloye JR, Kassir N, Litalien C, Theoret Y, et al. Limited sampling strategies for tacrolimus monitoring in pediatric liver transplant recipients. Am J Transplant 2009;9:535. PubMed. PMID: ISI:000265068801231.

[55] Miura M, Satoh S, Niioka T, Kagaya H, et al. Limited sampling strategy for simultaneous estimation of the area under the concentration-time curve of tacrolimus and mycophenolic acid in adult renal transplant recipients. Ther Drug Monit 2008;30(1):52–9.

[56] Barraclough KA, Isbel NM, Johnson DW, Hawley CM, et al. A limited sampling strategy for the simultaneous estimation of tacrolimus, mycophenolic acid and unbound prednisolone exposure in adult kidney transplant recipients. Nephrology 2012;17(3):294–9.

[57] Zhao W, Fakhoury M, Baudouin V, Maisin A, et al. Limited sampling strategy for estimating individual exposure of tacrolimus in pediatric kidney transplant patients. Ther
Drug Monit 2011;33(6):681–7.

[58] Zhu L, Wang H, Rao W, Qu W, et al. A limited sampling strategy for tacrolimus in liver
transplant patients. Int J Clin Pharmacol Ther 2013;51(6):509–12.

[59] Bentley R. Mycophenolic acid: a one hundred year odyssey from antibiotic to immunosuppressant. Chem Rev 2000;100(10):3801–26.

[60] Planterose DN. Antiviral and cytotoxic effects of mycophenolic acid. J Gen Virol
1969;4(4):629–30.

[61] Jones EL, Epinette WW, Hackney VC, Menendez L, et al. Treatment of psoriasis with
oral mycophenolic acid. J Invest Dermatol 1975;65(6):537–42.

[62] Marinari R, Fleischmajer R, Schragger AH, Rosenthal AL. Mycophenolic acid in the
treatment of psoriasis: long-term administration. Arch Dermatol 1977;113(7):930–2.

[63] Spatz S, Rudnicka A, McDonald CJ. Mycophenolic acid in psoriasis. Br J Dermatol
1978;98(4):429–35.

[64] Hager PW, Collart FR, Huberman E, Mitchell BS. Recombinant human inosine
monophosphate dehydrogenase type I and type II proteins. Purification and characterization of inhibitor binding. Biochem Pharmacol 1995;49(9):1323–9.

[65] Allison AC, Hovi T, Watts RW, Webster AD. Immunological observations on patients
with Lesch-Nyhan syndrome, and on the role of de-novo purine synthesis in lymphocyte
transformation. Lancet 1975;2(7946):1179–83.

[66] Eugui EM, Mirkovich A, Allison AC. Lymphocyte-selective antiproliferative
and immunosuppressive effects of mycophenolic acid in mice. Scand J Immunol
1991;33(2):175–83.

[67] Eugui EM, Almquist SJ, Muller CD, Allison AC. Lymphocyte-selective cytostatic and
immunosuppressive effects of mycophenolic acid in vitro: role of deoxyguanosine
nucleotide depletion. Scand J Immunol 1991;33(2):161–73.

[68] Allison AC, Eugui EM. Mycophenolate mofetil and its mechanisms of action.
Immunopharmacology 2000;47(2–3):85–118.

[69] Lee WA, Gu L, Miksztal AR, Chu N, et al. Bioavailability improvement of mycophenolic acid through amino ester derivatization. Pharm Res 1990;7(2):161–6.

[70] Novartis. Myfortic Package Insert. <https://http://www.pharma.us.novartis.com/prod-
uct/pi/pdf/myfortic.pdf>. Novartis; 2013.

[71] Granger DK, Group EBRTS 301 Group EBRTS 302. Enteric-coated mycophenolate sodium: results of two pivotal global multicenter trials. Transplant Proc
2001;33(7–8):3241–4.

[72] Nowak I, Shaw LM. Mycophenolic acid binding to human serum albumin: characterization and relation to pharmacodynamics. Clin Chem 1995;41(7):1011–7.

[73] Langman LJ, LeGatt DF, Yatscoff RW. Blood distribution of mycophenolic acid. Ther
Drug Monit 1994;16(6):602–7.

[74] Bernard O, Guillemette C. The main role of UGT1A9 in the hepatic metabolism of
mycophenolic acid and the effects of naturally occurring variants. Drug Metab Dispos
2004;32(8):775–8.

[75] Wang J, Figurski M, Shaw LM, Burckart GJ. The impact of P-glycoprotein and Mrp2 on
mycophenolic acid levels in mice. Transpl Immunol 2008;19(3–4):192–6.

[76] Takekuma Y, Kakiuchi H, Yamazaki K, Miyauchi S, et al. Difference between
pharmacokinetics of mycophenolic acid (MPA) in rats and that in humans is caused by
different affinities of MRP2 to a glucuronized form. J Pharm Pharm Sci 2007;10(1):
71–85.

[77] Westley IS, Brogan LR, Morris RG, Evans AM, et al. Role of Mrp2 in the hepatic disposition of mycophenolic acid and its glucuronide metabolites: effect of cyclosporine. Drug Metab Dispos 2006;34(2):261–6.

[78] Kobayashi M, Saitoh H, Kobayashi M, Tadano K, et al. Cyclosporin A, but not tacrolimus, inhibits the biliary excretion of mycophenolic acid glucuronide possibly mediated by multidrug resistance-associated protein 2 in rats. J Pharmacol Exp Ther 2004;309(3):1029–35.

[79] Bullingham RE, Nicholls AJ, Kamm BR. Clinical pharmacokinetics of mycophenolate mofetil. Clin Pharmacokinet 1998;34(6):429–55.

[80] Sollinger HW, Deierhoi MH, Belzer FO, Diethelm AG, et al. RS-61443—a phase I clinical trial and pilot rescue study. Transplantation 1992;53(2):428–32.

[81] Staatz CE, Tett SE. Clinical pharmacokinetics and pharmacodynamics of mycophenolate in solid organ transplant recipients. Clin Pharmacokinet 2007;46(1):13–58.

[82] Gillette JR. Overview of drug-protein binding. Ann N Y Acad Sci 1973;226:6–17.

[83] Hale MD, Nicholls AJ, Bullingham RE, Hene R, et al. The pharmacokinetic-pharmacodynamic relationship for mycophenolate mofetil in renal transplantation. Clin Pharmacol Ther 1998;64(6):672–83.

[84] Le Meur Y, Buchler M, Thierry A, Caillard S, et al. Individualized mycophenolate mofetil dosing based on drug exposure significantly improves patient outcomes after renal transplantation. Am J Transplant 2007;7(11):2496–503.

[85] van Gelder T, Silva HT, de Fijter JW, Budde K, et al. Comparing mycophenolate mofetil regimens for de novo renal transplant recipients: the fixed-dose concentration-controlled trial. Transplantation 2008;86(8):1043–51.

[86] Gaston RS, Kaplan B, Shah T, Cibrik D, et al. Fixed- or controlled-dose mycophenolate mofetil with standard- or reduced-dose calcineurin inhibitors: the Opticept trial. Am J Transplant 2009;9(7):1607–19.

[87] Mourad M, Malaise J, Chaib Eddour D, De Meyer M, et al. Correlation of mycophenolic acid pharmacokinetic parameters with side effects in kidney transplant patients treated with mycophenolate mofetil. Clin Chem 2001;47(1):88–94.

[88] Weber LT, Shipkova M, Armstrong VW, Wagner N, et al. The pharmacokinetic-pharmacodynamic relationship for total and free mycophenolic acid in pediatric renal transplant recipients: a report of the german study group on mycophenolate mofetil therapy. J Am Soc Nephrol 2002;13(3):759–68.

[89] van Gelder T, Le Meur Y, Shaw LM, Oellerich M, et al. Therapeutic drug monitoring of mycophenolate mofetil in transplantation. Ther Drug Monit 2006;28(2):145–54.

[90] Bennett WM. Immunosuppression with mycophenolic acid: one size does not fit all. J Am Soc Nephrol 2003;14(9):2414–6.

[91] Miller JL. Sirolimus approved with renal transplant indication. Am J Health Syst Pharm 1999;56(21):2177–8.

[92] Pfizer. Rapammune (sirolimus) Oral Solution and Tablets. Package Insert; 2010.

[93] Bierer BE, Mattila PS, Standaert RF, Herzenberg LA, et al. Two distinct signal transmission pathways in T lymphocytes are inhibited by complexes formed between an immunophilin and either FK506 or rapamycin. Proc Natl Acad Sci USA 1990;87(23):9231–5.

[94] Dumont FJ, Melino MR, Staruch MJ, Koprak SL, et al. The immunosuppressive macrolides FK-506 and rapamycin act as reciprocal antagonists in murine T cells. J Immunol 1990;144(4):1418–24.

[95] Dumont FJ, Staruch MJ, Koprak SL, Melino MR, et al. Distinct mechanisms of suppression of murine T cell activation by the related macrolides FK-506 and rapamycin. J Immunol 1990;144(1):251–8.

[96] Kuo CJ, Chung J, Fiorentino DF, Flanagan WM, et al. Rapamycin selectively inhibits interleukin-2 activation of p70 S6 kinase. Nature 1992;358(6381):70–3.

[97] Schreiber SL. Chemistry and biology of the immunophilins and their immunosuppressive ligands. Science 1991;251(4991):283–7.

[98] Heitman J, Movva NR, Hall MN. Targets for cell cycle arrest by the immunosuppressant rapamycin in yeast. Science 1991;253(5022):905–9.

[99] Li J, Kim SG, Blenis J. Rapamycin: one drug, many effects. Cell Metab 2014;19(3):373–9. 24508508.

[100] Shimobayashi M, Hall MN. Making new contacts: the mTOR network in metabolism and signalling crosstalk. Nat Rev Mol Cell Biol 2014;15(3):155–62.

[101] Araki K, Turner AP, Shaffer VO, Gangappa S, et al. mTOR regulates memory CD8 T-cell differentiation. Nature 2009;460(7251):108–12. 19543266.

[102] Kopf H, de la Rosa GM, Howard OM, Chen X. Rapamycin inhibits differentiation of Th17 cells and promotes generation of FoxP3+ T regulatory cells. Int Immunopharmacol 2007;7(13):1819–24. 17996694.

[103] Rao RR, Li Q, Odunsi K, Shrikant PA. The mTOR kinase determines effector versus memory CD8+ T cell fate by regulating the expression of transcription factors T-bet and Eomesodermin. Immunity 2010;32(1):67–78.

[104] Morrisett JD, Abdel-Fattah G, Hoogeveen R, Mitchell E, et al. Effects of sirolimus on plasma lipids, lipoprotein levels, and fatty acid metabolism in renal transplant patients. J Lipid Res 2002;43(8):1170–80.

[105] Hong JC, Kahan BD. Sirolimus-induced thrombocytopenia and leukopenia in renal transplant recipients: risk factors, incidence, progression, and management. Transplantation 2000;69(10):2085–90.

[106] Nashan B, Citterio F. Wound healing complications and the use of mammalian target of rapamycin inhibitors in kidney transplantation: a critical review of the literature. Transplantation 2012;94(6):547–61.

[107] Diekmann F, Andres A, Oppenheimer F. mTOR inhibitor-associated proteinuria in kidney transplant recipients. Transplant Rev 2012;26(1):27–9.

[108] Diekmann F, Budde K, Oppenheimer F, Fritsche L, et al. Predictors of success in conversion from calcineurin inhibitor to sirolimus in chronic allograft dysfunction. Am J Transplant 2004;4(11):1869–75.

[109] Schena FP, Pascoe MD, Alberu J, del Carmen Rial M, et al. Conversion from calcineurin inhibitors to sirolimus maintenance therapy in renal allograft recipients: 24-month efficacy and safety results from the CONVERT trial. Transplantation 2009;87(2):233–42.

[110] Naik MG, Heller KM, Arns W, Budde K, et al. Proteinuria and sirolimus after renal transplantation: a retrospective analysis from a large German multicenter database. Clin Transplant 2014;28(1):67–79.

[111] Letavernier E, Legendre C. mToR inhibitors-induced proteinuria: mechanisms, significance, and management. Transplant Rev 2008;22(2):125–30.

[112] Pfizer. Rapamune (Sirolimus) Package Insert. <https://http://www.pharma.us.novartis.com/product/pi/pdf/myfortic.pdf>. Novartis; 2011.

[113] Brattstrom C, Sawe J, Tyden G, Herlenius G, et al. Kinetics and dynamics of single oral doses of sirolimus in sixteen renal transplant recipients. Ther Drug Monit 1997;19(4):397–406.

[114] Zimmerman JJ, Kahan BD. Pharmacokinetics of sirolimus in stable renal transplant patients after multiple oral dose administration. J Clin Pharmacol 1997;37(5):405–15.

[115] Leung LY, Lim HK, Abell MW, Zimmerman JJ. Pharmacokinetics and metabolic disposition of sirolimus in healthy male volunteers after a single oral dose. Ther Drug Monit 2006;28(1):51–61.

[116] Kahan BD, Camardo JS. Rapamycin: clinical results and future opportunities. Transplantation 2001;72(7):1181–93.

[117] Zimmerman JJ, Ferron GM, Lim HK, Parker V. The effect of a high-fat meal on the oral bioavailability of the immunosuppressant sirolimus (rapamycin). J Clin Pharmacol 1999;39(11):1155–61.

[118] Kaplan B, Meier-Kriesche HU, Napoli KL, Kahan BD. The effects of relative timing of sirolimus and cyclosporine microemulsion formulation coadministration on the pharmacokinetics of each agent. Clin Pharmacol Ther 1998;63(1):48–53.

[119] Sattler M, Guengerich FP, Yun CH, Christians U, et al. Cytochrome P-450 3A enzymes are responsible for biotransformation of FK506 and rapamycin in man and rat. Drug Metab Dispos 1992;20(5):753–61.

[120] Paine MF, Leung LY, Watkins PB. New insights into drug absorption: studies with sirolimus. Ther Drug Monit 2004;26(5):463–7.

[121] Kahan BD, Napoli KL, Kelly PA, Podbielski J, et al. Therapeutic drug monitoring of sirolimus: correlations with efficacy and toxicity. Clin Transplant 2000;14(2):97–109.

[122] Napoli KL, Kahan BD. Routine clinical monitoring of sirolimus (rapamycin) whole-blood concentrations by HPLC with ultraviolet detection. Clin Chem 1996;42(12):1943–8.

[123] Zimmerman JJ. Exposure-response relationships and drug interactions of sirolimus. AAPS J 2004;6(4):e28. 15760093.

[124] Choi J, Chen J, Schreiber SL, Clardy J. Structure of the FKBP12-rapamycin complex interacting with the binding domain of human FRAP. Science 1996;273(5272):239–42.

[125] Zaza G, Tomei P, Ria P, Granata S, et al. Systemic and nonrenal adverse effects occurring in renal transplant patients treated with mTOR inhibitors. Clin Dev Immunol 2013;2013:403280.

[126] Jacobsen W, Serkova N, Hausen B, Morris RE, et al. Comparison of the in vitro metabolism of the macrolide immunosuppressants sirolimus and RAD. Transplant Proc 2001;33(1–2):514–5.

[127] Crowe A, Bruelisauer A, Duerr L, Guntz P, et al. Absorption and intestinal metabolism of SDZ-RAD and rapamycin in rats. Drug Metab Dispos 1999;27(5):627–32.

[128] Crowe A, Lemaire M. In vitro and in situ absorption of SDZ-RAD using a human intestinal cell line (Caco-2) and a single pass perfusion model in rats: comparison with rapamycin. Pharm Res 1998;15(11):1666–72.

[129] Kovarik JM, Kahan BD, Kaplan B, Lorber M, et al. Longitudinal assessment of everolimus in de novo renal transplant recipients over the first post-transplant year: pharmacokinetics, exposure-response relationships, and influence on cyclosporine. Clin Pharmacol Ther 2001;69(1):48–56.

[130] Serkova N, Hausen B, Berry GJ, Jacobsen W, et al. Tissue distribution and clinical monitoring of the novel macrolide immunosuppressant SDZ-RAD and its metabolites in monkey lung transplant recipients: interaction with cyclosporine. J Pharmacol Exp Ther 2000;294(1):323–32.

[131] Kovarik JM, Kaplan B, Silva HT, Kahan BD, et al. Pharmacokinetics of an everolimus-cyclosporine immunosuppressive regimen over the first 6 months after kidney transplantation. Am J Transplant 2003;3(5):606–13.

[132] Novartis. Zortress (Everolimus) Package Insert. <https://http://www.pharma.us.novartis. com/product/pi/pdf/zortress.pdf>. Novartis; 2013.

[133] Kovarik JM, Kaplan B, Tedesco Silva H, Kahan BD, et al. Exposure-response relationships for everolimus in de novo kidney transplantation: defining a therapeutic range. Transplantation 2002;73(6):920–5.

[134] Kovarik JM, Tedesco H, Pascual J, Civati G, et al. Everolimus therapeutic concentration range defined from a prospective trial with reduced-exposure cyclosporine in de novo kidney transplantation. Ther Drug Monit 2004;26(5):499–505.

[135] Budde K, Neumayer HH, Lehne G, Winkler M, et al. Tolerability and steady-state pharmacokinetics of everolimus in maintenance renal transplant patients. Nephrol Dial Transplant 2004;19(10):2606–14.

[136] Kovarik JM, Eisen H, Dorent R, Mancini D, et al. Everolimus in de novo cardiac transplantation: pharmacokinetics, therapeutic range, and influence on cyclosporine exposure. J Heart Lung Transplant 2003;22(10):1117–25.

[137] De Simone P, Nevens F, De Carlis L, Metselaar HJ, et al. Everolimus with reduced tacrolimus improves renal function in de novo liver transplant recipients: a randomized controlled trial. Am J Transplant 2012;12(11):3008–20.

[138] Saliba F, De Simone P, Nevens F, De Carlis L, et al. Renal function at two years in liver transplant patients receiving everolimus: results of a randomized, multicenter study. Am J Transplant 2013;13(7):1734–45.

Limitations of immunoassays used for therapeutic drug monitoring of immunosuppressants

Amitava Dasgupta

*Department of Pathology and Laboratory Medicine,
University of Texas–Houston Medical School, Houston, TX, USA*

2.1 INTRODUCTION

Immunosuppressive drugs nonspecifically diminish immune responses, and these agents are essential for preventing organ rejection after transplantation and must be taken lifelong. These drugs are also used to treat autoimmune disease, allergic disorders, and several other diseases. The discovery that cyclosporine has immunosuppressive activity that specifically targets T lymphocytes was a major breakthrough in organ transplantation because it dramatically reduced acute rejection and improved long-term graft and patient survival [1]. The identification of other immunosuppressive drugs that modulate immune responses by other molecular mechanisms provides a wide range of treatment options after solid organ transplant. Immunosuppressive agents used in organ transplantation can be categorized according to their mechanism of action in the following classes:

- Corticosteroids (prednisone, methylprednisolone, and dexamethasone)
- Antimetabolite/antiproliferative agents (azathioprine, cyclophosphamide, mycophenolate mofetil, and mycophenolate sodium)
- Calcineurin inhibitors (cyclosporine, voclosporin, and tacrolimus)
- Mammalian target of rapamycin (mTOR) inhibitors (sirolimus and everolimus)
- Costimulatory blocker (belatacept)
- Polyclonal and monoclonal antibodies against T lymphocyte cell surface antigens are also used in combination with other immunosuppressive agents.

Oral voclosporin, a novel calcineurin inhibitor, was developed to prevent organ graft rejection and to treat autoimmune disease. The chemical structure of voclosporine is similar to that of cyclosporine A, with a difference in one amino acid [2]. However, voclosporin is not approved by the US Food and Drug Administration (FDA) and has no future in transplantation. Belatacept was approved by the FDA in June 2011 for use as a prophylaxis against organ rejection in kidney transplant

M. Oellerich & A. Dasgupta (Eds): Personalized Immunosuppression in Transplantation.
DOI: http://dx.doi.org/10.1016/B978-0-12-800885-0.00002-3

recipients. This drug is a second-generation costimulation blocker (CD80 antagonism) and is a fusion protein structurally related to abatacept, which is currently used only in treating autoimmune disease. Belatacept-treated patients had improved renal function compared to cyclosporine-treated patients. Belatacept is effective and safe in renal transplant patients for preventing graft loss, and this drug is less nephrotoxic than calcineurin inhibitors [3]. Therefore, belatacept seems to be a promising drug for maintenance immunosuppression in kidney transplant patients, and it does not require therapeutic drug monitoring. Sotrastaurin, a protein kinase inhibitor, initially appeared to be an effective immunosuppressant, but its further development as an immunosuppressant was halted due to a high rejection rate in transplant recipients. Tofacitinib is a kinase inhibitor with immunosuppressant activity that was approved by the FDA in 2012 for treating patients with rheumatoid arthritis. Although this drug was investigated as a potential immunosuppressant instead of calcineurin inhibitors along with other antimetabolite agents, currently there is little interest in the development of this drug as a potential immunosuppressive agent [4]. This may be related to the association of tofacitinib therapy with more infection and more malignancies, although better renal function could be achieved by using this drug.

In general, therapeutic drug monitoring of corticosteroids, azathioprine, and cyclophosphamide is not needed, but other immunosuppressants, such as cyclosporine, tacrolimus, sirolimus, and everolimus, require routine therapeutic drug monitoring due to narrow therapeutic range and better correlation of blood levels of immunosuppressants with therapeutic efficacy and toxicity. In general, therapeutic drug monitoring of cyclosporine, tacrolimus, sirolimus, and everolimus is conducted using whole blood, whereas monitoring of mycophenolic acid can be conducted using serum or plasma. The rationale is that cyclosporine is distributed approximately 41–58% in erythrocytes, 33–47% in plasma, and the rest in other cellular components. Moreover, distribution of cyclosporine between erythrocytes and plasma is temperature dependent, and a 10% increase in hematocrit can decrease plasma concentration by 12–14% [5]. Similarly, approximately 15% of tacrolimus is found in plasma and the rest distributed in cellular components of blood. Sirolimus (rapamycin) is approximately 95% distributed to erythrocytes and only 3% in plasma. Therefore, whole blood concentration of sirolimus is substantially higher than plasma, and drug monitoring must be conducted using whole blood [6]. The in vitro distribution of [^{3}H] everolimus between red blood cells and plasma is concentration dependent between 5 and 5000 ng/mL in rats, monkeys, and humans, indicating full saturation of the high-affinity but low-capacity binding sites for everolimus in blood cells. For example, in rats at 5 ng/mL, an average of 33.6% of everolimus is distributed in plasma and 66.4% in erythrocytes. Therefore, whole blood is the preferred specimen for pharmacokinetic studies [7]. In contrast, mycophenolic acid is almost exclusively found in plasma, with no concentration-dependent or temperature-dependent distribution between plasma and blood cells. Therefore, plasma is the preferred matrix for therapeutic drug monitoring [8].

Although immunoassays are widely used for therapeutic drug monitoring of various immunosuppressants, major limitations of these immunoassays are significant cross-reactivities with various metabolites of the parent drug. Some immunosuppressants, such as cyclosporine, have more than 20 metabolites, which makes it difficult for the antibody used in an immunoassay to recognize only the parent drug without any metabolite cross-reactivity. For this reason, liquid chromatography combined with mass spectrometry (LC–MS) or tandem mass spectrometry (LC–MS/MS) is considered as the gold standard for therapeutic drug monitoring of various immunosuppressants.

2.2 METHODS FOR THERAPEUTIC DRUG MONITORING OF IMMUNOSUPPRESSANTS

For therapeutic drug monitoring of immunosuppressants, several immunoassays are available commercially. These assays are listed in Table 2.1. In general, for analysis of cyclosporine, tacrolimus, sirolimus, and everolimus, pretreatment of whole blood with an extraction solution (supplied with the assay kit) is needed, and clear supernatant is analyzed for determination of drug concentration using an appropriate automated analyzer. However, antibody conjugate magnetic immunoassay (ACMIA) is the only commercially available assay that does not require specimen pretreatment because extraction of the drug from whole blood is accomplished online. Because mycophenolic acid is analyzed using serum or plasma, no specimen pretreatment is needed.

The fluorescence polarization immunoassay, a homogenous immunoassay marketed by Abbott Laboratories for application on the TDx analyzer, is one of the oldest immunoassays developed for analysis of cyclosporine. The ACMIA assay marketed by Siemens Diagnostics (Deerfield, IL; formerly Dade Behring) includes CSA Flex (Cyclosporine), CSA-E Flex reagent cartridges (Cyclosporine Extended Range), and TAC-R Flex reagent cartridges (Tacrolimus) for application on the Dimension systems. This method relies on online mixing and ultrasonic lysing of whole blood followed by exposure to β-galactosidase–antibody conjugate, removal of free conjugate using analyte-coated magnetic particles, and detection via a spectrometric β-galactosidase reaction.

Cloned enzyme donor immunoassay (CEDIA) products are available commercially from Microgenics (now part of Thermo Fisher) as CEDIA Cyclosporine Plus Assay (also available are reagents for a High Range assay), CEDIA Mycophenolic Acid Assay, CEDIA Sirolimus Assay, and CEDIA Tacrolimus Assay. Analyses can be performed on a variety of instrument systems, including the Hitachi 917, Beckman SYNCHRON, Olympus, and other automated analyzers. The CEDIA method is based on recombinant DNA technology to produce a unique homogenous enzyme immunoassay system. The assay principle is based on the bacterial enzyme β-galactosidase, which has been genetically engineered into two inactive fragments. The small fragment is termed an enzyme donor (ED), which can freely associate in the solution with the larger part called an enzyme acceptor (EA), producing an active enzyme that is capable of cleaving a substrate and thus generating a color change in the medium that can be measured spectrophotometrically. In this assay, drug molecules in the specimen compete for limited antibody binding sites with drug molecules conjugated with ED fragment. If drug molecules are present in specimen, then they bind to antibody binding sites, leaving drug molecules conjugated with ED

Table 2.1 Commercially Available Common Immunoassays for Analysis of Various Immunosuppressants

Immunosuppressant	Immunoassay	Analytical Range
Cyclosporine	ACMIA cyclosporine flex	25–500 ng/mL
	ACMIA cyclosporine extended range flex	350–2000 ng/mL
	CEDIA cyclosporine plus	25–400 ng/mL
	CEDIA plus high range	450–2000 ng/mL
	CMIA cyclosporine	30–1500 ng/mL
	EMIT 2000 cyclosporine	25–500 ng/mL
	EMIT 2000 cyclosporine specific assay	350–2000 ng/mL
	ADVIA centaur cyclosporine immunoassay	30–1500 ng/mL
Tacrolimus	ACMIA TAC-R flex	1.2–30 ng/mL
	CEDIA tacrolimus assay	2.0–30 ng/mL
	CMIA tacrolimus assay	2.0–30 ng/mL
	MEIA tacrolimus assay	3.0–30 ng/mL
	EMIT 2000 tacrolimus assay	2.0–30 ng/mL
	QMS tacrolimus assay	0.7–30 ng/mL
Sirolimus	CEDIA sirolimus assay	5.0–30 ng/mL
	CMIA sirolimus assay	2.0–30 ng/mL
	MEIA sirolimus assay	2.5–30 ng/mL
	ACMIA sirolimus assay	2.0–39 ng/mL
Everolimus	QMS everolimus assay	1.5–20 ng/mL
	Fluorescence polarization immunoassay	2.0–40 ng/mL
Mycophenolic acid	CEDIA mycophenolic acid	0.3–10 µg/mL
	Roche total mycophenolic acid	0.4–15 µg/mL
	EMIT 2000 mycophenolic acid	0.1–15 µg/mL
	PETINIA assay	0.2–30 µg/mL

ACMIA: Antibody conjugated magnetic immunoassay from Dade Behring, now Siemens Diagnostics. CEDIA: Cloned enzyme donor immunoassay developed by Microgenics Corporation, now Thermo Fischer. CMIA: Chemiluminescent microparticle immunoassay developed by Abbott Laboratories. EMIT: Enzyme multiplied immunoassay developed by Syva, now in Siemens Diagnostics product line. Roche Diagnostics also marketed EMIT assay. QMS: A homogenous particle-enhanced turbidimetric immunoassay. PETINIA assay (particle enhanced immunoturbidimetric assay) from Siemens Diagnostics.

free to form active enzyme by binding with EA. A signal is generated, the intensity of which is proportional to the analyte concentration [9].

Chemiluminescent microparticle immunoassay (CMIA) is a relatively new product line from Abbott Diagnostics. Reagent kits are available for cyclosporine, sirolimus, and tacrolimus for analysis on the Abbott Diagnostics Architect *i* system. The principle of CMIA technology is to lyse whole blood with subsequent exposure to anti-analyte-coated paramagnetic particles, followed by addition of acridinium-labeled analyte conjugate and then pretrigger and trigger solutions to initiate a chemiluminescent reaction. The enzyme multiplied immunoassay technique (EMIT) was first introduced by the Syva Company, and it is a homogenous competitive immunoassay. In this immunoassay design, antigen is labeled with glucose 6-phosphate dehydrogenase enzyme. The active enzyme reduces nicotinamide adenine dinucleotide (NAD; no signal at 340 nm) to NADH (absorbs at 340 nm), and the absorbance is monitored at 340 nm. When labeled antigen binds with the antibody molecule, the enzyme becomes inactive. Therefore, signal is produced by free label, and the intensity of the signal is proportional to the analyte concentration. EMIT reagents are available commercially from Siemens as the Syva product line. EMIT 2000 reagent kits are available for cyclosporine, mycophenolic acid, and tacrolimus on Viva E or V-Twin drug testing systems. Roche Diagnostics also offers an EMIT assay for cyclosporine. EMIT methods require whole blood pretreatment except for mycophenolic acid assay because mycophenolic acid is analyzed using serum or plasma.

The enzymatic mycophenolic acid assay (total mycophenolic acid assay) commercialized by Roche Diagnostics for application on the COBAS INTEGRA systems is based on the principle of inhibition of an enzymatic reaction by mycophenolic acid. After sample addition to the reaction mixture, mycophenolic acid present in the serum inhibits inosine monophosphate dehydrogenase II (IMPDH II) catalyzed conversion of inosine monophosphate in the presence of NAD as a cofactor into xanthine monophosphate. In this reaction, NADH, which absorbs at 340 nm (NAD has no absorption at 340 nm), is generated. Therefore, the concentration of mycophenolic acid in the specimen is inversely proportional to the rate of NADH formation that is measured at 340 nm. The recently introduced particle-enhanced turbidimetric inhibition immunoassay (PETINIA) for application on the Dimension analyzer (Siemens Diagnostics) is a homogenous immunoassay method. This assay utilizes a synthetic particle conjugated with mycophenolic acid and monoclonal mycophenolic acid specific antibody. Mycophenolic acid present in the specimen competes with mycophenolic acid conjugated with synthetic particle for limited antibody binding sites, thereby decreasing the rate of aggregation. As a result, mycophenolic acid concentration in the specimen is inversely proportional to the rate of aggregation, which is measured using bichromatic turbidimetry reading at 340 and 700 nm.

For everolimus, only quantitative microsphere system (QMS) everolimus assay (Thermo Fischer) is approved by the FDA for use in the United States. QMS Everolimus assay is a homogenous PETINIA based on competition between everolimus present in the specimen and everolimus coated onto a microparticle for antibody binding sites of the everolimus antibody reagent. The everolimus-coated microparticle reagent is rapidly agglutinated in the presence of anti-everolimus antibody reagent in the absence of any competing drug in the sample. The rate of absorption change is measured photometrically. When a sample containing everolimus is added, the agglutination reaction is partly inhibited, slowing down the rate of absorption change. A concentration-dependent agglutination inhibition curve can be obtained with maximum rate of agglutination at the lowest everolimus concentration and the lowest agglutination rate at the highest everolimus concentration. This assay uses a 6-point calibration. A fluorescence polarization immunoassay for everolimus is also available but not FDA approved.

In addition to immunoassays, high-performance liquid chromatography combined with ultraviolet detection (HPLC-UV) is another well-developed technology for therapeutic drug monitoring of certain immunosuppressants. However, tacrolimus cannot be quantified by HPLC-UV because it lacks a significant chromophore. LC–MS or LC–MS/MS technology has been applied to therapeutic drug monitoring of all of the immunosuppressive drugs and is considered as the gold standard. In principle, analyte must be extracted from the biological matrix before application onto a short column where water-soluble substances are washed away, and then the compounds of interest are eluted (sometimes selectively) from the column using a methanol- or acetonitrile-based mobile phase. Per user-defined instrument specifications, column eluate is vaporized and compounds are ionized in the mass spectrometer source where specific ions are directed into the mass spectrometer. Because only ions with specific mass-to-charge ratios (e.g., analyte and internal standard) are permitted to pass through the quadrupoles to the photomultiplier for detection, this technology is highly selective and superior to immunoassays for therapeutic drug monitoring of various immunosuppressants.

2.3 CYCLOSPORINE MONITORING: TROUGH OR C2 MONITORING?

The timing of specimen collection has always been immediately before administration of the next dose (trough level or pre-dose level) for all immunosuppressants, and for standardization purposes, it has been suggested that the timing should be within 1 h before the next dose. However, only for cyclosporine, 2-h post-dosing cyclosporine concentrations (called C2 monitoring) have been proposed because it may improve the clinical outcome [10]. However, based on systematic review of 29 studies, Knight and Morris observed little evidence to support the benefit of C2 monitoring. The authors commented that the C2 monitoring strategy had no significant effect on rate of acute rejection. Furthermore, in stable transplant recipients, the majority of studies showed a reduction of mean cyclosporine dosage with adoption of C2 monitoring, but no obvious clinical benefit was derived from such dose reduction [11].

Therapeutic ranges for cyclosporine are often organ specific and vary widely between transplant types. In addition, target cyclosporine levels may be lower if cyclosporine is used in addition to another immunosuppressant. Trough whole blood cyclosporine levels following kidney transplant are typically between 150 and 250 ng/mL soon after transplant and are tapered down to less than 150 ng/mL during maintenance therapy. Recommended levels after liver and heart transplants are 250–350 ng/mL soon after transplant and less than 150 ng/mL during maintenance therapy. These target ranges were determined by HPLC. Min et al. demonstrated that up to 1 month after renal transplantation, cyclosporine therapeutic response threshold was 182 ng/mL, whereas nephrotoxicity threshold was 204 ng/mL. Between 1 and 3 months after transplantation, the therapeutic and toxic thresholds for cyclosporine were 175 and 189 ng/mL, respectively. However, between 3 and 12 months after transplantation, the therapeutic and toxic cyclosporine thresholds were 135 and 204 ng/mL, respectively [12]. Therefore, maintaining a cyclosporine level less than 150 ng/mL in stable transplant patients is justified. However, for C2 monitoring, target concentrations vary between 600 and 1700 ng/mL depending on the type of graft and the time after transplantation [13].

2.4 LIMITATIONS OF IMMUNOASSAYS USED FOR CYCLOSPORINE MONITORING

Cyclosporine, a cyclic undecapeptide, is extensively metabolized in the liver cells and intestine by cytochrome P450, producing more than 30 metabolites. The most prominent metabolites found in human blood are 2-hydroxylated products (AM1 and AM9) and N-demethylated product (AM4N). Further oxidation of AM1 and AM9 results in dehydroxylated AM19, AM49, and AM69 metabolites. Other metabolites found in blood include AM1A, AM1c, AMc9, and AM14N [14]. In general, AM1, AM9, and AM4N are considered as the primary metabolites of cyclosporine because these metabolites are derived directly from cyclosporine metabolism. Then other metabolites are formed that are considered as secondary and tertiary metabolites. It is assumed that CYP3A4 is the major isoform responsible for metabolism of cyclosporine, but CYP3A5 also has a modest contribution. However, CYP3A5 polymorphism may alter the cyclosporine metabolism pattern significantly [15]. Moreover, disease state may also alter metabolism of cyclosporine. Akhlaghi et al. reported that concentrations of cyclosporine metabolites were lower in kidney transplant recipients with diabetes compared to patients without diabetes [16].

Many investigators have reported positive bias in various immunoassays used for therapeutic drug monitoring of cyclosporine compared to chromatographic methods. It is desirable that if immunoassay is used for monitoring cyclosporine, an assay with the least metabolite cross-reactivity should be selected. If C2 monitoring is conducted, the specimen must be collected within ±10 min of 2-h post-dosage. Moreover, the laboratory should also state the bias in the cyclosporine assay used along with target cyclosporine level [17]. Morris et al. commented on behalf of the IFCC/IATDMCT Joint Working Group that a large percentage of laboratories use less specific monoclonal antibody-based method. In addition, for C2 monitoring, proper dilution protocol must be used for analysis of cyclosporine [18].

Polyclonal antibody-based fluorescence polarization immunoassay (p-FPIA) was one of the earliest immunoassays available for therapeutic drug monitoring of cyclosporine, and very significant positive bias in this method due to metabolite cross-reactivity was reported. In one study, the authors determined cyclosporine concentrations in 35 patient specimens using p-FPIA assay and HPLC and observed up to 12 times higher values using p-FPIA compared to HPLC [19]. Later, Abbott Laboratories introduced monoclonal antibody-based FPIA (m-FPIA) for cyclosporine for application on the TDx analyzer, followed by m-FPIA assay for application on the AxSYM analyzer. The m-FPIA showed substantially lower bias compared to the p-FPIA. For example, mean trough cyclosporine level obtained by the poly-clonal assay was 217 ng/mL, whereas that obtained by the monoclonal antibody-based assay was 80 ng/mL. For C2 monitoring, mean cyclosporine levels were 881 and 519 ng/mL, respectively, as determined by the polyclonal and monoclonal anti-body-based FPIA assays [20]. McBride et al. reported that based on the analysis of blood from 200 transplant recipients with various transplant types, average positive bias in cyclosporine values measured in whole blood using m-FPIA (TDx analyzer) was 31, 14, and 12%, respectively, with renal, liver, and heart transplant recipients compared to values observed using a more specific HPLC method [21]. Hamwi et al. studied performances of four cyclosporine immunoassays (EMIT, CEDIA, m-FPIA on the TDX analyzer, and m-FPIA on the AxSYM analyzer) by comparing results using blood from 127 patients after kidney, bone marrow, heart–lung, and liver trans-plantation and observed that all immunoassays showed positive bias compared to a reference method (HPLC-UV), regardless of transplant type. Despite dose reduc-tions, the authors observed higher cyclosporine levels measured by EMIT, CEDIA, and m-FPIA (using TDx and AxSYM analyzers) in the late post-transplant phase due to significantly increased levels of AM1 and AM19 metabolites over time after transplantation. Based on regression equation analysis, average bias compared to the HPLC-UV method was 25% for CEDIA assay, 12% for the EMIT assay, 15% for the m-FPIA/AxSYM assay, and 40% for the m-FPIA/TDx assay [22]. Steimer reported that mean differences compared with HPLC were as follows for cyclosporine analy-sis: 9–12% for EMIT, 18% for CEDIA, 29% for m-FPIA on AxSYM, and 57% for m-FPIA on TDx analyzer. In contrast to the mean differences, substantial (>200%) and variable overestimation of cyclosporine values using immunoassays compared to HPLC were observed in individual patient samples [23].

Significant positive bias observed in various immunoassays for cyclosporine compared to a corresponding value observed by a chromatographic method is mostly due to cross-reactivity of metabolites such as AM1, AM9, AM4N, AM19, and AM1c, which are present in blood. Newer immunoassays usually have improved specificity for cyclosporine due to reduced cross-reactivities with cyclosporine metabolites. For example, Abbott Laboratories has marketed a CMIA for application on the Architect analyzer. Wallemacq et al. reported findings from a multicenter evaluation of Abbott Architect cyclosporine assay involving seven clinical laboratories. Values obtained by the immunoassay were compared with corresponding values obtained by LC–MS/MS. The authors observed minimal cross-reactivity of cyclosporine metabolites in the CMIA cyclosporine immunoassay AM1 and AM9, the two major cyclosporine metabolites, exhibited −2.5–0.2% and 0.8–2.2% cross-reactivity, respectively, with the cyclosporine immunoassay. Comparison testing with Roche Integra assay (Integra 800) showed 2.4% cross-reactivity for AM1c metabolite, 10.7% cross-reactivity with the AM9 metabolite, and 2.9% cross-reactivity with the AM19 metab-olite. Dade Dimension's (now Siemens Diagnostics) Xpand assay showed 6.4–6.8% cross-reactivity with the AM4N metabolite, whereas cross-reactivity of AM9 was 2.6–3.6% [24]. Brate et al. reported that cross-reactivities of each of the cyclosporine metabolites (AM1, AM9, AM4N, AM19, and AM1c) were less than 1% with the

CMIA assay for application on the Architect analyzer [25]. Nevertheless, Hetu et al. reported an average 15.6% positive bias with CMIA cyclosporine assay compared to values obtained by LC–MS/MS [26]. Soldin et al. evaluated the performance of a new ADVIA Centaur cyclosporine immunoassay that requires a single-step extraction and observed excellent correlation between cyclosporine values obtained by the LC–MS/MS assay and ADVIA Centaur cyclosporine assay. The authors concluded that the ADVIA Centaur assay compared favorably to the LC–MS/MS assay [27].

Although all cyclosporine immunoassays showed positive bias with values obtained by HPLC, in general, use of C2 concentration for therapeutic drug monitoring of cyclosporine provided better performance than cyclosporine trough level monitoring (C0 monitoring) because values obtained by immunoassays showed less bias compared to corresponding values obtained by HPLC using C2 specimens compared to C0 specimens. This may be due to significantly lower concentrations of cyclosporine metabolites in C2 specimens than in C0 specimens. In addition, ACMIA is the only immunoassay affected by the presence of endogenous antibody, such as rheumatoid factor, and heterophilic antibody. De Jonge et al. reported a falsely elevated cyclosporine level of 492 ng/mL in a 77-year-old patient using ACMIA assay on the Dimension analyzer. However, using LC–MS, the cyclosporine level was undetectable. In addition, Architect cyclosporine assay also yielded a value lower than the detection limit. Treating specimen with polyethylene glycol and remeasuring cyclosporine in the supernatant by the same ACMIA assay showed no detectable level of cyclosporine, confirming that the interfering substance was a protein, most likely an endogenous antibody [28]. Issues with therapeutic drug monitoring of cyclosporine using immunoassays are summarized in Table 2.2.

CASE REPORT

A 23-month-old pediatric patient underwent allogeneic hematopoietic stem cell transplantation from cord blood obtained from an unrelated donor for familial hemophagocytic lymphohistiocytosis with a homozygous 284–285 mutation in the perforin gene; both parents were heterozygous for this molecular defect. The patient received oral cyclosporine before transplant and then for prevention of graft-versus-host disease. Blood cyclosporine levels were routinely tested by ACMIA assy. Two months after transplantation, a trend toward increasing cyclosporine blood concentration was observed. Cyclosporine treatment was discontinued on day 58 and restarted on day 68 (5 mg/kg per day). However, cyclosporine concentration increased from 222 ng/mL on day 58 to 312 ng/mL on day 60. The highest value observed was 850 ng/mL on day 67, and then after restarting cyclosporine on day 68, the observed value was 1034 ng/mL. The cyclosporine value increased to 1146 ng/mL on day 72. In contrast, using EMIT cyclosporine assay, all cyclosporine values were less than 40 ng/mL, the detection limit of the assay between days 65 and 68 (no values available before day 65). On day 72, the corresponding value obtained by EMIT was 64 ng/mL, which was significantly lower than the 1146 ng/mL value observed by the ACMIA assay. When five of the blood samples that showed high cyclosporine levels using the ACMIA assay were purified by protein A-sepharose chromatography to remove endogenous IgG, the cyclosporine values re-assayed by the same ACMIA assay showed values less than 25 ng/mL, the detection limit of the assay. Therefore, falsely high cyclosporine values as determined by the ACMIA assay were due to interference by an endogenous antibody in the assay [29].

Table 2.2 Issues with Therapeutic Drug Monitoring of Cyclosporine Using Immunoassays

- Reference method for cyclosporine monitoring is HPLC-UV or preferable LC–MS or liquid chromatography combined with tandem mass spectrometry (LC–MS/MS) using EDTA whole blood.
- In general, less bias between immunoassays and HPLC is observed if C2 specimen is used instead of C0 (trough) specimen for therapeutic drug monitoring of cyclosporine. This is due to significantly lower concentrations of metabolites in C2 specimens compared to C0 specimens.
- Significant positive bias in cyclosporine immunoassays is due to cyclosporine metabolite cross-reactivities with antibodies used in immunoassays. In general, AM1, AM9, AM4N, AM19, and AM1c metabolites of cyclosporine are present in blood, but major interferences are due to AM1, AM9, AMN4, and AM1c metabolites, which are also present in blood in significant amounts.
- Monoclonal antibody-based FPIA assay for application on the AxSYM analyzer showed less bias (average 29%) than FPIA assay on the TDx analyzer, although both assays used the same antibody. This may be related to different wash step.
- EMIT cyclosporine assay in general showed less bias than FPIA. Nevertheless 9–12% positive bias may be observed compared to HPLC values. In one report, average positive bias was 43% in C0 specimens and 34% in C2 specimens.
- CMIA assay for application on the Architect analyzer has minimal cross-reactivity with cyclosporine metabolites. Nevertheless, estimated 15.6% positive bias with LC–MS/MS has been reported.
- Recently introduced ADVIA Centaur cyclosporine assay showed minimal bias compared to LC–MS/MS assay.
- ACMIA assay for application on the Dimension analyzer is the only immunoassay affected by endogenous antibodies. Detectable cyclosporine level in patients after discontinuation of cyclosporine by this assay has been reported. This assay also showed average bias of 12% compared to HPLC. In one report, average bias was 23% for C2 specimen but 31% in C0 specimens.

2.5 LIMITATIONS OF IMMUNOASSAYS USED FOR TACROLIMUS MONITORING

Tacrolimus, a 23-membered macrolide lactone, is monitored in whole blood using trough specimen. Tacrolimus is also metabolized but less extensively than cyclosporine. Tacrolimus is metabolized by CYP3A4 and CYP3A5, and it is also a substrate of P-glycoprotein. Homozygous carriers of the CYP3A5*3 allele require a lower dose of tacrolimus than do carriers of the CYP3A5*1 allele. Tacrolimus undergoes O-demethylation, hydroxylation, and oxidative metabolic reactions in the liver and intestine and is eliminated mostly through bile. Four primary metabolites (M-I, M-II, M-III, and M-IV) are produced during tacrolimus metabolism, which may be further metabolized to secondary metabolites (Table 2.3). CYP3A5 genetic polymorphism is associated with individual differences in tacrolimus pharmacokinetics and pharmacodynamics and affects trough cyclosporine level as well as metabolite concentrations [30,31]. Interestingly, seasonal variation in tacrolimus and sirolimus levels due to changes in vitamin D levels in patients receiving such drugs had been

Table 2.3 Major Tacrolimus Metabolites

Abbreviation	Name	Immunosuppressive Activity
Primary metabolites		
M-I	13-*O*-demethylated tacrolimus	Minimal
M-II	31-*O*-demethylated tacrolimus	Significant
M-III	15-*O*-demethylated tacrolimus	Negligible
M-IV	12-Hydroxylated tacrolimus	Minimal
Secondary metabolites		
M-V	15- and 31-*O*-demethylated	None
M-VI	13- and 31-*O*-demethylated	Minimal
M-VII	13- and 15-*O*-demethylated	None
M-VIII	31-*O*-demethylated and ring formation	Minimal

reported. For same dosage (concentration:dosage ratio), sirolimus and tacrolimus drug levels were significantly lower during July–September than January–March. This may be due to higher levels of vitamin D during the summer months, which may upregulate the CYP3A4 gene. However, no such seasonal variation was observed for mycophenolic acid [32].

Although HPLC-based assays are considered as the reference method for analysis of tacrolimus in whole blood, immunoassays are routinely used in clinical laboratories due to speed and ease of operation. Studies have reported false-positive tacrolimus concentrations in patients with low hematocrit values and high imprecision at tacrolimus value less than 9 ng/mL with the microparticle enzyme immunoassay (MEIA) for tacrolimus for application on the AxSYM platform (Abbott Laboratories). However, the EMIT assay was not affected. In one study, when specimens were divided into three groups (group A, hematocrit <25%; group B, hematocrit 25–35%; group C, hematocrit >35%), the difference between methods (MEIA vs. EMIT 2000) increased as hematocrit values were decreased. Moreover, false-positive results were reported in 63% of specimens with MEIA, for which patients did not receive any tacrolimus, but only 2.2% of specimens showed false-positive tacrolimus values using EMIT. The false-positive values ranged from 0.0 to 3.7 ng/mL using MEIA in patients who never received tacrolimus. In addition, the median difference between tacrolimus results was 2.2 ng/mL using MEIA assay compared to corresponding values using EMIT assay in patients with hematocrit equal to or less than 25%. In contrast, no difference was observed in tacrolimus values measured by MEIA and EMIT assays in patients with hematocrit greater than 35% [33].

Immunoassays for tacrolimus are also affected by the cross-reactivity from tacrolimus metabolites. Ansermont et al. reported on average 30% overestimation of tacrolimus concentrations with EMIT tacrolimus assay compared to a reference liquid chromatography–electrospray mass spectrometric method due to significant metabolite cross-reactivity with the immunoassay [34]. Guilhaumou et al. reported an average positive bias of 28.2% in tacrolimus levels determined by the EMIT assay compared to the LC–MS/MS method [35]. Westely et al. evaluated CEDIA tacrolimus assay by measuring values obtained by CEDIA assay, LC–MS/MS, and MEIA assay. The authors observed 33.1% bias with the CEDIA assay and 20.1% bias with the MEIA assay compared to the tacrolimus values measured by the LC–MS/MS method in renal transplant recipients [36]. The relatively new Architect tacrolimus assay (CMIA tacrolimus assay), although free from interferences of low hematocrit that affect the MEIA assay manufactured by the same company, still shows positive bias in tacrolimus values measured by this assay compared to the more specific LC–MS/MS [37]. However, one advantage of CMIA assay is that the limit of quantitation is less than 1 ng/mL, which is consistent with recommendations issued at the European consensus conference. Bazin et al. also evaluated CMIA Architect tacrolimus assay and observed an average bias of 20% between values determined by the CMIA assay and LC–MS/MS [38]. Hetu et al. reported that CMIA tacrolimus assay for application on the Architect analyzer on average overestimates tacrolimus levels by 18.1% compared to the LC–MS/MS method [26]. Hirano et al. evaluated tacrolimus levels in whole blood collected from patients with rheumatoid arthritis and renal transplant using Architect tacrolimus immunoassay and LC–MS/MS assay. In general, the authors observed a mean bias of 45% in rheumatoid arthritis patients and 35% in renal transplant patients in tacrolimus values measured by the immunoassay on the Architect analyzer compared to LC–MS/MS assay. In the spiked samples, 13-*O*-demethylated tacrolimus (M-I) did not show any cross-reactivity with the immunoassay, but 31-*O*-demethylated tacrolimus (M-II) metabolite showed 120% cross-reactivity [39]. Other studies have shown that active M-II metabolite and inactive M-III metabolite have 94% and 45% cross-reactivity with CMIA assay, respectively. The active M-II metabolite can represent up to 15% of tacrolimus level in trough specimen in renal transplant recipients. Moreover, bias between immunoassay and LC–MS/MS is in general lower with lower tacrolimus levels (1–15 ng/mL) than with higher tacrolimus levels (20 ng/mL or higher) [40]. In another study, the authors observed an average 35% positive bias with the CMIA assay compared to the LC–MS/MS reference method, but specimens were collected in the morning 12 h after evening dosage of tacrolimus (trough tacrolimus monitoring). In addition, genetic polymorphism of the *CYP3A5* gene affected metabolite profile and therefore magnitude of cross-reactivity with the CMIA tacrolimus assay. The ratio of 13-*O*-demethylated tacrolimus to tacrolimus was significantly lower in the *CYP3A5*3/*3* genotype than the *CYP3A5*1/*3* genotype. A higher cross-reactivity was observed in patients with tacrolimus level less than 3 ng/mL and *CYP3A5*1/*3* genotype [41].

QMS tacrolimus assay is now commercially available for therapeutic drug monitoring of tacrolimus. QMS tacrolimus assay is a homogenous particle-enhanced turbidimetric assay that can be adopted on an open channel chemistry analyzer such as the Roche P-modular analyzer. Based on analysis of 145 specimens collected from patients who received kidney, liver, stem cell, lung, and islet cell transplantation,

Leung et al. observed a statistically significant positive proportional positive bias of 17% based on Passing–Bablok regression analysis ($y = 1.17x + 0.03$) with QMS tacrolimus assay compared to the LC–MS/MS method. However, in subgroup analysis using liver and kidney transplant patients, proportional positive biases were 22 and 31%, respectively, with QMS tacrolimus assay compared to the LC–MS/LS reference method [42].

ACMIA assay is the only assay commercially available for which no sample pretreatment is necessary. This assay shows an average positive bias of 16.6% compared to LC–MS/MS. However, samples from liver transplant recipients in the early post-surgery phase showed a higher bias with ACMIA assay compared to LC–MS/MS. In addition, these patients also had low plasma albumin. Therefore, low plasma albumin in the early post-surgery phase may lead to higher positive bias with the ACMIA assay [43]. Moreover, like cyclosporine ACMIA assay, the tacrolimus ACMIA assay is also affected by rheumatoid factors and endogenous heterophilic antibodies. In one study, the authors analyzed blood sample from patients who never received tacrolimus but had various concentrations of rheumatoid factors in their blood. No positive tacrolimus value was observed (above 2.3 ng/mL, the detection limit of the assay) in patients with rheumatoid factor concentrations less than 20 U/mL. However, 2 patients out of 50 analyzed showed false-positive tacrolimus values, and the concentration range of rheumatoid factors in these patients varied from 110 to 2650 U/mL. When two specimens that showed positive tacrolimus values were treated with immunoglobin blocking agent, the tacrolimus values were not detected after reanalysis with the same ACMIA assay, indicating that rheumatoid factor may interfere with the ACMIA tacrolimus assay [44]. Altinier et al. also described the interference of heterophilic antibody in the ACMIA tacrolimus assay. A sample of a patient showed tacrolimus values in the range of 49 to 12.5 ng/mL even after interruption of the treatment. The authors confirmed that the elevated tacrolimus levels were due to the presence of heterophilic antibody by treating samples with heterophilic blocking tubes and protein G resin that removed such interference [45]. In another report, the authors observed a high tacrolimus value (79.7 ng/mL) in a liver transplant recipient using ACMIA tacrolimus assay despite discontinuation of tacrolimus therapy. The authors identified β-galactosidase antibodies as the cause of interference because in this assay, anti-tacrolimus antibody conjugated to β-galactosidase is used [46]. Rostaing et al. observed a falsely elevated tacrolimus level of 24 ng/mL using the ACMIA tacrolimus assay, but tacrolimus was not detected using LC–MS/MS as well as EMIT tacrolimus assay. The authors identified positive anti-double-stranded DNA autoantibodies as the cause of interference in the ACMIA assay [47]. Moscato et al. commented that in their medical center, abnormally high tacrolimus results measured by the ACMIA method had been observed in 1% of patients who were followed up. The authors suggested that because falsely elevated tacrolimus results may lead to erroneous adjustment of drug dosage, elevated tacrolimus values observed by the ACMIA method that cannot be explained clinically must be checked by other methods [48]. Issues with therapeutic drug monitoring of tacrolimus using immunoassays are summarized in Table 2.4.

Table 2.4 Issues with Therapeutic Drug Monitoring of Tacrolimus Using Immunoassays

- Tacrolimus is monitored usually in trough whole blood (EDTA-whole blood).
- Tacrolimus cannot be monitored using HPLC-UV method due to lack of absorption of tacrolimus in UV region. Reference method is LC–MS or liquid chromatography combined with tandem mass spectrometry (LC–MS/MS)
- Tacrolimus metabolite M-II (active metabolite) has significant cross-reactivity with antibodies used in tacrolimus immunoassays. M-III metabolite may also have some cross-reactivity, but M-I metabolite usually has negligible cross-reactivity.
- MEIA assay for application on the AxSYM analyzer may produce false-positive tacrolimus result if hematocrit is low (<25%). No other immunoassays suffers from this problem.
- MEIA assay shows an average positive bias of 20% compared to LC–MS method.
- Average positive bias reported for CEDIA assay is 33.1% compared to LC–MS method
- Relatively new CMIA assay for application on the Architect analyzer has average positive bias of 18% compared to LC–MS. However, in one report, the authors observed 35% positive bias in renal transplant recipients.
- Recently introduced QMS tacrolimus assay has an overall average bias of 17% compared to LC–MS/MS method. However, liver and kidney transplant patients showed slope bias of 22 and 31%, respectively.
- ACMIA assay shows an average positive bias of 16.6% compared to LC–MS/MS method. However, samples from liver transplant recipients early post-surgery showed a higher bias with ACMIA assay compared to LC–MS/MS.
- ACMIA tacrolimus assay for application on the Dimension analyzer is the only immunoassay affected by endogenous antibodies such as heterophilic antibodies. As much as 1% of patients may show abnormally high tacrolimus due to such interferences.

There is a need for standardization of tacrolimus assay. Because of a lack of tacrolimus reference material, currently available LC–MS and immunoassays for tacrolimus are not standardized. Data from the International Proficiency Scheme of tacrolimus (http://www.bioanalytics.co.uk) indicate that interlaboratory variability of results is typically 6.2% with the Architect assay, 8.1% with LC–MS/MS assay, but 18.1% with the EMIT assay. Such significant variations, especially with the EMIT assay, may have clinical significance. Levine et al. sent blinded whole blood tacrolimus proficiency specimens to 22 clinical laboratories in 14 countries and observed a coefficient of variation (CV) range between 11.4% and 18.7% when LC–MS methods were used for analysis. The ranges of CVs were 3.9–9.5% with the Architect analyzer and 5.0–48.1% with the Dade Dimension analyzer. The authors concluded that tacrolimus assay standardization is necessary to compare patient results obtained between laboratories. In addition, improved assay accuracy is needed to provide optimized drug dosing and consistent care across transplant centers globally [49].

CASE REPORT

A 59-year-old man underwent kidney transplant and was treated with tacrolimus and corticosteroids. In the post-transplant period, he experienced recurrent bacterial and fungal infection and was treated with antibiotics. For the first 3 weeks after transplant, the patient's tacrolimus whole blood concentrations were consistent with dosage and were less than 12 ng/mL. Twenty-five days after transplant, his tacrolimus level was measured by the ACMIA tacrolimus assay and Dimension analyzer and was found to be highly elevated to 21.5 ng/mL. The whole blood tacrolimus levels were monitored continuously, but values, although reduced, were discordant with the discontinuation of tacrolimus therapy. The tacrolimus values measured by the ACMIA assay after discontinuation of tacrolimus were all greater than 10 ng/mL, whereas corresponding tacrolimus values measured by the MEIA assay were less than 2 ng/mL, indicating interference in tacrolimus measurement with the ACMIA assay. The authors diluted whole blood samples showing high tacrolimus concentrations with zero calibrator and then remeasured tacrolimus values using the ACMIA assay and observed nonlinearity, thus further confirming the interference in the ACMIA assay. However, washed erythrocytes showed significantly lower tacrolimus values as measured by the ACMIA assay compared to those of the corresponding whole blood specimens. The authors concluded that the interference with the ACMIA tacrolimus assay was method specific and was due to a factor present in the plasma because plasma tacrolimus values as measured by the ACMIA assay were higher than whole blood values. The authors also suggested that if the tacrolimus value measured by the ACMIA assay does not match the clinical picture, tacrolimus must be measured by an alternative method before any clinical intervention [50].

CASE REPORT

An abnormally elevated trough tacrolimus level of 78.5 ng/mL was observed in a 52-year-old male renal transplant recipient 2 days post-transplant. Because of the abnormally high tacrolimus value, tacrolimus therapy was discontinued. Despite discontinuation of therapy, his tacrolimus level was 59.1, 52.4, 45.6, and 41.1 ng/mL on days 3, 4, 5 and 6, respectively. Suspecting interference, the authors measured the tacrolimus level at the pre-transplant phase before administration of tacrolimus, and the value was falsely elevated at 43 ng/mL. At that time, blood specimen at day 7 was analyzed by ACMIA and EMIT assay. Whereas ACMIA assay showed a value of 42.8 ng/mL, EMIT assay showed a value of 0.89 ng/mL, confirming that the falsely elevated tacrolimus value obtained using the ACMIA assay was due to interference. At that point, tacrolimus therapy was restarted, and eventually the authors replaced tacrolimus therapy with cyclosporine therapy. Interestingly, using ACMIA cyclosporine assay, the authors did not observe any interference [51].

2.6 LIMITATIONS OF IMMUNOASSAYS USED FOR SIROLIMUS MONITORING

Sirolimus, a macrocyclic lactone with immunosuppressive properties, requires routine therapeutic drug monitoring. Sirolimus has UV absorption and can be analyzed by HPLC-UV. However, LC–MS/MS is a more desirable method for therapeutic drug monitoring of sirolimus. Sirolimus is metabolized in the intestine and liver by cytochrome P450 enzymes (CYP3A). The multidrug efflux pump P-glycoprotein in the gastrointestinal tract also controls metabolism by regulating bioavailability. Sirolimus is hydroxylated and demethylated to more than seven metabolites, with the hydroxyl forms being the most abundant. Metabolites represent approximately 55% of whole blood sirolimus levels [52]. Leung et al. observed that 41-*O*-demetyl sirolimus, 7-*O*-demethyl sirolimus, and several hydroxy, dihydroxy, hydroxy-dimethyl, and didemethyl sirolimus metabolites can be detected in whole blood [53]. Pediatric patients may show complex patterns of metabolism, with different metabolic patterns from those of adults. The pharmacological activity of all metabolites has not been fully investigated due to difficulties associated with their isolation. However, preliminary studies indicate that the immunosuppressive activity of metabolites is less than 30% of that observed for the parent compound. Sirolimus is eliminated primarily by biliary and fecal pathways, with small quantities appearing in urine. As with the calcineurin inhibitors, dosage adjustments are needed in patients with hepatic dysfunction. EDTA anticoagulated whole blood is the recommended specimen matrix [54]. Although LC–MS/MS methods should be used for routine therapeutic drug monitoring of sirolimus in whole blood, immunoassays are widely used for routine therapeutic drug monitoring of sirolimus. As expected, immunoassays for sirolimus suffer from many limitations, including significant cross-reactivity from sirolimus metabolites producing falsely elevated sirolimus concentrations.

Colantonio et al. compared the suitability of CEDIA and MEIA sirolimus immunoassays for therapeutic drug monitoring of sirolimus. The limit of detection was 1.1 ng/mL and the limit of quantitation was found to be 1.5 ng/mL for the MEIA assay. In contrast, the limit of detection was much higher with the CEDIA assay (4.8 ng/mL). Comparison of sirolimus values obtained by these assays and a specific LC–MS analytical method for measuring sirolimus concentration showed average positive bias of 0.9 ng/mL with the MEIA assay and a larger average positive bias of 2.1 ng/mL with the CEDIA sirolimus assay. The authors concluded that whereas the MEIA assay is suitable for therapeutic drug monitoring of sirolimus, the CEDIA assay based on a higher limit of quantitation that falls within the therapeutic range is not [55]. Westley et al. evaluated the performance of CEDIA sirolimus assay for application on the Hitachi 917 analyzer and observed a mean positive bias of 20.4% with the CEDIA sirolimus assay compared to a reference LC–MS/MS method. The authors used specimens collected predominately from renal transplant recipients [56].

Morris et al. compared values obtained by the MEIA sirolimus assay with the values obtained using a specific LC–MS/MS assay and observed a mean bias of 49.2% in sirolimus values obtained by the MEIA assay with the corresponding values obtained by the LC–MS/MS assay. Although the authors did not investigate the cause of the large and variable bias between the MEIA assay and the specific LC–MS/MS assay, they speculated that sirolimus metabolite cross-reactivity with the MEIA assay could be a substantive contributing factor [57]. Wilson et al. also reported results of a multicenter trial of performance evaluation of the MEIA sirolimus assay. The authors observed an overall 25% positive slope bias in the MEIA assay compared to specific chromatographic methods (LC–MS/MS as well as HPLC-UV). Such positive bias was mostly attributable to metabolite cross-reactivity with the antibody used in the MEIA assay. The authors also reported that 41-*O*-demethyl sirolimus, the major metabolite present in whole blood, had 58% cross-reactivity with the MEIA assay. Another metabolite, 7-*O*-demethyl sirolimus, which is also present in significant amounts in whole blood of patients treated with sirolimus, has 63% cross-reactivity. However, 41-*O*-demethyl hydroxy sirolimus and 11-hydroxy sirolimus, which are present in very low amounts (11-hydroxy sirolimus may not be detectable), have 6% and 37% cross-reactivity, respectively. In addition, hematocrit may affect sirolimus values determined by the MEIA assay. The authors also observed a 21% difference in sirolimus results (lower values with higher hematocrit) for hematocrit when it increased from 25 to 45%. The difference was more significant at lower sirolimus values (approximately 5 ng/mL). In the upper therapeutic range, hematocrit bias may be less significant. This effect may be related to incomplete extraction of sirolimus from endogenous binding proteins in specimens with high hematocrit because sirolimus is primarily sequestered in red blood cells. The experiments discussed here were performed by supplementing sirolimus in pooled specimens with various hematocrit values [58].

Schmidt et al. evaluated the CMIA sirolimus assay for application on the Architect analyzer and concluded that the assay only cross-reacts with sirolimus metabolites F4 (11-hydroxy sirolimus) and F5 (41-*O*-demethyl sirolimus), showing 36.8% and 20.3% cross-reactivity, respectively. In a multisite clinical trial, the authors observed an average mean bias of 14, 25, and 39% with the CMIA assay compared to LC–MS/MS for determination of sirolimus at three different sites. However, higher biases were observed if sirolimus concentrations were low in certain specimens. The authors concluded that although the CMIA assay correlated well with LC–MS/M, it still showed significant positive bias in sirolimus values compared to values determined by more specific LC–MS/MS assays [59]. Holt et al. reported that the mean percentage bias of sirolimus values measured by the CMIA assay was 21.9% compared to LC–MS/MS values [60]. ACMIA sirolimus assay for application on the Dimension analyzer is also commercially available. Using 119 specimens collected from two sites from kidney transplant recipients, Cervinski et al. observed a mean positive difference of 0.95 ng/mL between values obtained by ACMIA assay and a reference LC–MS/MS method using Bland–Altman comparison. The authors used least square regression equation analysis and observed a slope of 1.20 with a correlation coefficient of 0.95 between ACMIA and LC–MS/MS assay [61]. Issues with therapeutic drug monitoring of sirolimus using immunoassays are summarized in Table 2.5.

2.7 LIMITATIONS OF IMMUNOASSAYS USED FOR EVEROLIMUS MONITORING

Everolimus, a hydroxyethyl derivative of sirolimus, has a pharmacokinetic profile that is better than that of the other popular mTOR inhibitor, sirolimus. Everolimus has higher bioavailability than sirolimus and also has a shorter half-life. Everolimus

Table 2.5 Issues with Therapeutic Drug Monitoring of Sirolimus Using Immunoassays

- Sirolimus is monitored usually using trough whole blood (EDTA-whole blood).
- Sirolimus has UV absorption and can be detected by both HPLC-UV and LC–MS/MS methods. However, LC–MS/MS methods are more analyte specific.
- Sirolimus metabolite 41-O-demethyl sirolimus, the major metabolite present in the whole blood, has significant cross-reactivity with various sirolimus immunoassays. Other metabolites, such as 7-O-demethyl sirolimus, 41-O-demethyl hydroxy sirolimus, and 11-hydroxy sirolimus, also have cross-reactivities with sirolimus immunoassays.
- MEIA sirolimus assay is affected by hematocrit, with lower values observed in the presence of higher hematocrit. This is particularly important for sirolimus value around 5 ng/mL.
- MEIA sirolimus assay shows an average 49% positive bias compared to LC–MS assay, although other investigators observed a mean bias of 25%.
- Average positive bias reported for CEDIA tacrolimus assay is 20.4% compared to LC–MS method, but the limit of quantitation of this assay is 4.8 ng/ml, which approaches the lower end of the therapeutic range of sirolimus.
- Relatively new CMIA assay for application on the Architect analyzer has average positive bias of 20% compared to LC–MS.
- ACMIA assay shows an average positive bias of 20% compared to LC–MS/MS method.

is primarily metabolized by the liver cytochrome P450 enzymes (CYP3A4, CYP3A5, and CYP2C8) to major metabolites such as 46-hydroxy, 24-hydroxy, and 25-hydroxy everolimus. Minor *O*-demethylated metabolites have also been described [62]. Strom et al. investigated everolimus metabolite pattern in trough blood specimens collected from kidney transplant recipients. The median concentrations of major metabolites 46-hydroxy, 24-hydroxy, and 25-hydroxy everolimus were 44.1, 7.7, and 14.4%, respectively. Minor metabolites detected included 11-hydroxy, 12-hydroxy, 14-hydroxy, 49-hydroxy, two hydroxy-piperidine everolimus metabolites, 16-*O*-desmethyl, 16,39-*O*-didesmethyl, 16,27-*O*-didesmethyl, and 27,39-*O*-didesmethyl everolimus [63].

Quantitative Microparticle System (QMS) everolimus assay received FDA approval for clinical use in 2011, and the assay can be adopted on an automated analyzer using open channel. QMS everolimus assay is linear between 1.5 and 20 ng/mL, covering the entire therapeutic range of everolimus. The limit of quantitation for this assay is 1.3 ng/mL. Dasgupta et al. adopted QMS everolimus assay on Hitachi 917 analyzer and reported that this assay is not affected by 70 commonly used drugs, but structurally similar sirolimus exhibited an average 46% cross-reactivity. In addition, the average bias for everolimus values determined by the QMS everolimus assay and corresponding values obtained by a specific LC–MS/MS method was 11% based on comparison of 90 specimens obtained from patients receiving everolimus. The authors concluded that QMS everolimus assay showed adequate sensitivity and specificity and can be used for routine therapeutic drug monitoring of everolimus [64]. Shu et al. adopted the QMS everolimus assay on Vitros 5, 1 FS Fusion Analyzer (Ortho

Diagnostics, Rochester, NY) and observed a slope of 1.271 in Deming regression analysis when values obtained by the QMS everolimus assay were compared with corresponding values obtained by a reference LC–MS/MS method [65]. Sallustio et al. observed an average bias of greater than 30% in everolimus concentration as determined by the FPIA of everolimus developed by Seradyn (Indianapolis, IN; Innofluor Certican assay) and a specific LC–MS/MS for everolimus, and they concluded that further investigation is needed before this assay can be used for routine therapeutic monitoring of everolimus [66]. Moes et al. also compared everolimus values obtained by the Innofluor Certican FPIA assay (on TDx analyzer) and LC–MS/MS method and observed on average a 23% positive bias with the FPIA everolimus assay. Moreover, everolimus concentration lower than 15 ng/mL could produce higher bias (up to twofold) using the FPIA assay. This variability could affect dosage adjustment of everolimus up to 1.25 mg despite using a correction factor of 23%. In addition, higher intrapatient variability was also observed using the FPIA assay compared to LC–MS/MS [67]. Strom et al. reported that major metabolites of everolimus, 46-hydroxy and 24-hydroxy everolimus, showed 1% or less cross-reactivity with the Innofluor Certican assay, whereas 25-hydroxy everolimus showed 6% or less cross-reactivity. Cross-reactivity testing with minor metabolites showed 16.3% cross-reactivity with 45-hydroxy, 33.0% with 12-hydroxy, 18.3% with 11-hydroxy, 15.3% with 14-hydroxy, 43% with 39-*O*-desmethyl, 142% with 27-*O*-desmethyl, and 68.0% with 40-*O*-desmethyl everolimus (sirolimus). Two hydroxy-piperidine everolimus metabolites showed 46.3 and 43% cross-reactivity [68]. Because sirolimus significantly cross-reacts with everolimus assay, if a patient also has sirolimus in the blood, everolimus immunoassays are invalid for therapeutic drug monitoring of everolimus.

Currently, the QMS everolimus assay is the only FDA-approved immunoassay commercially available for therapeutic drug monitoring of everolimus. Therefore, several investigators have attempted to measure everolimus concentration in specimens using sirolimus immunoassays, taking advantage of high cross-reactivity of everolimus with sirolimus immunoassays due to structural similarity between sirolimus and everolimus. In one report, the authors observed concentration-dependent cross-reactivity of everolimus with CMIA sirolimus assay on the Architect analyzer. The cross-reactivity was higher at lower concentration of everolimus (100% cross-reactivity at 1.0 ng/mL and 78% cross-reactivity at 25.0 ng/mL). Using curve fitting, the authors derived a polynomial equation ($y = -0.0042x^2 + 1.3985x - 0.4322$, where x is the observed sirolimus concentration obtained by the CMIA assay, and y is the calculated everolimus value) [69]. Hermida-Cadahia and Tutor also described determination of everolimus in blood samples of kidney and liver transplant recipients using the CMIA sirolimus assay and Architect i 1000 analyzer [70]. Bouzas and Tutor determined blood everolimus concentrations in kidney and liver transplant recipients using the sirolimus ACMIA assay (Siemens Diagnostics) [71]. However, in the opinion of this author, such indirect measurement may cause significant errors in calculated everolimus values in certain patients, and it is always advisable to use a chromatographic method for direct determination of everolimus concentration in

Table 2.6 Issues with Therapeutic Drug Monitoring of Everolimus Using Immunoassays

- Everolimus is monitored usually using through whole blood (EDTA-whole blood).
- Everolimus has UV absorption and can be detected by both HPLC-UV and LC–MS/MS methods. However, LC–MS/MS methods are more analyte specific.
- QMS everolimus assay is FDA approved, and this assay can be adopted on an automated analyzer with open channel capability.
- Major everolimus metabolites are 46-hydroxy, 24-hydroxy, and 25-hydroxy everolimus.
- In one report, QMS everolimus assay showed an average positive bias of 11% compared to LC–MS/MS assay, although in another report, the authors observed a slope of 1.271 using Deming regression analysis when everolimus values obtained by the QMS analyzer (adopted on Vitros 5, 1 FS Fusion Analyzer) were compared with values obtained by LC–MS/MS.
- Average positive bias reported for Innofluor Certican assay (fluorescence polarization assay for everolimus developed and marketed by Seradyn, Indianapolis, IN) was greater than 30% in one report compared to LC–MS/MS assay. In another report, the average bias was 23%, but specimens containing 15 ng/mL or lower concentrations of everolimus may show higher positive bias using Innofluor Certican assay.
- Major metabolites of everolimus 46-hydroxy and 24-hydroxy everolimus showed 1% or less cross-reactivity with the Innofluor Certican assay, whereas 25-hydroxy everolimus showed 6% or less cross-reactivity. However, minor metabolites of everolimus showed higher cross-reactivity, with highest cross-reactivity of 142% observed with 27-O-desmethyl everolimus.

whole blood. If such a method is not available in the clinical laboratory, an everolimus immunoassay should be used or the specimen should be send to a reference laboratory that provides therapeutic drug monitoring of everolimus using a specific chromatography-based method. Issues with therapeutic drug monitoring of everolimus using immunoassays are summarized in Table 2.6.

2.8 LIMITATIONS OF IMMUNOASSAYS USED FOR MYCOPHENOLIC ACID MONITORING

Mycophenolate mofetil and mycophenolate sodium are two available formulations of the immunosuppressant agent mycophenolic acid. Mycophenolate mofetil, a prodrug, is rapidly converted after oral administration into the active drug mycophenolic acid by esterases present in the gut wall, blood, liver, and tissues. Oral bioavailability is high (80–94%), and the drug is strongly bound to serum albumin (97–99%). Because free mycophenolic acid is biologically active, monitoring free mycophenolic acid concentration may be beneficial for a certain subset of patients (see Chapter 4). Mycophenolic acid is metabolized in the liver, gastrointestinal tract, and kidney by uridine diphosphate glucosyltransferase, forming 7-O-phenolic glucuronide (7-O-mycophenolic acid β-glucuronide; MPAG). This is the major metabolite of mycophenolic acid present in plasma at a concentration 20- to 100-fold higher than that of the parent drug mycophenolic acid. Mycophenolic acid metabolite

MPAG is inactive, but mycophenolic acid acyl-glucuronide, a minor metabolite of mycophenolic acid, has pharmacological potency. At least two other minor metabolites have been characterized. MPAG is excreted in the urine via active tubular secretion and also is secreted into the bile by multidrug resistance protein 2. Then MPAG is de-conjugated back into mycophenolic acid by gut bacteria and reabsorbed in the colon [72]. Kuypers et al. published a consensus report on the therapeutic drug monitoring of mycophenolic acid in solid organ transplantation. In general, mycophenolic acid area under the curve 0–12h (AUC_{0-12h}) is more strongly correlated with acute rejection than trough mycophenolic acid serum level [73]. Mycophenolic acid is 97–99% protein bound, and for certain patients, monitoring free mycophenolic acid concentration has clinical significance (see Chapter 4).

Mycophenolic acid is monitored in serum or plasma. Mycophenolic acid has UV absorption and can be monitored by HPLC-UV, although LC–MS and LC–MS/MS are superior techniques. Mycophenolic acid can also be determined using immunoassays. Although MPAG, the major metabolite of mycophenolic acid, usually does not cross-react with immunoassays for mycophenolic acid, mycophenolic acid acyl glucuronide, the minor metabolite, may show significant cross-reactivity with certain immunoassays, causing falsely elevated mycophenolic acid levels. Hosotsubo et al. studied the analytical performance of EMIT mycophenolic acid immunoassay and observed no interference from major metabolite MPAG. In addition, the EMIT assay also correlated well with a HPLC-UV for determination of mycophenolic acid [74]. In contrast, Martiny et al. observed significant overestimation of mycophenolic acid concentrations (30%) in the early post-transplant period. Moreover, an approximately 45% overestimation of mycophenolic acid concentrations compared to HPLC-UV was observed in patients who in addition to mycophenolic acid also received cyclosporine. The authors concluded that EMIT mycophenolic acid assay is not suitable for therapeutic drug monitoring of mycophenolic acid in the early post-transplant phase as well as in patients also receiving cyclosporine. For these patients, a chromatographic method must be used [75]. Brown et al. observed a mean positive bias of 14.6% between mycophenolic acid levels measured by the EMIT assay and those measured by a reference LC–MS/MS method [76].

Decavele et al. investigated the analytical performance of Roche total mycophenolic acid assay for application on Cobas Integra 400 and Cobas 6000 analyzers by comparing these methods with a specific LC–MS/MS method for determination of mycophenolic acid in specimens obtained from liver transplant recipients. The authors observed no significant bias between values obtained by Roche total mycophenolic acid immunoassay and values determined by LC/MS/MS. Passing–Bablok regression analysis showed a slope of 1.02 using the Cobas Integra 400 analyzer and a slope of 0.98 using the Cobas 6000 analyzer when values were compared with corresponding values obtained by LC–MS/MS. All specimens analyzed by the authors were collected from liver transplant patients. Due to excellent correlation with LC–MS/MS values, the authors concluded that the Roche immunoassay is suitable for therapeutic drug monitoring of mycophenolic acid [77]. The good agreement between Roche total mycophenolic acid assay and LC–MS/MS is due to very low

Table 2.7 Issues with Therapeutic Drug Monitoring of Mycophenolic Acid Using Immunoassays

- Mycophenolic acid is the only immunosuppressant drug that is monitored in serum or plasma.
- Mycophenolic acid has UV absorption and can be detected by both HPLC-UV and LC–MS/MS methods. However, LC–MS/MS methods are more analyte specific.
- Major mycophenolic acid metabolite is MPAG, which is inactive. Other three minor metabolites have been characterized. A minor metabolite mycophenolic acid acyl glucuronide has pharmacological activity.
- EMIT 2000 mycophenolic acid assay may overestimate mycophenolic acid level by 14.6% on average, but significant positive bias may be observed in early post-transplant phase (30%) and in patients receiving cyclosporine (45%). Therefore, for these patients, the chromatographic method should be used for therapeutic drug monitoring.
- CEDIA mycophenolic acid assay showed a mean positive bias of 15% with samples obtained from patients after heart transplantation, but mean bias was 41.7% and 52.3%, respectively, in specimens obtained from kidney transplant recipients and liver transplant. This is due to high cross-reactivity of mycophenolic acid acyl glucuronide metabolite (up to 215%) with the CEDIA assay.
- Roche total mycophenolic acid assay (enzymatic assay based on inhibition of monophosphate dehydrogenase inhibition by mycophenolic acid) has little cross-reactivity (<5%) with mycophenolic acid acyl glucuronide metabolite. This assay shows a very good correlation with LC–MS/MS method.
- A PETINIA mycophenolic acid is now available from Siemens Diagnostics for application on the Dimension EXL analyzer. Although this assay showed an average 12% positive bias compared to values obtained by HPLC-UV method, the average positive bias was 22.4% in liver transplant patients and 8.3% in kidney transplant patients. The highest positive bias observed in one specimen was 45.5%.

cross-reactivity of mycophenolic acid acyl glucuronide metabolite (<5%) with the Roche total mycophenolic acid assay [78].

Westley et al. observed approximately 18% positive bias in mycophenolic acid determined by the CEDIA assay on a Hitachi 911 analyzer compared to a chromatographic method (HPLC-UV) [79]. Shipkove et al. observed a mean positive bias of 15% with samples obtained from patients after heart transplantation, but mean bias was 41.7% and 52.3% in specimens obtained from kidney transplant recipients and liver transplant recipients, respectively, using the CEDIA mycophenolic acid immunoassay compared to values obtained by the more specific HPLC-UV method. The CEDIA mycophenolic acid assay in general showed a mean positive bias of 36.3%. The significant positive bias observed in the CEDIA mycophenolic acid assay is due to significant cross-reactivity of mycophenolic acid acyl glucuronide metabolite (192% cross-reactive according to the package insert). The authors observed concentration-dependent cross-reactivity of mycophenolic acid acyl glucuronide with the CEDIA assay, reaching a maximum cross-reactivity of 215%. However, the major metabolite MPAG showed no cross-reactivity with the CEDIA assay. The authors concluded that positive bias observed in the CEDIA assay was mostly due to cross-reactivity of mycophenolic acid acyl glucuronide with the antibody used in the assay [80].

Dasgupta and Johnson also observed an overall 15.6% positive bias with CEDIA mycophenolic acid assay compared to a HPLC-UV method for mycophenolic acid. However, the positive bias was less (11.8%) with kidney transplant recipients but much higher (33.4%) with liver transplant recipients. The highest positive bias of 102.6% was observed in mycophenolic acid level determined by the CEDIA assay in a liver transplant recipient (CEDIA value, 7.7 µg/mL; HPLC-UV value, 3.8 µg/mL). The authors concluded that caution must be used when interpreting therapeutic drug monitoring results of mycophenolic acid obtained with the CEDIA assay [81].

PETINIA mycophenolic acid assay is available from Siemens Diagnostics for application on the Dimension EXL analyzer. Although this assay showed an average 12% positive bias compared to values obtained by HPLC-UV, the average positive bias was 22.4% in liver transplant patients and 8.3% in kidney transplant patients. However, 7 out of 60 specimens analyzed showed positive bias greater than 20% when values obtained by the PETINIA assay were compared to corresponding values obtained by HPLC-UV. The highest positive bias observed in one specimen was 45.5% [82]. Issues with therapeutic drug monitoring of mycophenolic acid using immunoassays are summarized in Table 2.7.

2.9 CONCLUSIONS

Although immunoassays are used for therapeutic drug monitoring of cyclosporine, tacrolimus, sirolimus, everolimus, and mycophenolic assay, LC–MS or LC–MS/MS are considered as the gold standard for therapeutic drug monitoring of immunosuppressants because all immunoassays show significant positive bias compared to reference LC–MS or LC–MS/MS. Whereas cyclosporine, sirolimus, everolimus, and mycophenolic acid can also be determined using HPLC-UV, tacrolimus cannot be analyzed by HPLC-UV because it does not absorb at UV wavelength. Nevertheless, LC–MS and LC–MS/MS offer more specificity than HPLC-UV. However, care must be taken in selecting proper internal standards for chromatographic method. In addition, ion suppression and isobaric ion may interfere with LC–MS- or LC–MS/MS-based methods; therefore, caution must be taken to develop a robust method for monitoring of immunosuppressant. Moreover, multiple immunosuppressants can be monitored in a single run using chromatographic methods.

REFERENCES

[1] Lindholm A, Albrechtsen D, Tufveson G, Karlberg I, et al. A randomized trial of cyclosporine and prednisolone versus cyclosporine, azathioprine, and prednisolone in primary cadaveric renal transplantation. Transplantation 1992;54:624–31.

[2] Roese M, Tappeiner C, Heiligenhaus A, Heinz C. Oral voclosporin: novel calcineurin inhibitor for treatment of noninfectious uveitis. Clin Ophthalmol 2011;5:1309–13.

[3] Grannas G, Schrem H, Klempnauer J, Lehner F. Ten years' experience with belatacept based immunosuppression after kidney transplantation. J Clin Med 2014;6:98–110.

[4] Hardinger KL, Brennan DC. Novel immunosuppressive agents in kidney transplantation. World J Transplant 2013;3:68–77.

[5] Rosano TG. Effect of hematocrit on cyclosporine (cyclosporine A) in whole blood and plasma of renal transplant recipient. Clin Chem 1985;31:410–2.

[6] Yatscoff RW, Wang P, Chan K, Hicks D, et al. Rapamycin: distribution, pharmacokinetics, and therapeutic range investigations. Ther Drug Monit 1995;17:666–71.

[7] Laplanche R, Meno-Tetang GM, Kawai R. Physiological based pharmacokinetic modelling of everolimus (RAD 001) in arts involving non-linear tissue uptake. J Pharmacokinet Pharmacodyn 2007;34:373–400.

[8] Langman LJ, LeGatt DF, Yatscoff RW. Blood distribution of mycophenolic acid. Ther Drug Monit 1994;16:602–7.

[9] Jeon SI, Yang X, Andrade JD. Modeling of homogeneous cloned enzyme donor immunoassay. Anal Biochem 2004;333:136–47.

[10] Kokuhu T, Fukushima K, Ushigome H, Yoshimura N, et al. Dose adjustment strategy of cyclosporine A in renal transplant patients: evaluation of anthropometric parameters for dose adjustment and Co vs C2 monitoring in Japan, 2001–2010. Int J Med Sci 2013;10:1665–73.

[11] Knight SR, Morris PJ. The clinical benefits of cyclosporine C2 level monitoring: a systematic review. Transplantation 2007;83:1525–35.

[12] Min DI, Perry PJ, Chen HY, Hunsicker LG. Cyclosporine trough concentrations in pediatric allograft rejection and renal toxicity up to 12 months after renal transplantation. Pharmacotherapy 1998;18:282–7.

[13] Sukhavasharin NH, Praditpornsilpa K, Avihingsanon Y, Kuoatawintu P, et al. Study of cyclosporine level at 2 hours after administration in preoperative kidney transplant recipients for prediction of postoperative optimal cyclosporine dose. J Med Assoc Thai 2006;89(Suppl. 2):S15–20.

[14] Maurer G, Lemaire M. Biotransformation and distribution in blood of cyclosporine and its metabolites. Transplant Proc 1986;18:25–34.

[15] Zheng S, Tasnif Y, Hebert MF, Davis CL, et al. CYP3A5 gene variation influences cyclosporine A metabolite formation and renal cyclosporine disposition. Transplantation 2013;95:821–7.

[16] Akhlaghi F, Dostalek M, Falck P, Mendonza A, et al. The concentration of cyclosporine metabolites is significantly lower in kidney transplant recipients with diabetes mellitus. Ther Drug Monit 2012;34:38–45.

[17] Morris RG, Ilett KF, Tett SE, Ray JE, et al. Cyclosporine monitoring in Australia: 2002 update of consensus document. Ther Drug Monit 2002;24:677–88.

[18] Morris RG, Holt DW, Armstrong VW, Griesmacher A, et al. Analytical aspects of cyclosporine monitoring, on behalf of IFCC/IATDMCT joint working group. Ther Drug Monit 2004;26:227–30.

[19] Rondanelli R, Regazzi MB, Gastaldi L, Legnazzi P, et al. Measurement of cyclosporine in plasma of cardiac allograft recipients by fluorescence polarization immunoassay. Ther Drug Monit 1990;12:182–6.

[20] Vyzantiadis T, Belechri AM, Memmos D, Axiotou M, et al. Cyclosporine and its metabolites before and 2 h post-dose: comparative measurements of a monoclonal and polyclonal immunoassay. Clin Transplant 2003;17:231–3.

[21] McBride JH, Kim SS, Rodgerson DO, Reyes AF, et al. Measurement of cyclosporine by liquid chromatography and three immunoassays in blood from liver, cardiac and renal transplant recipients. Clin Chem 1992;38:2300–6.

[22] Hamwi A, Salomon A, Steinbrugger R, Frirzer-Szekeres M, et al. Cyclosporine metabolism in patients after kidney, bone marrow, heart-lung and liver transplantation in the early and late posttransplant period. Am J Clin Pathol 2000;114:536–43.

[23] Steimer W. Performance and specificity of monoclonal immunoassays for cyclosporine monitoring: how specific is specific? Clin Chem 1999;45:371–81.

[24] Wallemacq P, Maine GT, Berg K, Rosiere T, et al. Multisite analytical evaluation of Abbott Architect cyclosporine assay. Ther Drug Monit 2010;32:145–51.

[25] Brate EM, Finley DM, Grote J, Holets-McCormack S, et al. Development of an Abbott Architect cyclosporine immunoassay without metabolite cross-reactivity. Clin Biochem 2010;43:1152–7.

[26] Hetu PO, Robitaille R, Vinet B. Successful and cost effective replacement of immunoassays by tandem mass spectrometry for the quantification of immunosuppressants in the clinical laboratory. J Chromatogr B 2012;883:95–101.

[27] Soldin SJ, Hardy RW, Wians FH, Balko JA, et al. Performance evaluation of the new ADVIA Centaur system cyclosporine assay (single-step extraction). Clin Chim Acta 2010;411:806–911.

[28] De Jonge H, Geerts I, Declercq P, de Loor H, et al. Apparent elevation of cyclosporine whole blood concentration in a renal allograft recipient. Ther Drug Monit 2010;32:529–31.

[29] Bartoli A, Molinaro M, Visal L. Falsely elevated whole blood cyclosporine concentrations measured by an immunoassay with automated pretreatment. Ther Drug Monit 2010;32:791–2.

[30] Yoon SH, Cho JH, Kwon O, Choi JY, et al. CYP3A4 and ABCB1 genetic polymorphism on the pharmacokinetic and pharmacodynamics of tacrolimus and its metabolites (MI and M III). Transplantation 2013;95:828–34.

[31] Cusinato DA, Lacchini R, Romao EA, Moyses-Neto M, et al. Relationship of CYP3A5 genotype and Abcb diplotype to tacrolimus disposition in Brazilian kidney transplant patients. Br J Clin Pharmacol 2014 Feb 17 [e-pub ahead of print].

[32] Lindh JD, Andersson ML, Eliasson E, Bjorkhem-Bergman L. Season variation in blood concentrations and potential relationship to vitamin D. Drug Metab Dispos 2011;39:933–7.

[33] Armedariz Y, Garcia S, Lopez R, Pou L, et al. Hematocrit influences immunoassay performance for the measurement of tacrolimus in whole blood. Ther Drug Monit 2005;27:766–9.

[34] Ansermot N, Fathi M, Veuthey JL, Desmeules J, et al. Quantification of cyclosporine and tacrolimus in whole blood. Comparison of liquid chromatography-electrospray mass spectrometry with enzyme multiplied immunoassay technique. Clin Biochem 2008;41:910–3.

[35] Guilhaumou R, Lacarelle B, Sampol-Manos E. A rapid, simple and sensitive liquid chromatography-tandem mass spectrometric method for routine clinical monitoring of tacrolimus with the Waters Masstrak immunosuppressant kit. Methods Find Exp Clin Pharmacol 2010;32:737–43.

[36] Westley IS, Taylor PJ, Salm P, Morris RG. Cloned enzyme donor immunoassay tacrolimus assay compared with high-performance liquid chromatography-tandem mass spectrometry in liver and renal transplant recipients. Ther Drug Monit 2007;29:584–91.

[37] Wallemacq P, Goffinet JS, O'Morchoe S, Rosiere T, et al. Multi-site analytical evaluation of the Abbott Architect tacrolimus assay. Ther Drug Monit 2009;31:198–204.

[38] Bazin C, Guinedor A, Barau C, Gozalo C, et al. Evaluation of the Architect tacrolimus assay in kidney, liver and heart transplant recipients. J Pharm Biomed Appl 2010;53:997–1002.

[39] Hirano K, Maruyama S, Mino Y, Naito T. Suitability of chemiluminescent enzyme immunoassay for the measurement of blood tacrolimus concentrations in rheumatoid arthritis. Clin Biochem 2011;44:397–402.

[40] Bazin C, Guinedor A, Barau C, Gozalo C, et al. Evaluation of the Architect tacrolimus assay in kidney, liver and heart transplant recipients. J Pharm Biomed Anal 2010;33:997–1002.

[41] Hirano K, Naito T, Mino Y, Takayama T, et al. Impact of CYP3A5 genetic polymorphism on cross-reactivity in tacrolimus chemiluminescent immunoassay in kidney transplant recipients. Clin Chim Acta 2012;414:120–4.

[42] Leung EK, Yi X, Gloria C, Yeo KT. Clinical evaluation of the QMS tacrolimus immunoassay. Clin Chim Acta 2014;431:270–5.

[43] Tempestilli M, Di Stasio E, Basile MR, Elisei F, et al. Low plasma concentrations of albumin influence the affinity column-mediated immunoassay method for the measurement of tacrolimus in blood during the early period after liver transplantation. Ther Drug Monit 2013;35:96–100.

[44] Barcelo-Martin B, Marquet P, Ferrer JM, Castanyer Puig B, et al. Rheumatoid factor interference in a tacrolimus immunoassay. Ther Drug Monit 2009;31:743–5.

[45] Altinier S, Varagnolo M, Zaninotto M, Boccagni P, et al. Heterophilic antibody interference in a non-endogenous molecule assay: an apparent elevation in the tacrolimus concentration. Clin Chim Acta 2009;402:193–5.

[46] Knorr JP, Grewal KS, Balasubramanian M, Zaki R, et al. Falsely elevated tacrolimus levels caused by immunoassay interference secondary to beta-galactosidase antibodies in an infected liver transplant recipient. Pharmacotherapy 2010;30:954.

[47] Rostaing L, Cointault O, Marquet P, Josse AG, et al. Falsely elevated whole blood tacrolimus concentrations in a kidney transplant patient: potential hazards. Transplant Int 2010;23:227–30.

[48] Moscato D, Nonnato A, Adamo R, Vancheri M, et al. Therapeutic monitoring of tacrolimus: aberrant results by an immunoassay with automated pretreatment. Clin Chim Acta 2010;411:77–80.

[49] Levine DM, Maine GT, Armbruster DA, Mussell C, et al. The need for standardization of tacrolimus assay. Clin Chem 2011;57:1739–47.

[50] D'Alessandro M, Mariani P, Mennini G, Severi D, et al. Falsely elevated tacrolimus concentrations measures using the ACMIA method due to circulating endogenous antibodies in a kidney transplant recipient. Clin Chim Acta 2011;412:245–8.

[51] Toraishi T, Takeuchi H, Nakamura Y, Konno O, et al. Falsely abnormally elevated blood trough concentration of tacrolimus measured by antibody conjugated magnetic immunoassay in a renal transplant recipient: a case study. Transplant Proc 2012;44:134–6.

[52] Yatscoff R, LeGatt D, Keenan R, Chackowsky P. Blood distribution of rapamycin. Transplantation 1993;56:1202–6.

[53] Leung LY, Lim HK, Abell MW, Zimmerman JJ. Pharmacokinetics and metabolic disposition of sirolimus in healthy male volunteers after a single oral dose. Ther Drug Monit 2006;28:51–61.

[54] Gallant-Haidner HL, Trepanier DJ, Freitag DG, Yatscoff RW. Pharmacokinetics and metabolism of sirolimus. Ther Drug Monit 2000;22:31–5.

[55] Colantonio DA, Borden KK, Clarke W. Comparison of the CEDIA and MEIA assays for the measurement of sirolimus in organ transplant recipients. Clin Biochem 2007;40:680–7.

[56] Westley IS, Morris RG, Taylor PJ, Salm P, et al. CEDIA sirolimus assay compared with HPLC-Ms/MS and HPLC-UV in transplant recipient specimens. Ther Drug Monit 2005;27:309–14.

[57] Morris RG, Salm P, Taylor PJ, Wicks FA. Comparison of the reintroduced MEIA assay with HPLC-Ms/MS for the determination of whole blood sirolimus from transplant recipients. Ther Drug Monit 2006;28:164–8.

[58] Wilson D, Johnston F, Holt D, Moreton M, et al. Multi-center evaluation of analytical performance of the microparticle enzyme immunoassay for sirolimus. Clin Biochem 2006;39:378–86.

[59] Schmidt RW, Lotz J, Schweigert R, Lackner K, et al. Multi-site analytical evaluation of a chemiluminescent magnetic microparticle immunoassay (CMIA) for sirolimus on the Abbott ARCHITECT analyzer. Clin Biochem 2009;42:1543–8.

[60] Holt DW, Mandelbrot DA, Tortorici MA, Korth-Bradley JM, et al. Long term evaluation of analytical methods used in sirolimus therapeutic drug monitoring. Clin Transplant 2014;28:243–51.

[61] Cervinski MA, Duh SH, Hock KG, Gray J, et al. Performance characteristics of a no pre-treatment random access sirolimus assay for the Dimension RxL clinical chemistry analyzer. Clin Biochem 2009;42:1123–7.

[62] Kirchner GI, Meier-Wiedenbach I, Manns MP. Clinical pharmacokinetics of everolimus. Clin Pharmacokinet 2004;43:83–95.

[63] Strom T, Haschke M, Zhang YL, Bendrick-Peart J, et al. Identification of everolimus metabolite pattern in trough blood samples of kidney transplant patients. Ther Drug Monit 2007;29:592–9.

[64] Dasgupta A, Davis B, Chow L. Evaluation of QMS everolimus assay using Hitachi 917 analyzer: comparison with liquid chromatography/mass spectrometry. Ther Drug Monit 2011;33:149–54.

[65] Shu I, Wright AM, Chandler WL, Bernard DW, et al. Analytical performance of QMS everolimus assay on Ortho Vitros 5, 1 FS fusion analyzer: measuring everolimus trough levels for solid organ transplant recipients. Ther Drug Monit 2014;36:264–8.

[66] Sallustio BC, Noll BD, Morris RG. Comparison of blood sirolimus, tacrolimus and everolimus concentrations measured by LC-Ms/MS, HPLC-UV and immunoassay methods. Clin Biochem 2011;44:231–6.

[67] Moes DJ, Press RR, de Fijter JW, Guchelaar HJ, et al. Liquid chromatography-tandem mass spectrometry outperforms fluorescence polarization immunoassay in monitoring everolimus therapy in renal transplantation. Ther Drug Monit 2010;32:413–9.

[68] Strom T, Haschke M, Boyd J, Roberts M, et al. Cross-reactivity of isolated everolimus metabolites with the Innofluor Certican immunoassay for therapeutic drug monitoring of everolimus. Ther Drug Monit 2007;29:743–9.

[69] Dasgupta A, Moreno V, Balak S, Smith A, et al. Rapid estimation of whole blood everolimus concentrations using Architect sirolimus immunoassay and mathematical equations: comparison with everolimus values determined by liquid chromatography/ mass spectrometry. J Clin Lab Anal 2011;25:207–11.

[70] Hermida-Cadahia EF, Tutor JC. Determination of everolimus in blood samples from kidney and liver transplant recipients using the sirolimus chemiluminescence magnetic microparticle immunoassay (CMIA) on the Architect i1000 system. Scand J Lab Invest 2012;72:180–3.

[71] Bouzas L, Tutor JC. Determination of blood everolimus concentrations in kidney and liver transplant recipients using the sirolimus antibody conjugated magnetic immunoassay (ACMIA). Clin Lab 2011;57:403–6.

[72] Staatz CE, Tett SE. Clinical pharmacokinetics and pharmacodynamics of mycophenolate in solid organ transplant recipients. Clin Pharmacokinet 2007;46:13–58.

[73] Kuypers DR, Le Meur Y, Cantarovich M, Tredger MJ, et al. Consensus report on therapeutic drug monitoring of mycophenolic acid in solid organ transplantation. Clin J Am Soc Nephrol 2010;5:341–58.

[74] Hosotsubo H, Takahara S, Imamura R, Kyakuno M, et al. Analytical validation of the enzyme multiplied immunoassay technique for the determination of mycophenolic acid in plasma from renal transplant recipients compared with a high performance liquid chromatographic assay. Ther Drug Monit 2001;23:669–74.

[75] Martiny D, Macours P, Cotton F, Thiry P, et al. Reliability of mycophenolic acid monitoring by an enzyme multiplied immunoassay technique. Clin Lab 2010;56:345–53.

[76] Brown NW, Franklin ME, Einarsdottir EN, Gonde CE. An investigation into the bias between liquid chromatography-tandem mass spectrometry and an enzyme multiplied immunoassay technique for the measurement of mycophenolic acid. Ther Drug Monit 2010;32:420–6.

[77] Decavele AS, Favoreel N, Heyden FV, Verstraete AG. Performance of the Roche total mycophenolic acid assay on the Cobas Integra 400, Cobas 6000 and comparison to LC-Ms/MS in liver transplant patients. Clin Chem Lab Med 2011;49:1159–65.

[78] Brandhorst G, Marquet P, Shaw LM, Liebisch G, et al. Multicenter evaluation of a new inosine monophosphate dehydrogenase inhibition assay for quantification of total mycophenolic acid in plasma. Ther Drug Monit 2008;30:428–33.

[79] Westley IS, Ray JE, Morris RG. CEDIA mycophenolic acid assay compared with HPLC-UV in specimens from transplant recipients. Ther Drug Monit 2006;28:632–6.

[80] Shipkova M, Schutz E, Besenthal I, Fraunberger P, et al. Investigation of the crossreactivity of mycophenolic acid glucuronide metabolites and of mycophenolic acid mofetil in the Cedia MPA assay. Ther Drug Monit 2010;32:79–85.

[81] Dasgupta A, Johnson M. Positive bias in mycophenolic acid concentrations determined by the CEDIA assay compared to HPLC-UV method: is CEDIA assay suitable for therapeutic drug monitoring of mycophenolic acid? J Clin Lab Anal 2013;27:77–80.

[82] Dasgupta A, Tso G, Chow L. Comparison of mycophenolic acid concentrations determined by a new PETINIA assay on the Dimension EXL analyzer and a HPLC-UV method. Clin Biochem 2013;46:685–7.

Application of liquid chromatography combined with mass spectrometry or tandem mass spectrometry for therapeutic drug monitoring of immunosuppressants

Kamisha L. Johnson-Davis and Gwendolyn A. McMillin

*Department of Pathology, University of Utah Health Sciences Center, Salt Lake City, UT, USA,
and ARUP Institute for Clinical and Experimental Pathology, Salt Lake City, UT, USA*

3.1 INTRODUCTION

Therapeutic drug monitoring (TDM) is routinely performed to optimize efficacy and to minimize toxicity. Therapeutic ranges for immunosuppressant drugs obtained by immunoassay may be inappropriate when results are determined by chromatographic methods. As discussed in Chapter 2, several immunoassays produce results that have a positive bias compared to chromatographic methods, due to metabolite cross-reactivity of the detection antibodies. The actual bias will vary per patient and time post-transplant, among other variables, but on average, immunoassay results may be 20–60% higher than those obtained by chromatographic techniques [1–4]. Immunoassays are not validated for alternative matrices that may have clinical utility for special populations, and they may not provide analytical measurement ranges sufficient to support selected sparing protocols or pharmacokinetic studies. Chromatographic methods, coupled to several different detectors, have been developed to overcome concerns about specificity and performance of immunoassays, relative to TDM of immunosuppressants. Direct injection mass spectrometric assays have also been described, with a primary advantage of a faster time to result in comparison with mass spectrometry methods that utilize chromatographic separation. Some of these approaches to testing are discussed here. In general, however, liquid

M. Oellerich & A. Dasgupta (Eds): Personalized Immunosuppression in Transplantation.
DOI: http://dx.doi.org/10.1016/B978-0-12-800885-0.00003-5

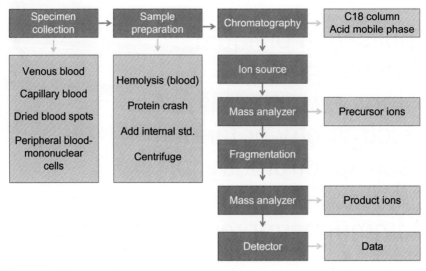

FIGURE 3.1

Schematic diagram of LC–MS/MS workflow for immunosuppressive drug TDM.

chromatography combined with tandem mass spectrometry (LC–MS/MS) is considered to be the gold standard for TDM of cyclosporine A, tacrolimus, mycophenolic acid (MPA), sirolimus, and everolimus. Application of LC–MS/MS to immunosuppressant TDM has improved specificity of results because of the several opportunities to separate the components of the matrix and separate drugs and drug metabolites from one another. A typical workflow for immunosuppressant TDM by LC–MS/MS is illustrated in Figure 3.1.

CASE REPORT

A 48-year-old male recipient of a renal transplant was treated with cyclosporine A and sirolimus. The patient was clinically stable, with pre-dose concentrations targeted at 50 ng/mL for cyclosporine A and 8 ng/mL for sirolimus. The patient had been monitored at his local hospital, where the transplant was performed, but was forced to move to another state 3 years post-transplant due to a change in employment. TDM results obtained through a community clinic in his new city were confusing because whereas the sirolimus result was consistent with previous testing results, the cyclosporine A was substantially higher than expected, at 83 ng/mL. Investigation of the provider revealed that the original hospital lab performed TDM for cyclosporine A with an LC–MS/MS method, whereas the community clinic performed TDM using a monoclonal immunoassay with fluorescent polarization detection (FPIA) for cyclosporine A and a chemiluminescent magnetic microparticle immunoassay (CMIA) for sirolimus. Overestimations of cyclosporine A concentrations when determined by FPIA, relative to LC–MS/MS, are well documented, and they are exaggerated when a patient is also treated with sirolimus [5]. In contrast, the MEIA for sirolimus has little bias with LC–MS/MS [6].

3.2 EVOLUTION OF NON-IMMUNOASSAY METHODS FOR IMMUNOSUPPRESSANTS

Examples of published non-immunoassay methods that could support TDM of immunosuppressants are summarized in Table 3.1. Most of these methods include chromatographic methods that are typically developed by individual laboratories and vary relative to sample preparation methods, chemistry of related solid (e.g., column) and mobile (e.g., gas or liquid) phases, flow rates, temperatures, instrument platforms and associated capabilities, detection technologies, methods of data collection, extent of data analysis, and analytical performance. Traditional chromatographic methods for detection and quantification of cyclosporine A employed liquid chromatography combined with ultraviolet light absorption (UV) detector. A UV detector is not appropriate for detecting tacrolimus due to the weak chromophore group in this molecule, without special sample preparation [7]. As such, traditional chromatographic methods for detection and quantification of tacrolimus are performed with mass spectrometry. Chromatographic separation is also applied to separate sirolimus and everolimus because currently available immunoassays for these drugs cannot distinguish the two drugs [8]. Several mass spectrometric methods have been published for cyclosporine A, tacrolimus, sirolimus, everolimus, and MPA. One advantage of mass spectrometric methods is that they can be designed for the quantification of many drug analytes in a single method [9]. Organ transplant patients may be prescribed multiple immunosuppressant therapies to reduce the incidence of organ rejection or may transition from one therapy to another. A multianalyte method can provide quantitative results of more than one drug in a single specimen.

Mass spectrometry is a highly selective detection technology that detects mass-to-charge ratios of ionized molecules and fragments. This detection technology is most commonly coupled to liquid chromatography, although gas chromatography, capillary electrophoresis, and direct injection methods are also published for immunosuppressant TDM. Ions are produced by protonation, deprotonation, removing an electron through fragmentation, capturing an electron, or adduct formation with another molecule. Ions

Table 3.1 Non-Immunoassay Approaches for Therapeutic Drug Monitoring of Immunosuppressants

- High-performance liquid chromatography coupled to ultraviolet detection (HPLC-UV)
- Liquid chromatography coupled to mass spectrometry (LC–MS)
- Liquid chromatography coupled to tandem mass spectrometry (LC–MS/MS)
- Ultra-high-performance liquid chromatography coupled to tandem mass spectrometry (UPLC–MS/MS)
- Turbulent flow chromatography coupled to tandem mass spectrometry (direct injection)
- Liquid chromatography coupled to high-resolution mass spectrometry (LC–HR-MS)
- Solid phase extraction coupled to tandem mass spectrometry (SPE–MS/MS)
- Laser diode thermal desorption coupled to tandem mass spectrometry (LDTD–MS/MS)

enter the mass spectrometer by the use of thermospray, electrospray, atmospheric pressure chemical ionization, or atmospheric pressure ionization. Then they are guided along by electric, radio frequency, or magnetic fields to the mass analyzer. The mass analyzer functions to separate or isolate ions by their ratio between the mass and the charge on the molecule versus time. Analyzers may also be designed to detect all ions over a mass range, such as in time-of-flight mass spectrometry, wherein ions are projected into a flight tube and are identified by exact mass and the time it takes to hit the detector. Ion trap, magnetic sector, ion cyclotron resonance mass spectrometers, and Fourier transform are other forms of analyzers for mass selection. These mass analyzers can be further coupled together to form hybrid technologies such as quadrupole time-of-flight (QTOF). When the ions are detected, the detector converts the amount of ions for a specific mass-to-charge ratio into a signal. Detectors can consist of photon or electron multipliers. Mass analyzers have limitations with regard to the highest mass-to-charge ratio that can be detected, resolution of two peaks by mass units, scanning speeds for mass detection, and the number of ions that can reach the detector.

3.3 LC–MS/MS METHODS FOR ANALYSIS OF IMMUNOSUPPRESSANTS

Numerous mass spectrometry methods have been published for the analysis of immunosuppressive drugs [10–15]. Some of the common features for sample preparation include hemolysis, protein precipitation with zinc sulfate, methanol, and acetonitrile, followed by the addition of internal standard to the sample, centrifugation, and analysis. The internal standards used in various methods include ascomycin, cyclosporine D, rapamune-d3, everolimus-d4, tacrolimus-C^{13}-d2, and cyclosporine A-d12. General chromatographic separation is performed by HPLC or ultra-high-pressure liquid chromatography (UPLC) with a C_{18} reverse-phase column. A binary step gradient mobile phase can be used, which generally consists of the following solvents in combination: ammonium acetate, ammonium formate, formic acid, acetonitrile, methanol, and water. The pH of the mobile phase is acidified to enhance positive ionization of the ammonium adduct $[M + NH_4]^+$ of the molecule for cyclosporine A, tacrolimus, sirolimus, and everolimus. The inactive and active metabolites are not usually monitored for these drugs.

For MPA, sample preparation may consist of protein precipitation with zinc sulfate, methanol, or acetonitrile, followed by centrifugation and analysis. The internal standards for MPA may include MPA-d3 and the isotopically labeled form of the inactive metabolite, 7-*O*-mycophenolic acid β-glucuronide (MPAG). General chromatographic separation is performed by HPLC or UPLC with a C_{18} reverse-phase column. A binary step gradient mobile phase can be used, which generally consists of the following solvents in combination: ammonium acetate, ammonium formate, formic acid, acetonitrile, methanol, and water. The pH of the mobile phase is acidified to enhance positive ionization of the ammonium adduct $[M + NH_4]^+$ of the molecule for MPA [16]. Analytical methods may also include the transitions for the ammonium adducts of the

Table 3.2 Common Analyte Transitions (*m/z*) for LC–MS/MS

Analyte	Precursor	Product Ion (Quantitative)
Ascomycin	809.5	756.5
Cyclosporine A	1219.9	1203.1
Cyclosporine A-d12	1231.9	1215.1
Cyclosporine D	1234.0	1217.0
Everolimus	975.6	908.6
Everolimus-d4	979.6	912.6
Rapamune	931.6	864.5
Rapamune-d3	934.6	864.6
Tacrolimus	821.5	768.5
Tacrolimus-C13-d2	825.5	772.5
MPA	338.1	207.1
MPAG	514.2	207.1
AcMPAG	514.2	207.1
MPA-d3	341.1	210.0
MPAG-d3	517.2	210.1

metabolites, MPAG, and the active metabolite, acyl-glucuronide (AcMPAG). MPAG and AcMPAG are isobaric (identical mass) and must be chromatographically separated for identification. Table 3.2 is a general summary of the *m/z* transitions used in mass spectrometry methods to monitor each analyte. Of note, laboratories should monitor two product ions for analyte identification and quantification. A typical analytical measurement range (AMR) for these methods is 5–2000 ng/mL for cyclosporine A and 0.5–100 ng/mL for tacrolimus, sirolimus, and everolimus [10,11]. The AMR for MPA is typically 0.1–50 μg/mL, that for MPAG is 1–500 μg/mL, and that for AcMPAG is 0.05–10 μg/mL [16]. Accuracy for laboratory-developed tests usually falls between 85 and 115%, and imprecision (percentage coefficient of variation (%CV)) is less than 15%. As such, precision may be better with immunoassays.

Laboratory-developed tests for TDM may be a limitation for some laboratories that do not have the personnel with mass spectrometry experience to develop and validate a method for routine testing. As a result, commercial kits from Waters Corporation (MassTrak Immunosuppressants for tacrolimus) and Chromsystems (MassTox Immunosuppressants in whole blood—ONEMinute Test—LC–MS/MS) were created to meet this need. These kits provide liquid chromatography and mass spectrometry parameters for an instrument, sample preparation procedure, calibrators, controls, internal standards, analytical column, and a quantitation method. Published method comparison studies to existing laboratory-developed methods have shown that the commercial kits are comparable with regard to accuracy (range, 85–115%), imprecision (<15% CV), and analytical measurement range for the various immunosuppressive drugs [17–19].

Analytical methods have been developed to reduce the analytical runtime by eliminating chromatographic separation and direct injection of the sample into the source of a mass spectrometer. Direct injection methods can perform comparable to traditional LC–MS/MS methods, but they cannot separate isobaric compounds [20] Turbulent flow chromatography coupled to tandem mass spectrometry is another form of the direct injection technique. Sample preparation includes hemolysis and protein precipitation of whole blood prior to online matrix removal through turbulent flow chromatography [21]. The reported AMR was 4.5–1000 ng/mL for cyclosporine A, 0.2–100 ng/mL for tacrolimus, and 0.4–100 ng/mL for sirolimus. Within- and between-run imprecision was less than 10% CV [21].

Solid phase extraction coupled to tandem mass spectrometry (SPE–MS/MS) has reduced the analysis time of cyclosporine A, tacrolimus, sirolimus, and everolimus to 13 s per sample (Application Note, Agilent Technologies, Wakefield, MA). This method requires lysing the red blood cells (RBCs) prior to extraction by online SPE. The AMR was 0.8–50 ng/mL for tacrolimus, sirolimus, and everolimus. Cyclosporine A has an AMR of 7.8–1000 ng/mL. Linearity was reported with an R^2 value greater than 0.995 for all drugs, accuracy within ±15%, and imprecision of less than 10% CV for all concentrations within the AMR. This methodology can analyze 270 samples per hour and drastically reduce the use of mobile phase solvent with a run time of less than 15 s per sample. A 96-well plate of patient samples can be analyzed in less than 20 min. The limitation of this methodology is that isobaric interferences cannot be resolved because the technology does not employ chromatographic separation. In addition, the method may require larger specimen volume for extraction in order to compensate for the loss of analyte from SPE.

Laser Diode Thermal Desorption (LDTD; Phytronix, Quebec, Canada) is another technology that has eliminated the use of liquid chromatography for rapid quantitative analysis. The ion source on the mass spectrometer is replaced with the LDTD source. Sample preparation is usually performed on whole blood and serum/plasma to remove matrix interference, and 2–10 μL of sample is placed into a specialized 96-well plate (LazWell) and dried by evaporation with or without heat onto the well. The drying step may add additional time to the sample preparation. An infrared laser is used to heat the bottom of the LazWell plate to cause thermal desorption of the sample into the mass spectrometer. Analysis of four immunosuppressant drugs in less than 10 s has been reported with comparable analytical performance to that of traditional liquid chromatography-based methods [22]. Accuracy of results were within ±15%, and imprecision was 3.4–13.1% CV [22]. This technology may have limitations with low-end sensitivity resolution of isobaric compounds and requires a more sensitive mass spectrometer for analysis that is similar in performance to an AB Sciex 5500 LC–MS/MS [22]. High-resolution mass spectrometry instruments have been developed and can be utilized for TDM of immunosuppressive drugs that have the advantage of accurate mass determination. Methods have been developed using the Orbitrap [23] and TOF technologies. Mass accuracy using high-resolution mass spectrometry can range within 5–10 parts per million.

3.3.1 PREANALYTICAL VARIABLE: SPECIMENS

Cyclosporine A, tacrolimus, sirolimus, and everolimus are highly bound to RBCs and proteins, and TDM is best performed with whole blood. The percentage binding to RBCs is 50–55% for cyclosporine A [24], 95–98% for tacrolimus [25], and 95% for sirolimus and everolimus [26]. Consequently, changes in hematocrit and severe hemolysis may affect accuracy of whole blood testing results [27]. Specifically, low hematocrit values (25%) are associated with overestimated tacrolimus concentrations by some immunoassays, and the overestimation can be accounted for by correcting for hematocrit [28]. In addition, intracellular concentrations of calcineurin inhibitors display high interpatient and intrapatient variability [29].

Plasma concentrations for these drugs are severalfold lower than that of whole blood, and the concentrations may fall below the limit of quantification of the method. Another limitation of using plasma for TDM for cyclosporine A, tacrolimus, sirolimus, and everolimus is that the unbound drug can passively diffuse inside RBCs [30]. Mycophenolate mofetil is not bound to RBCs but is highly bound to plasma proteins [31]; therefore, TDM is performed with plasma [32].

Capillary blood sampling onto dried blood spots (DBS) can also be used as a specimen type for TDM of immunosuppressant drugs [27,33–41]. Blood from a finger prick is applied to sampling paper and then dried. The DBS must be completely dried before storage or transportation to the laboratory to minimize bacterial growth. The sampling paper is sent to the laboratory, where a circular disk is punched out of the blood spot and then the drug is extracted from the matrix for analysis [42]. The benefits of using DBS are that the collection does not require the use of a phlebotomist, sampling time can occur at convenience and without travel to a clinic facility for blood draw, the biohazard risk is reduced, and drug stability can be maintained within the DBS [42]. Some of the limitations of using DBS as a specimen type include the effects from heat or moisture buildup, which can impact the integrity of the specimen. Plasticizers can leach from the plastic packaging onto the DBS and may interfere with analysis. There must be reproducibility with punching the disk from the DBS for consistently accurate results [33]. Fresh normal blood should be used for calibrators and controls when preparing them as DBS. Hemolyzed blood or blood specimens with an abnormal hematocrit will impact the accuracy of results. Of note, the quality of the sampling paper and the analytical method will also affect the reliability of results [42]. Capillary blood can also be utilized for TDM in pediatric patients. Cyclosporine A concentrations in capillary blood are comparable to drug concentrations in venous sampling and can be used as an alternative specimen [43–45]. Lastly, another specimen type for the analysis of immunosuppressive drugs is peripheral blood mononuclear cells, which may require cell separation by centrifugation, purification, extraction, and analysis using a highly sensitive mass spectrometer with quantification below 1 ng/mL [46–49]. Therapeutic ranges for DBS and peripheral blood mononuclear cells are not well established.

3.3.2 PREANALYTICAL VARIABLE: SPECIMEN COLLECTION

Timing of specimen collection is typically performed before the next dose administration (pre-dose, trough) for immunosuppressants as an indicator of drug exposure [50]. EDTA is a preferred anticoagulant for whole blood and plasma specimens for analysis of immunosuppressants [51–53]. Plasma specimens for MPA analysis should be centrifuged and separated from RBCs within 2h of collection. If the specimen cannot be centrifuged within 2h, then it should be kept at ambient temperature to reduce the risk of hemolysis. Of note, gel separator tubes have the potential to decrease total drug recovery through adsorption of the drug to the gel material. Consequently, gel separator tubes should not be used as collection tubes for TDM unless validated to be appropriate [54]. Immunosuppressive drug concentrations are stable in whole blood and plasma between a few hours [55] to several days at ambient temperature [56,57]. These drugs are also stable between 7 and 30 days when the specimens are refrigerated at 4°C [51,57–61] and up to 3 years when stored at −20° to −70°C [51,56,58–60].

3.3.3 PREANALYTICAL VARIABLE: DRUG–DRUG INTERACTIONS

Another preanalytical variable is drug–drug interactions. Patients receiving organ transplants may be prescribed multiple medications that could inhibit or induce drug metabolism. In addition, combination therapy could lead to synergistic effects or may exacerbate toxicity. Immunosuppressive drugs are metabolized primarily by the cytochrome P450 isoenzyme CYP3A4/5 liver enzyme and excreted via the kidneys. This isozyme is part of the superfamily of CYP enzymes associated with drug metabolism and is involved in metabolism of approximately 50% of all drugs. Drugs such as calcium channel blockers, antifungal agents, antibiotics, glucocorticoids, and HIV drugs, which inhibit CYP 3A4, will increase immunosuppressant concentrations in blood. Anticonvulsants, antituberculosis medications, and St. John's wort, which induce CYP3A4, will increase metabolism of immunosuppressive drugs and decrease drug concentrations and may lead to subtherapeutic concentrations in blood. Synergistic drug–drug interactions can potentiate nephrotoxicity and hepatotoxicity, and overdose of immunosuppressants can lead to opportunistic infections and malignancy.

Drug–drug interactions can also occur with MPA. The rate-limiting step for the clearance of MPA is conversion to the inactive MPAG metabolite, which is cleared via the kidneys. MPAG undergoes enterohepatic recirculation to prolong MPA exposure. The clearance of MPA is affected by glucuronidation, the free fraction of MPA, and enterohepatic circulation. In addition, clearance of MPA can also be affected in patients with impaired kidney function, which can lead to the accumulation of MPAG concentrations in plasma to several hundredfold higher than MPA. Enterohepatic recirculation of MPAG is inhibited by a drug–drug interaction with cholestyramine, and it may cause a 40% decrease in MPA exposure [62]. Inhibition of MPAG transportation from liver into bile is the likely mechanism for the significant decrease of MPA concentration and increase of MPAG concentration by the coadministration of cyclosporine A [63]. Antacids containing Mg^{2+} and aluminum hydroxide can cause an interaction to decrease peak concentration of MPA by 33% [64]. Furthermore, drug–drug interaction with ganciclovir can increase the area under the concentration curve (AUC) for MPAG and promote enterohepatic recirculation of MPA.

CASE REPORT

A 54-year-old male kidney recipient was treated with everolimus with a target pre-dose whole blood concentration between 3 and 8 ng/mL due to a previous history of tuberculosis and pulmonary aspergillosis. Prophylaxis against the aspergillosis and other infections was initiated 14 days post-transplant with voriconazole, isoniazid, acyclovir, and oral amphotericin B. Voriconazole is a known inhibitor of cytochrome CYP3A4, which would be expected to inhibit metabolic inactivation of everolimus. As such, everolimus dose was tapered based on TDM that was performed at 2, 7, and 10 days post initiation of voriconazole. Everolimus concentrations were 18.6, 14.1, and 12.0 ng/mL, respectively. Voriconazole was discontinued after 1 month, and the dose of everolimus was again adjusted to achieve a pre-dose concentration that fell within the therapeutic range. This case demonstrates that TDM is critical to manage dosing when drug–drug interactions are anticipated. Adjustment of everolimus dose, and possibly the doses of anti-infectious or other medications being coprescribed, based on appropriately timed TDM, will help ensure stability of the patient and success of the graft [65].

CASE REPORT

A 57-year-old male kidney recipient was treated with prednisolone, mycophenolate mofetil, and losartan. The patient was stable for approximately 4 years, being monitored by MPA monitoring with a well-tolerated AUC_{0-12} of approximately 50 mg·h/L. While traveling out of the country, the patient was diagnosed with tuberculosis and was treated with rifampicin. He scheduled a follow-up appointment at the transplant center when he arrived back in his home country. The MPA AUC_{0-12} had dropped to approximately 14 mg·h/L. Due to the known drug–drug interaction, leading to decreased enterohepatic recirculation of MPA, the transplant center physician discontinued the rifampicin and prescribed ofloxacin instead. The mycophenolate mofetil dose was not adjusted, and the MPA AUC_{0-12} was gradually restored to target. This case demonstrates the significant impact of enterohepatic recirculation of MPA on the AUC and the requirement to monitor by TDM in vulnerable patients [66,67].

3.3.4 PREANALYTICAL VARIABLE: GENETIC POLYMORPHISMS

Polymorphisms in the genes that code for drug-metabolizing enzymes will also affect an individual's ability to biotransform drugs for activation or elimination. Genetic mutations can cause a patient to be a slow or rapid drug metabolizer. Moreover, rapid metabolizers are at risk of therapeutic failure due to suboptimal dosing and will require higher doses to achieve optimal therapy. For example, *CYP3A5*1* is associated with low blood concentrations of tacrolimus compared to those of patients who do not express *CYP3A5* (e.g., *CYP3A5*3*) [68]. A single nucleotide polymorphism in the promoter region of the uridine diphosphate-glucuronosyltransferase 1A9 (*UGT1A9*) gene can have an impact on the pharmacokinetics for the metabolism of

MPA [69]. Transplant patients with polymorphisms in *CYP3A4*1B* and *-3A5*1* may require a higher dose of sirolimus to reach therapeutic concentrations in blood [70]. Thus, accurate TDM is an important tool for optimizing dosing under conditions of unpredictable pharmacokinetics, such as pharmacogenetic variants.

3.3.5 PREANALYTICAL VARIABLE: CLINICAL STATUS OF THE PATIENT

TDM results can also be affected by a patient's lifestyle or clinical status, such as diet, smoking, alcohol use, and comorbidities. Food and fluid intake can alter the pharmacokinetics of a drug by impacting gastric pH and emptying time, which can affect drug absorption. Food–drug interactions with grapefruit can inhibit CYP3A4 and increase immunosuppressive drug concentrations [71].

Bioavailability is highly variable with most immunosuppressant drugs. Orally administered drugs that are lipid soluble or non-ionized are absorbed into the bloodstream through the gastrointestinal tract by passive diffusion. Factors that affect intestinal motility, hepatic blood flow, and bile flow will also have an impact on the pharmacokinetics of a drug. Patients with impaired hepatic, renal, or gastrointestinal function are subject to unpredictable pharmacokinetics. For instance, liver transplant patients with hyperbilirubinemia will accumulate tacrolimus metabolites, which leads to a positive bias in tacrolimus results by immunoassay [72].

In critically ill patients, impaired cardiovascular, hepatic, renal, or gastrointestinal function are factors that contribute to variable pharmacokinetics. Renal disease will decrease the glomerular filtration rate and reduce the clearance of drugs that are eliminated through the kidneys. Kidney disease will also influence drug–protein binding in patients with uremia. Uremia toxins will compete for drug binding sites to albumin and increase the concentration of non-protein-bound (free) drug and therapeutic effect. Liver disease or toxicity will reduce the production of albumin and other proteins that bind to drugs. Hypoalbuminemia will cause an increase in the free (unbound) fraction of pharmacologically active drugs and may increase the risk of toxicity. Impaired liver function will decrease first-pass metabolism and also affect the expression of CYP450 isozymes. Gastrointestinal disease or a history of bariatric surgery, malabsorptive disorders, or intestinal disease may impact absorption of drugs [73]. Cardiovascular disease will reduce cardiac output, tissue perfusion, drug disposition, and absorption. Decreased blood flow to the liver will reduce drug metabolism.

3.3.6 PREANALYTICAL VARIABLE: PREGNANCY

TDM is necessary in pregnant or nursing women to factor in the changes that will occur in maternal physiology to protect the fetus or infant from toxicity. Pregnant women have increased body fat, plasma volume, and total body water, which will decrease plasma protein concentration and drug–protein binding. Bioavailability is reduced when lipophilic drugs distribute and accumulate in fat tissues. Drugs that are water soluble will have a lower volume of distribution in the body and may have increased clearance and decreased bioavailability in patients with excessive percentage body fat content. Cardiac output in pregnant women is increased, which will enhance drug metabolism. TDM is recommended to carefully monitor pregnant or nursing women to ensure safety and efficacy for both mother and unborn child [74].

CASE REPORT

A 32-year-old female recipient of a liver transplant, who had been stable for 5 years, underwent a successful pregnancy and wanted to breast-feed her child. The safety of the breast milk to the infant was questioned. Timed breast milk and whole blood samples were collected and evaluated for tacrolimus pre-dose and more than 12 h following a morning dose of tacrolimus. The whole blood pre-dose target concentration of tacrolimus was maintained at 6.5 ng/mL. The milk-to-blood ratios at pre-dose and 1-h post-dose were 0.08 and 0.09, suggesting minimal exposure of tacrolimus to the infant. The infant was developing well both physiologically and neurologically after 2.5 months of breast-feeding, and the mother continued to be successfully managed with tacrolimus. This case suggests that breast-feeding is safe under conditions of maternal tacrolimus therapy [75].

CASE REPORT

A 28-year-old female recipient of a renal transplant was successfully managed with 5 mg bid tacrolimus and a target whole blood pre-dose concentration of 10 ng/mL. Two years post-transplant, she becomes pregnant. The first trimester TDM was stable, but in the second trimester, the concentrations of tacrolimus began to decrease and eventually fell below 5 ng/mL. The dose was doubled, but the total tacrolimus concentration increased only to 8 ng/mL throughout the rest of the pregnancy. Pregnancy produces many unique challenges for monitoring immunosuppressant therapy. For example, the mean oral clearance for tacrolimus is 39% higher during mid- to late pregnancy compared to postpartum values. In addition, the free fraction of tacrolimus increases by 91% in plasma during pregnancy, largely explained by the decrease in albumin anticipated with pregnancy. As such, TDM and careful monitoring for signs of toxicity due to a high proportion of unbound tacrolimus is recommended [76,77].

3.3.7 ANALYTICAL STEP: SPECIMEN PREPARATION

Most automated immunoassays do not incorporate any sample preparation methods and are consequently at higher risk for interferences. For mass spectrometry methods, specimen preparation is frequently utilized to remove proteins and cellular debris in order to minimize matrix effects. Some interfering substances may be eliminated through sample preparation methods such as sample dilution, protein precipitation, and liquid–liquid or solid phase extraction. Physical separation techniques (e.g., chromatography, ultrafiltration, and ultracentrifugation) may also help minimize matrix effects. Protein precipitation can be used as a means for sample cleanup; however, it has been shown that this technique may cause clumping in whole blood samples, which can lead to a decrease in drug recovery, especially for sirolimus, and variable imprecision for the assay [78]. In addition, protein precipitation may not be sufficient to remove lipids that cause suppression of the ion intensity during mass spectrometry analysis [78]. Specimen cleanup using liquid–liquid, solid phase, or supported liquid extraction can be utilized to remove the presence of interfering substances, such as phospholipids, and improve the analyte signal at the detector to minimize ion suppression and chromatographic interferences [78]. Sample preparation with water/zinc sulfate/methanol provides better sample cleanup than protein precipitation. Lysing the sample with water will minimize the clumping that occurs with rapid precipitation of proteins. In addition, zinc sulfate/methanol helps remove the drug from the cellular debris for more uniform and consistent analysis [78].

3.3.8 ANALYTICAL STEP: REAGENTS

Mass spectrometry methods for immunosuppressant analysis employ reagents for sample preparation and instrument analysis that are different from reagents used when testing by immunoassay. Internal standards are used in mass spectrometry to assist with the quantification of an analyte, to serve as a measure of recovery during the extraction of the analyte from the matrix, and to compensate for matrix effects and ion suppression. The internal standard is added to the sample either before the extraction or at a step during the extraction. The internal standard should be structurally similar to the analyte of interest and mimic its chemical and ionization characteristics and retention time, where it co-elutes with the analyte of interest. Internal standards may consist of analogs with isotopic labels, such as deuterium or carbon-13, for distinction from the target analyte. These analogs must be stable to maintain the isotopic labels during storage, exposure to low and high temperatures, sample preparation, ionization, and fragmentation, in order to prevent breakdown during processing. The internal standard should be chemically pure (>95%) and not contaminated with the target analyte that does not have the isotopic label. The rapamycin-d3 internal standard is documented to contain approximately 2% unlabeled compound (rapamycin-d0). The presence of significant quantities of unlabeled impurities, such as rapamycin-d0, is always a concern when using deuterated internal standards because it may introduce a positive bias into the method at low analyte concentrations. The representation of d0 may become a significant contributor to the signal at low analyte concentrations when using the peak area ratio. The higher value for the limit of quantification using the deuterated sirolimus internal standard may be explained by the presence of unlabeled compound in the formulation.

Before the development of isotopically labeled internal standard for each of the drugs, cyclosporine-D was used as an internal standard for chromatographic methods for cyclosporine A [79], ascomycin was traditionally used as an internal standard for tacrolimus [80], and 32-desmethoxyrapamycin was used as the internal standard for sirolimus and everolimus [81,82]. Studies have performed comparisons between stable isotope-labeled and analog internal standard, and the results demonstrate that isotope-labeled internal standards have a more favorable agreement with accuracy and imprecision compared to analog internal standards [83,84].

3.3.9 ANALYTICAL STEP: SOLVENTS

Solvents used in the extraction and analysis can have an impact on ionization efficiency and internal standard stability. Annesley et al. demonstrated that the solvent grade can impact the area response for the internal standard where ion intensities could vary 10-fold between various grades of methanol solvents. It was also demonstrated that 32-desmethoxyrapamycin, which was used as an internal standard for sirolimus, had a decrease in ion formation (ionization), along with a 50–77% reduction in the ion signal for MPA (Figure 3.2) [85]. Acetonitrile was also shown to degrade ascomycin within a few hours [86]. Solvents may also affect the formation of sodium, ammonium, and formate ion [87]. Thus, it is important to evaluate the matrix effects of various reagents for optimal assay performance [88]. The chromatography conditions of the mobile phase during the analytical run can be utilized to separate the matrix from the analyte of interest. The mobile phase can be a consistent concentration (isocratic) or variable throughout the run (gradient). The pH of the mobile phase can also affect the ionization and the retention time on column to optimize chromatographic separation.

3.3.9.1 Proficiency testing

Proficiency testing programs for immunosuppressive drug testing include the International Proficiency Testing Schemes (IPTS) from Analytical Services International (ASI; London) and testing from the College of American Pathologists (CAP). The CAP CSM 2013 PT survey consists of three 5.0-mL whole blood

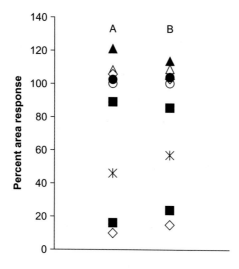

FIGURE 3.2

Relative LC–MS/MS area response for (A) 32-desmethoxyrapamycin and (B) ascomycin versus methanol brand or grade.

Reproduced from Annesley [85].

specimens that are shipped twice per year for cyclosporine A, tacrolimus, and sirolimus (rapamycin). In addition, the 2013 CSM survey for MPA consists of three 5.0-mL lyophilized serum specimens that are shipped twice per year. The 2013 CAP EV survey for everolimus consists of three 5.0-mL whole blood specimens that are shipped twice per year. The proficiency testing material is spiked to a known concentration in blood or other source material obtained from human donors or animals. The percentage of laboratories that perform testing by immunoassay and mass spectrometry, along with their respective interlaboratory %CV from the 2013 CAP CSM-B, are summarized in Table 3.3.

The ASI survey consists of three spiked whole blood samples that are shipped each month for cyclosporine A, tacrolimus, and sirolimus. For everolimus, three samples are shipped six times per year. The survey consists of two spiked MPA samples in plasma that are supplied four times per year. The proficiency testing material is either spiked to a known concentration or pooled samples from patients receiving the target drug. The percentage of laboratories that perform testing by immunoassay and mass spectrometry, along with their respective interlaboratory %CV from the 2013 ASI proficiency testing for immunosuppressive drugs, are summarized in Table 3.3.

According to the IPTS survey, the results of mass spectrometry methods tend to be closest in accuracy to the spiked values. However, assay performance can vary across different laboratories with lab-developed tests because the sample preparation, liquid chromatography conditions, mass spectrometry parameters, sources of calibrators, control material, and internal standards will vary among labs. Proficiency testing samples are not like real patient specimens because they are prepared by spiking the drug of interest into either artificial, whole blood-like matrices or sometimes pooled patient blood, which may not represent the metabolic profile of the drug. Global proficiency testing programs for cyclosporine A [89,90], tacrolimus [91], sirolimus [53], and MPA [51] have highlighted the issue with variation in results among labs and instrumentation (immunoassay vs. mass spectrometry) and have stressed the importance of standardization of analytical methods and processes for consistent TDM results [92–94]. In 2007, a consortium from the European consensus conference made the following recommendations for tacrolimus testing: (i) Promote the use of analytical methods with a limit of quantification of 1 ng/mL, (ii) incorporate extensive validation of new methods, (iii) participate in external proficiency testing programs, (iv) develop certified material for calibrators, and (v) take into consideration intermethod bias in results [91].

3.4 LIMITATION OF MASS SPECTROMETRIC METHODS

Table 3.4 is a summary of factors that can impact analysis by mass spectrometry. Mass spectrometry methods are susceptible to interferences from co-eluting compounds that may or may not be structurally similar to the compounds of interest [95]. The impact of a co-eluting substance depends on whether that substance interferes with

Table 3.3 Summary Data from Proficiency Survey Testing

	MPA	Cyclosporine A	Tacrolimus	Sirolimus	Everolimus
2013 CAP CSM-B and EV-B surveys					
Immunoassays (% used in surveys)	~63–65	~85–86	~82.1–82.5	~75–76	~23–33
Immunoassay (%CV)	~7.7	~6.2–16.6	~5.6–38.2	~10.4–13.4	~7.9–8.3
Mass spectrometry (% used in surveys)	~35–37	~14–15	~16.2–16.6	~24–25	~67–77
			~1.3, Waters MassTrak kit		
Mass spectrometry (%CV)	~8.3–17.0	~9.6–10.6	~7.9–9.4	~17.4–20	~14–14.5
2013 ASI immunosuppressive drug survey					
Immunoassays (% used in surveys)	~24	~65	~60	~32	~30
Immunoassay (%CV)	~5.5–6.3	~5.4–18.5	~5.4–18.6	~6.6–8.0	~10.3–18.2
Mass spectrometry (% used in surveys)	~28	~35	~40	~68	~70
Mass spectrometry (%CV)	~10	~7.1–7.5	~7.9–8.2	~11.5–13.1	~9.2–11.4

Table 3.4 Limitations of Mass Spectrometry

- Matrix effects
- Endogenous and exogenous interference
- Ion suppression/enhancement
- Cross talk
- In-source fragmentation
- Isobaric interference

the analyte signal that is generated, which is based on the signal-to-noise ratio, and on the detection method [96]. Interferences can come from endogenous compounds, commonly used over-the-counter drugs, drugs that are frequently coprescribed, metabolites (active and inactive), collection tube preservatives, anticoagulants, and matrix effects.

3.4.1 ION SUPPRESSION/ENHANCEMENT

Ion suppression or enhancement from components in the matrix alters ion intensity/ abundances, desolvation, charge on the ion, and signal-to-noise ratios, and it may be difficult to identify when isolated to a single patient specimen. Ion suppression can decrease the number of ions that reach the mass detector and may be caused by the presence of compounds that are less volatile than the analyte of interest or the specimen matrix, which can affect the ionization of the analyte. Ion enhancement will increase the number of ions that reach the mass detector.

Whole blood matrix is composed of a variety of different components, of which red cells, white cells, platelets, and plasma are the most important. The average total circulating volume of whole blood is approximately 8%. The plasma compartment is approximately 55% of the component of whole blood and is composed of 91.5% water, 7.5% proteins (albumin and other plasma proteins, globulins, fibrinogen and other clotting factors, and trace substances), and 1% electrolytes, vitamins, hormones, gases, and waste products [30]. When whole blood is lysed, phospholipid cell membranes and hemoglobin can be contributing factors causing ion suppression or assay interference. The matrix of serum does not contain blood cells, clotting factors, or fibrinogen, but it consists of protein, electrolytes, antibodies, antigens, hormones, and exogenous substances that may contribute to ion suppression or enhancement if not removed before analysis by mass spectrometry [30].

In electrospray ionization, the main source of ion suppression is due to changes in spray droplet formation in the presence of nonvolatile compounds [97,98]. Anions, salts, ion-pairing agents (trifluoroacetic acid), drugs/metabolites, uncharacterized sample matrix components and co-eluting compounds, and reagent impurities are known to produce ion suppression or enhancement. To minimize the effects of ion suppression, ion pair agents such as trifluoroacetic acid can be substituted for weak acids such as formic or acetic acid, or the concentration of the ion pairing agent can be reduced in order to maintain chromatographic separation and peak shape. Plasticizers, reagents, and anticoagulants in blood collection tubes are known to introduce matrix effects, which can cause either suppression or enhancement of the analytical response [99]. Furthermore, changing the ionization source or adjusting the liquid chromatography mobile phase conditions may also provide chromatographic separation to alleviate co-eluting substances. Consequently, ion suppression experiments should be performed during assay development and validation for the analyte of interest in blank matrix, before and after extraction, to evaluate the change in ion counts. To evaluate ion suppression, a matrix that has undergone extraction is injected onto the mass spectrometer while there is a flow of the analyte infused into the effluent flow. Another method to assess ion suppression is to perform a post-extraction spike of the analyte and compare the effect of the matrix to the analyte spiked in mobile phase, a buffer, or solvent [100]. In addition, internal standards, such as stable isotope-labeled compounds, are used to help minimize the effects of ion suppression and improve the analytical accuracy of mass spectrometry when the compound of interest and the analyte co-elute [95]. The internal standard should have ionization characteristics that are similar to those of the analyte, and both compounds should have a similar magnitude of ion suppression. Ion suppression and enhancement should also be monitored as part of routine assay performance metrics. Once areas of suppression or enhancement are identified, the chromatography can be modified or optimized to avoid or minimize the potential impact on the signal of the analytes. Furthermore, the internal standards should co-elute close to or at the same time as the analytes of interest, and the signal for the analytes should be divided by the signal for the internal standard to normalize the suppression or enhancement.

3.4.1.1 Cross talk and in-source fragmentation

Cross talk is another type of interference that occurs when the precursor ions fragment, produce identical product ion masses, and the fragment ion of one precursor transition is lingering in the collision cell when the next transition is being monitored [87]. Cross talk can occur with isotopically labeled internal standards, compound analogs, and unrelated compounds that are structurally similar. This form of interference can be minimized by diluting the specimen, reducing the sample volume that is injected onto the mass spectrometer, or by chromatographic separation of analytes [101]. Fragmentation of the molecule with weak bonds, such as sulfate and glucuronide conjugates, can also occur within the source of the mass spectrometer and cause an interference by forming the precursor molecule and lead to a falsely elevated precursor result [87]. Column overload can cause an interference with chromatographic separation when the matrix from the sample has not been sufficiently removed through extraction or eluted from the LC column. This can lead to abnormal analyte peak shape or tailing, suboptimal chromatographic separation, and high back pressure on the column. To resolve this interference, a wash step with a high percentage of organic solvent can be used to clean the column, the sample injection volume can be utilized, or the LC column can be replaced.

3.4.1.2 Isobaric interferences

Compounds that are isobaric to the analyte of interest are another source of interference in mass spectrometry. This is a limitation of traditional LC–MS, in which several compounds may have similar mass-to-charge ratios for the precursor ion. The progression to LC–MS/MS and the increase in mass resolution have resulted in dramatic improvement to specificity by the fragmentation pattern of the precursor ion. There are instances in which some precursor ions have the same product ion and chromatographic separation required to distinguish between the two compounds. Examples of isobaric interferences for immunosuppressive drugs include the MPA metabolites such as MPAG and mycophenolic acid acyl glucuronide, which have similar precursor and product transitions and require chromatographic separation by retention time to distinguish the compounds from one another.

Analytical methods should be designed to detect, minimize, or compensate for predictable interferences. Despite these limitations, chromatographic methods, particularly coupled with mass spectrometric detection, are recognized to resolve many of the interferences that are encountered with immunoassay methods, and they are generally regarded as gold standard platforms for TDM.

3.5 TURNAROUND TIME

Turnaround time to obtain concentrations of immunosuppressant drugs is relevant for clinicians to optimize dosing. The time to result may be longer in laboratories that perform testing in batch mode, which is typical for mass spectrometry methods, in comparison to random access mode for testing performed by immunoassay. The difference in immunoassay and mass spectrometry methods is relevant for single-point analyses and freshly collected blood that are intended for rapid assessment of dosing. AUC analyses and DBS testing may not require the same expectation for rapid time to result. Immunoassays may provide an advantage, with automation of sample preparation and analysis, compared to mass spectrometry. However, there are efforts to automate mass spectrometry methods through online sample preparation and multiplexing for sample analysis. These improvements to automate analysis by mass spectrometry will help streamline workflow in the laboratory and may reduce cost [102].

3.6 CONCLUSIONS

TDM is a critical tool for optimizing drug therapy. The accuracy of laboratory testing to support TDM depends on minimizing both preanalytical and analytical sources of interferences. Sources of interferences may be endogenous or exogenous, and they may interfere with specific technologies in a direct or indirect manner. By understanding vulnerabilities in various analytical technologies to interferences, some of the common sources of interferences can be identified and either managed or prevented. Patient history, timing of specimen collection, and performance characteristics of analytical techniques are pertinent information to help guide the interpretation of a TDM result.

Although immunoassays are frequently used in the United States for TDM of cyclosporine A, tacrolimus, sirolimus, everolimus, and mycophenolic assay, LC–MS/MS is considered as the gold standard for TDM because immunoassay results tend to show significant positive bias due to cross-reactivity to inactive metabolites. Moreover, multiple immunosuppressants can be monitored in a single method using this approach. Despite the benefits of employing LC–MS/MS for TDM, there are several limitations that can impact patient results. Ion suppression and isobaric ions may interfere with mass spectrometry-based methods; therefore, caution must be taken in selecting proper reagents, solvents, internal standards, and extraction techniques to develop a robust method for monitoring immunosuppressants.

REFERENCES

[1] Johnston A, Holt DW. Therapeutic drug monitoring of immunosuppressant drugs. Br J Clin Pharmacol 1999;47:339–50.

[2] Fillee C, Mourad M, Squifflet JP, Malaise J, et al. Evaluation of a new immunoassay to measure sirolimus blood concentrations compared to a tandem mass-spectrometric chromatographic analysis. Transplant Proc 2005;37:2890–1.

[3] Sallustio BC, Noll BD, Morris RG. Comparison of blood sirolimus, tacrolimus and everolimus concentrations measured by LC-Ms/MS, HPLC-UV and immunoassay methods. Clin Biochem 2011;44:231–6.

[4] Shipkova M, Schutz E, Besenthal I, Fraunberger P, et al. Investigation of the crossreactivity of mycophenolic acid glucuronide metabolites and of mycophenolate mofetil in the Cedia MPA assay. Ther Drug Monit 2010;32:79–85.

[5] Napoli KL. 12-hour area under the curve cyclosporine concentrations determined by a validated liquid chromatography-mass spectrometry procedure compared with fluorescence polarization immunoassay reveals sirolimus effect on cyclosporine pharmacokinetics. Ther Drug Monit 2006;28:726–36.

[6] Johnson-Davis KL, De S, Jimenez E, McMillin GA, et al. Evaluation of the Abbott ARCHITECT i2000 sirolimus assay and comparison with the Abbott IMx sirolimus assay and an established liquid chromatography-tandem mass spectrometry method. Ther Drug Monit 2011;33:453–9.

[7] Amardeep MS, Bande SA. Validated spectrophotometric method for determination of Tacrolimus in marketed formulation. IOSR J Pharm 2012;2:317–21.

[8] Bouzas L, Tutor JC. Determination of everolimus in whole blood using the Abbott IMx sirolimus microparticle enzyme immunoassay. Clin Biochem 2007;40:132–6.

[9] Buchwald A, Winkler K, Epting T. Validation of an LC–MS/MS method to determine five immunosuppressants with deuterated internal standards including MPA. BMC Clin Pharmacol 2012;12:2.

[10] Karapirli M, Kizilgun M, Yesilyurt O, Gul H, et al. Simultaneous determination of cyclosporine A, tacrolimus, sirolimus, and everolimus in whole-blood samples by LC–MS/MS. ScientificWorldJournal 2012;2012:571201.

[11] Koster RA, Dijkers EC, Uges DR. Robust, high-throughput LC–MS/MS method for therapeutic drug monitoring of cyclosporine, tacrolimus, everolimus, and sirolimus in whole blood. Ther Drug Monit 2009;31:116–25.

[12] Hammett-Stabler CA, Geis DC, Ritchie JC, Papadea C. Monitoring of mycophenolate acid in serum or plasma using LC tandem mass spectrometry. Methods Mol Biol 2010;603:379–87.

[13] Kuhn J, Gotting C, Kleesiek K. Sample cleanup-free determination of mycophenolic acid and its glucuronide in serum and plasma using the novel technology of ultra-performance liquid chromatography-electrospray ionization tandem mass spectrometry. Talanta 2010;80:1894–8.

[14] Kuhn J, Prante C, Kleesiek K, Gotting C. Measurement of mycophenolic acid and its glucuronide using a novel rapid liquid chromatography-electrospray ionization tandem mass spectrometry assay. Clin Biochem 2009;42:83–90.

[15] Garg U, Munar A, Frazee III CC. Simultaneous determination of cyclosporine, sirolimus, and tacrolimus in whole blood using liquid chromatography-tandem mass spectrometry. Methods Mol Biol 2012;902:167–73.

[16] Brandhorst G, Streit F, Goetze S, Oellerich M, et al. Quantification by liquid chromatography tandem mass spectrometry of mycophenolic acid and its phenol and acyl glucuronide metabolites. Clin Chem 2006;52:1962–4.

[17] Napoli KL, Hammett-Stabler C, Taylor PJ, Lowe W, et al. Multi-center evaluation of a commercial Kit for tacrolimus determination by LC/MS/MS. Clin Biochem 2010;43:910–20.

[18] Ji M, Kim S, Chung HJ, Lee W, et al. Evaluation of the MassTrak Immunosuppressant XE Kit for the determination of everolimus and cyclosporin A in human whole blood employing isotopically labeled internal standards. Clin Chem Lab Med 2011;49:2021–7.

[19] Becker S, Thiery J, Ceglarek U. Evaluation of a novel commercial assay for the determination of cyclosporine A, tacrolimus, sirolimus, and everolimus by liquid chromatography-tandem mass spectrometric assay. Ther Drug Monit 2013;35:129–32.

[20] Pitt JJ. Principles and applications of liquid chromatography-mass spectrometry in clinical biochemistry. Clin Biochem Rev 2009;30:19–34.

[21] Ceglarek U, Lembcke J, Fiedler GM, Werner M, et al. Rapid simultaneous quantification of immunosuppressants in transplant patients by turbulent flow chromatography combined with tandem mass spectrometry. Clin Chim Acta 2004;346:181–90.

[22] Jourdil JF, Picard P, Meunier C, Auger S, et al. Ultra-fast cyclosporin A quantitation in whole blood by Laser Diode Thermal Desorption-tandem mass spectrometry: comparison with high performance liquid chromatography-tandem mass spectrometry. Anal Chim Acta 2013;805:80–6.

[23] Henry H, Sobhi HR, Scheibner O, Bromirski M, et al. Comparison between a high-resolution single-stage Orbitrap and a triple quadrupole mass spectrometer for quantitative analyses of drugs. Rapid Commun Mass Spectrom 2012;26:499–509.

[24] Yatscoff RW, Honcharik N, Lukowski M, Thliveris J, et al. Distribution of cyclosporin G (NVa2 cyclosporin) in blood and plasma. Clin Chem 1993;39:213–7.

[25] Nagase K, Iwasaki K, Nozaki K, Noda K. Distribution and protein binding of FK506, a potent immunosuppressive macrolide lactone, in human blood and its uptake by erythrocytes. J Pharm Pharmacol 1994;46:113–7.

[26] Yatscoff R, LeGatt D, Keenan R, Chackowsky P. Blood distribution of rapamycin. Transplantation 1993;56:1202–6.

[27] Wilhelm AJ, den Burger JC, Chahbouni A, Vos RM, et al. Analysis of mycophenolic acid in dried blood spots using reversed phase high performance liquid chromatography. J Chromatogr B Analyt Technol Biomed Life Sci 2009;877:3916–9.

[28] Doki K, Homma M, Hori T, Tomita T, et al. Difference in blood tacrolimus concentration between ACMIA and MEIA in samples with low haematocrit values. J Pharm Pharmacol 2010;62:1185–8.

[29] Falck P, Asberg A, Guldseth H, Bremer S, et al. Declining intracellular T-lymphocyte concentration of cyclosporine a precedes acute rejection in kidney transplant recipients. Transplantation 2008;85:179–84.

[30] Hinderling PH. Red blood cells: a neglected compartment in pharmacokinetics and pharmacodynamics. Pharmacol Rev 1997;49:279–95.

[31] Langman LJ, LeGatt DF, Yatscoff RW. Blood distribution of mycophenolic acid. Ther Drug Monit 1994;16:602–7.

[32] Holt DW. Monitoring mycophenolic acid. Ann Clin Biochem 2002;39:173–83.

[33] Hoogtanders K, van der Heijden J, Christiaans M, Edelbroek P, et al. Therapeutic drug monitoring of tacrolimus with the dried blood spot method. J Pharm Biomed Anal 2007;44:658–64.

[34] Hoogtanders K, van der Heijden J, Christiaans M, van de Plas A, et al. Dried blood spot measurement of tacrolimus is promising for patient monitoring. Transplantation 2007;83:237–8.

[35] Cheung CY, van der Heijden J, Hoogtanders K, Christiaans M, et al. Dried blood spot measurement: application in tacrolimus monitoring using limited sampling strategy and abbreviated AUC estimation. Transpl Int 2008;21:140–5.

[36] van der Heijden J, de Beer Y, Hoogtanders K, Christiaans M, et al. Therapeutic drug monitoring of everolimus using the dried blood spot method in combination with liquid chromatography-mass spectrometry. J Pharm Biomed Anal 2009;50:664–70.

[37] den Burger JC, Wilhelm AJ, Chahbouni A, Vos RM, et al. Analysis of cyclosporin A, tacrolimus, sirolimus, and everolimus in dried blood spot samples using liquid chromatography tandem mass spectrometry. Anal Bioanal Chem 2012;404:1803–11.

[38] Koster RA, Alffenaar JW, Greijdanus B, Uges DR. Fast LC–MS/MS analysis of tacrolimus, sirolimus, everolimus and cyclosporin A in dried blood spots and the influence of the hematocrit and immunosuppressant concentration on recovery. Talanta 2013;115:47–54.

[39] Wilhelm AJ, den Burger JC, Vos RM, Chahbouni A, et al. Analysis of cyclosporin A in dried blood spots using liquid chromatography tandem mass spectrometry. J Chromatogr B 2009;877:1595–8.

[40] Wilhelm AJ, Klijn A, den Burger JC, Visser OJ, et al. Clinical validation of dried blood spot sampling in therapeutic drug monitoring of ciclosporin A in allogeneic stem cell transplant recipients: direct comparison between capillary and venous sampling. Ther Drug Monit 2013;35:92–5.

[41] Arpini J, Antunes MV, Pacheco LS, Gnatta D, et al. Clinical evaluation of a dried blood spot method for determination of mycophenolic acid in renal transplant patients. Clin Biochem 2013;46:1905–8.

[42] Edelbroek PM, van der Heijden J, Stolk LM. Dried blood spot methods in therapeutic drug monitoring: methods, assays, and pitfalls. Ther Drug Monit 2009;31:327–36.

[43] Merton G, Jones K, Lee M, Johnston A, et al. Accuracy of cyclosporin measurements made in capillary blood samples obtained by skin puncture. Ther Drug Monit 2000;22:594–8.

[44] Pettersen MD, Driscoll DJ, Moyer TP, Dearani JA, et al. Measurement of blood serum cyclosporine levels using capillary "fingerstick" sampling: a validation study. Transpl Int 1999;12:429–32.

[45] Profumo RJ, Foy TM, Kane RE. Correlation between venous and capillary blood samples for cyclosporine monitoring in pediatric liver transplant patients. Clin Transplant 1995;9:424–6.

[46] Capron A, Musuamba F, Latinne D, Mourad M, et al. Validation of a liquid chromatography-mass spectrometric assay for tacrolimus in peripheral blood mononuclear cells. Ther Drug Monit 2009;31:178–86.

[47] Roullet-Renoleau F, Lemaitre F, Antignac M, Zahr N, et al. Everolimus quantification in peripheral blood mononuclear cells using ultra high performance liquid chromatography tandem mass spectrometry. J Pharm Biomed Anal 2012;66:278–81.

[48] Nguyen Thi MT, Capron A, Mourad M, Wallemacq P. Mycophenolic acid quantification in human peripheral blood mononuclear cells using liquid chromatography-tandem mass spectrometry. Clin Biochem 2013;46:1909–11.

[49] Ansermot N, Fathi M, Veuthey JL, Desmeules J, et al. Quantification of cyclosporine A in peripheral blood mononuclear cells by liquid chromatography-electrospray mass spectrometry using a column-switching approach. J Chromatogr B 2007;857:92–9.

[50] Holt DW. Therapeutic drug monitoring of immunosuppressive drugs in kidney transplantation. Curr Opin Nephrol Hypertens 2002;11:657–63.

[51] Shaw LM, Holt DW, Oellerich M, Meiser B, et al. Current issues in therapeutic drug monitoring of mycophenolic acid: report of a roundtable discussion. Ther Drug Monit 2001;23:305–15.

[52] Holt DW, Armstrong VW, Griesmacher A, Morris RG, et al. International Federation of Clinical Chemistry/International association of therapeutic drug monitoring and clinical toxicology working group on immunosuppressive drug monitoring. Ther Drug Monit 2002;24:59–67.

[53] Yatscoff RW, Boeckx R, Holt DW, Kahan BD, et al. Consensus guidelines for therapeutic drug monitoring of rapamycin: report of the consensus panel. Ther Drug Monit 1995;17:676–80.

[54] Dasgupta A, Yared MA, Wells A. Time-dependent absorption of therapeutic drugs by the gel of the Greiner Vacuette blood collection tube. Ther Drug Monit 2000;22:427–31.

[55] Tsina I, Chu F, Hama K, Kaloostian M, et al. Manual and automated (robotic) high-performance liquid chromatography methods for the determination of mycophenolic acid and its glucuronide conjugate in human plasma. J Chromatogr B 1996;675:119–29.

[56] Annesley TM, Hunter BC, Fidler DR, Giacherio DA. Stability of tacrolimus (FK 506) and cyclosporin G in whole blood. Ther Drug Monit 1995;17:361–5.

[57] Alak AM, Lizak P. Stability of FK506 in blood samples. Ther Drug Monit 1996;18:209–11.

[58] Smith MC, Sephel GC. Long-term in vitro stability of cyclosporine in whole-blood samples. Clin Chem 1990;36:1991–2.

[59] Freeman DJ, Stawecki M, Howson B. Stability of FK 506 in whole blood samples. Ther Drug Monit 1995;17:266–7.

[60] Yatscoff RW, Faraci C, Bolingbroke P. Measurement of rapamycin in whole blood using reverse-phase high-performance liquid chromatography. Ther Drug Monit 1992;14:138–41.

[61] Jones K, Saadat-Lajevard S, Lee T, Horwatt R, et al. An immunoassay for the measurement of sirolimus. Clin Ther 2000;22(Suppl. B):B49–61.

[62] van Gelder T, Klupp J, Barten MJ, Christians U, et al. Comparison of the effects of tacrolimus and cyclosporine on the pharmacokinetics of mycophenolic acid. Ther Drug Monit 2001;23:119–28.

[63] van Gelder T, Le Meur Y, Shaw LM, Oellerich M, et al. Therapeutic drug monitoring of mycophenolate mofetil in transplantation. Ther Drug Monit 2006;28:145–54.

[64] Bullingham R, Shah J, Goldblum R, Schiff M. Effects of food and antacid on the pharmacokinetics of single doses of mycophenolate mofetil in rheumatoid arthritis patients. Br J Clin Pharmacol 1996;41:513–6.

[65] Billaud EM, Antoine C, Berge M, Abboud I, et al. Management of metabolic cytochrome P450 3A4 drug-drug interaction between everolimus and azole antifungals in a renal transplant patient. Clin Drug Investig 2009;29:481–6.

[66] Annapandian VM, Fleming DH, Mathew BS, John GT. Mycophenolic acid area under the curve recovery time following rifampicin withdrawal. Indian J Nephrol 2010;20:51–3.

[67] Kuypers DR, Le Meur Y, Cantarovich M, Tredger MJ, et al. Consensus report on therapeutic drug monitoring of mycophenolic acid in solid organ transplantation. Clin J Am Soc Nephrol 2010;5:341–58.

[68] Haufroid V, Mourad M, Van Kerckhove V, Wawrzyniak J, et al. The effect of CYP3A5 and MDR1 (ABCB1) polymorphisms on cyclosporine and tacrolimus dose requirements and trough blood levels in stable renal transplant patients. Pharmacogenetics 2004;14:147–54.

[69] Hesselink DA, van Gelder T. Genetic and nongenetic determinants of between-patient variability in the pharmacokinetics of mycophenolic acid. Clin Pharmacol Ther 2005;78:317–21.

[70] Anglicheau D, Le Corre D, Lechaton S, Laurent-Puig P, et al. Consequences of genetic polymorphisms for sirolimus requirements after renal transplant in patients on primary sirolimus therapy. Am J Transplant 2005;5:595–603.

[71] Hanley MJ, Cancalon P, Widmer WW, Greenblatt DJ. The effect of grapefruit juice on drug disposition. Expert Opin Drug Metab Toxicol 2011;7:267–86.

[72] Gonschior AK, Christians U, Winkler M, Linck A, et al. Tacrolimus (FK506) metabolite patterns in blood from liver and kidney transplant patients. Clin Chem 1996;42:1426–32.

[73] Edwards A, Ensom MH. Pharmacokinetic effects of bariatric surgery. Ann Pharmacother 2012;46:130–6.

[74] Best BM, Capparelli EV. Implications of gender and pregnancy for antiretroviral drug dosing. Curr Opin HIV AIDS 2008;3:277–82.

[75] French AE, Soldin SJ, Soldin OP, Koren G. Milk transfer and neonatal safety of tacrolimus. Ann Pharmacother 2003;37:815–8.

[76] Zheng S, Easterling TR, Umans JG, Miodovnik M, et al. Pharmacokinetics of tacrolimus during pregnancy. Ther Drug Monit 2012;34:660–70.

[77] Hebert MF, Zheng S, Hays K, Shen DD, et al. Interpreting tacrolimus concentrations during pregnancy and postpartum. Transplantation 2013;95:908–15.

[78] Annesley TM, Clayton L. Simple extraction protocol for analysis of immunosuppressant drugs in whole blood. Clin Chem 2004;50:1845–8.

[79] Giesbrecht EE, Soldin SJ, Wong PY. A rapid, reliable high-performance liquid chromatographic micromethod for the measurement of cyclosporine in whole blood. Ther Drug Monit 1989;11:332–6.

[80] Zhang Q, Simpson J, Aboleneen HI. A specific method for the measurement of tacrolimus in human whole blood by liquid chromatography/tandem mass spectrometry. Ther Drug Monit 1997;19:470–6.

[81] Connor E, Sakamoto M, Fujikawa K, Law T, et al. Measurement of whole blood sirolimus by an HPLC assay using solid-phase extraction and UV detection. Ther Drug Monit
2002;24:751–6.

[82] Deters M, Kirchner G, Resch K, Kaever V. Simultaneous quantification of sirolimus,
everolimus, tacrolimus and cyclosporine by liquid chromatography-mass spectrometry
(LC-Ms). Clin Chem Lab Med 2002;40:285–92.

[83] Heideloff C, Payto D, Wang S. Comparison of a stable isotope-labeled and an analog
internal standard for the quantification of everolimus by a liquid chromatography-
tandem mass spectrometry method. Ther Drug Monit 2013;35:246–50.

[84] Korecka MA, Patel R, Shaw LM. Evaluation of performance of new, isotopically
labeled internal standard ([13c2d4]RAD001) for everolimus using a novel high-
performance liquid chromatography tandem mass spectrometry method. Ther Drug
Monit 2011;33:460–3.

[85] Annesley TM. Methanol-associated matrix effects in electrospray ionization tandem
mass spectrometry. Clin Chem 2007;53:1827–34.

[86] Napoli KL. Organic solvents compromise performance of internal standard (ascomycin) in proficiency testing of mass spectrometry-based assays for tacrolimus. Clin Chem
2006;52:765–6.

[87] Vogeser M, Seger C. Pitfalls associated with the use of liquid chromatography-tandem
mass spectrometry in the clinical laboratory. Clin Chem 2010;56:1234–44.

[88] Napoli KL. More on methanol-associated matrix effects in electrospray ionization mass
spectrometry. Clin Chem 2009;55:1250–2.

[89] Morris RG, Holt DW, Armstrong VW, Griesmacher A, et al. Analytic aspects of cyclosporine monitoring, on behalf of the IFCC/IATDMCT Joint Working Group. Ther Drug
Monit 2004;26:227–30.

[90] Shaw LM, Yatscoff RW, Bowers LD, Freeman DJ, et al. Canadian Consensus Meeting
on cyclosporine monitoring: report of the consensus panel. Clin Chem 1990;36:1841–6.

[91] Wallemacq P, Armstrong VW, Brunet M, Haufroid V, et al. Opportunities to optimize
tacrolimus therapy in solid organ transplantation: report of the European consensus conference. Ther Drug Monit 2009;31:139–52.

[92] Levine DM, Maine GT, Armbruster DA, Mussell C, et al. The need for standardization
of tacrolimus assays. Clin Chem 2011;57:1739–47.

[93] Annesley TM, McKeown DA, Holt DW, Mussell C, et al. Standardization of LC-Ms for
therapeutic drug monitoring of tacrolimus. Clin Chem 2013;59:1630–7.

[94] Agrawal YP, Cid M, Westgard S, Parker TS, et al. Transplant patient classification and
tacrolimus assays: more evidence of the need for assay standardization. Ther Drug
Monit 2014;36:706–9.

[95] Keller BO, Sui J, Young AB, Whittal RM. Interferences and contaminants encountered
in modern mass spectrometry. Anal Chim Acta 2008;627:71–81.

[96] Bonfiglio R, King RC, Olah TV, Merkle K. The effects of sample preparation methods
on the variability of the electrospray ionization response for model drug compounds.
Rapid Commun Mass Spectrom 1999;13:1175–85.

[97] Guo X, Lankmayr E. Phospholipid-based matrix effects in LC-Ms bioanalysis.
Bioanalysis 2011;3:349–52.

[98] Honour JW. Development and validation of a quantitative assay based on tandem mass
spectrometry. Ann Clin Biochem 2011;48:97–111.

[99] Guo X, Bruins AP, Covey TR. Characterization of typical chemical background inter-
      ferences in atmospheric pressure ionization liquid chromatography-mass spectrometry.
      Rapid Commun Mass Spectrom 2006;20:3145–50.

[100] Hall TG, Smukste I, Bresciano KR, Wang Y, et al. Identifying and overcoming matrix
      effects in drug discovery and development. In: Dr. Prasain J, editor. Tandem mass spetrom-
      etry — applications and principles. ISBN: 978-953.51-0141-3. In Tech, India; 2012.
      p. 389–20.

[101] Morin LP, Mess JN, Furtado M, Garofolo F. Reliable procedures to evaluate and repair
      crosstalk for bioanalytical MS/MS assays. Bioanalysis 2011;3:275–83.

[102] Brandhorst G, Oellerich M, Maine G, Taylor P, et al. Liquid chromatography-tandem
      mass spectrometry or automated immunoassays: what are the future trends in therapeu-
      tic drug monitoring? Clin Chem 2012;58:821–5.

Monitoring free mycophenolic acid concentration: Is there any clinical advantage?

4

Amitava Dasgupta

Department of Pathology and Laboratory Medicine,
University of Texas–Houston Medical School, Houston, TX, USA

4.1 INTRODUCTION

Therapeutic drug monitoring is defined as the management of a patient's drug regime based on serum, plasma, or whole blood concentration of a drug. The International Association for Therapeutic Drug Monitoring and Clinical Toxicology adopted the following definition [1]:

Therapeutic drug monitoring is defined as the measurement made in the labora-tory of a parameter that, with appropriate interpretation, will directly influence prescribing procedures. Commonly, the measurement is in a biological matrix of a prescribed xenobiotic, but it may also be of an endogenous compound prescribed as a replacement therapy in an individual who is physiologically or pathologi-cally deficient in that compound.

Immunosuppressant drugs cyclosporine, tacrolimus, sirolimus, everolimus, and mycophenolic acid fulfill the criteria for therapeutic drug monitoring and are routinely monitored in solid organ transplant recipients. Although all these immunosuppres-sants are strongly protein bound, currently clinical utility of free mycophenolic acid monitoring has been documented for certain special patient populations, and some clinical laboratories offer free mycophenolic acid monitoring service. However, to the knowledge of this author, free concentrations of cyclosporine, tacrolimus, siroli-mus, or everolimus are not monitored in the clinical laboratories, although there are published reports dealing with free fraction determination of both cyclosporine and tacrolimus. In this chapter, emphasis is placed on clinical utility of free mycophe-nolic acid monitoring, but a brief review of monitoring free cyclosporine and tacroli-mus is also included. One of the reasons why many investigators have focused on free mycophenolic acid monitoring is that mycophenolic acid is monitored in serum or plasma, whereas cyclosporine, tacrolimus, sirolimus, and everolimus are moni-tored using whole blood. Therefore, ultrafiltrate of serum or plasma could be easily

M. Oellerich & A. Dasgupta (Eds): Personalized Immunosuppression in Transplantation.
DOI: http://dx.doi.org/10.1016/B978-0-12-800885-0.00004-7

prepared in the clinical laboratory using commercially available filtration device, but preparing ultrafiltrate of whole blood is technically difficult.

4.2 MONITORING FREE DRUG CONCENTRATION

The free concentration of a drug represents the fraction of a drug not bound to serum proteins (unbound drug fraction) that is freely diffusible and immediately available to distribute in the body, pass through biological membranes, and bind to receptors. Therefore, the free drug concentration correlates with clinical efficacy and drug toxicity better than total drug concentration because the fraction of drug bound to serum proteins has no pharmacological activity. However, the vast majority of decisions in clinical pharmacokinetics and research continue to be made based on the sum of free plus bound drug molecules, which is conventionally monitored as total drug concentration. Moreover, some investigators claim that free drug monitoring is unnecessary because the free drug fraction within and between individuals is constant for a particular drug. However, this phenomenon is not applicable to all patients. Although the free fraction is fairly constant when drug concentrations are much lower than protein concentrations, the free fraction always depends on the concentration of binding protein, which may vary widely between individuals with various pathophysiological conditions. Furthermore, the binding characteristics of proteins can change dramatically in genetic or metabolic diseases, as well as in patients who suffer from burns or malnutrition. In all these cases, total drug concentration is not necessarily proportional to pharmacodynamic activity, and the free drug concentration should be monitored instead for better patient management [2].

Levy and Moreland commented that free drug monitoring should be considered for drugs for which the usefulness of plasma level monitoring has been established, drugs that are strongly protein bound, and drugs that exhibit a variable free fraction. In terms of drug distribution, free drug concentration is independent of free fraction for drugs with low extraction ratio, but total drug concentration is a resultant of free concentration and free fraction. For drugs with high extraction ratio, the free drug concentration depends on free fraction but only after parenteral administration. There are many drugs that are highly protein bound and also exhibit large variations in free fractions. Pathophysiological conditions that alter the concentration of drug binding proteins in serum such as albumin and α_1 acid glycoprotein as well as changes in concentrations of endogenous compounds that compete with drug binding sites may significantly alter free drug concentrations. Binding interactions due to polytherapy may also result in variable free fraction [3].

Drug distribution throughout the body is mostly influenced by the flow of blood, which contains two main drug binding proteins: albumin (normal concentration in serum: 3.5–5.2 g/dL; 527–783 μmol/L, assuming molecular weight of albumin as 66,437) and α_1 acid glycoprotein (AGP; with a normal concentration of 50–120 mg/dL; 12.5–30 μmol/L, assuming molecular weight of AGP as 40,000). If the free drug concentration cannot be measured, the concentration of these binding proteins should be determined in addition to total drug concentration. Subsequently, the normalized drug concentration or the free drug concentration can be calculated from total drug concentration and the concentration of the binding protein. There are mathematical models to calculate the free drug fraction based on total drug concentration and plasma protein concentration that binds the drug. In order to calculate the free drug fraction (f_u) and the plasma protein binding (PPB), most models are based on the assumption that plasma contains a binding protein P (representing the active binding sites on all proteins) with the concentration C_p and the binding constant K between drug (D) and protein. The binding equilibrium can then be described as

$$[P] + [D] = [PD]$$

Therefore, equilibrium constant K can be defined as

$$K = \frac{[PD]}{[D] \cdot [P]} = \frac{C_{total} - C_{free}}{C_{free} \cdot (C_p - C_{total} + C_{free})}$$

where C_{total} is the total drug concentration, and C_{free} is the free drug concentration.

When the concentration of the drug is much lower than the concentration of proteins, the bound drug concentration ($C_{total} - C_{free}$) is negligible with respect to C_p, and the equation becomes

$$K = \frac{C_{total} - C_{free}}{C_{free} \cdot C_p} = \frac{C_{total}/C_{free} - 1}{C_p}$$

Because most drugs are active at low micromolar concentrations, this assumption is certainly applicable in the case of binding to albumin that is present in plasma at a concentration of 660–750 µmol/L. Furthermore, some studies suggest that the binding sites are not limited even at drug concentrations higher than 2000 µmol/L [4]. The values of the unbound fraction and that of PPB% can easily be derived:

$$f_u = 1 - \frac{PPB}{100} = \frac{C_{free}}{C_{total}} = \frac{1}{1 + C_p \cdot K} \Rightarrow PPB = \frac{100}{1 + 1/(C_p \cdot K)}$$

Drugs with high plasma protein binding tend to be confined mostly in the central compartment, have a low volume of distribution, and are mostly eliminated by metabolism. In order for these drugs to be active, they must achieve total blood concentrations significantly higher than those required for receptor activation in tissues. Such drugs, with low free concentration and high total concentration in serum, require routine free concentration monitoring; examples are phenytoin, valproic acid, and, to some extent, carbamazepine. The immunosuppressant drug mycophenolic acid also falls in this category. Drugs that have similar plasma and tissue binding distribute relatively homogeneously throughout the body, and for these drugs, plasma concentration is a good indicator of target site concentration. In general, it is assumed that if protein binding of a drug is less than 80%, free drug monitoring may not be necessary.

4.3 MONITORING FREE (UNBOUND) FRACTION OF CYCLOSPORINE

Cyclosporine, a cyclic polypeptide of fungal origin, was approved for use as an immunosuppressant in 1983. Cyclosporine is very lipophilic and extensively bound to blood cells and plasma proteins, mainly lipoproteins. Cyclosporine is distributed approximately 41–58% in erythrocytes, 33–47% in plasma, and the rest in other cellular components. Cyclosporine present in plasma is bound to lipoproteins, including very low-density lipoprotein (VLDL; 10%), low-density lipoprotein (LDL; 35%), and high-density lipoprotein (HDL, 33%), leaving approximately 1 or 2% unbound cyclosporine in plasma, although the free fraction is highly variable (Table 4.1). Therefore, free cyclosporine level present in plasma represents only a small fraction of the total cyclosporine level measured in whole blood for the purpose of therapeutic drug monitoring. Based on analysis of 1878 blood specimens collected from renal transplant recipients, Lindholm and Henricsson observed that free fraction in plasma ranged from 0.5 to 4.2%, with a median of 1.30%. The authors observed a significant decline in the free fraction of cyclosporine prior to acute rejection episodes compared

Table 4.1 Plasma Protein Binding of Cyclosporine, Tacrolimus, Sirolimus, and Everolimus

Immunosuppressant	% Free	Comments
Cyclosporine	Approximately 2% of plasma cyclosporine is unbound.	In whole blood, cyclosporine is distributed approximately 41–58% in erythrocytes, 33–47% in plasma, and the rest in other cellular components. In plasma, cyclosporine is bound to lipoproteins, mainly low-density lipoprotein (LDL: 35%) and high density lipoprotein (HDL: 33%).
Tacrolimus	Approximately 1.2% of plasma tacrolimus is unbound.	In whole blood, tacrolimus is mostly bound to cellular components of blood such as erythrocytes, and approximately 14.3% is found in plasma. In plasma, tacrolimus is bound mainly to soluble proteins such as albumin and also to HDL and, to a lesser extent, VLDL and LDL.
Sirolimus	Approximately 2% of sirolimus is unbound in plasma.	Sirolimus (rapamycin) is approximately 94.5% distributed to erythrocytes, 3.1% in plasma, 1.01% in lymphocytes, and 1.0% in granulocytes. In plasma, approximately 2% sirolimus is unbound (free), and the rest is bound to plasma proteins.
Everolimus	Approximately 25% of plasma everolimus is unbound.	Approximately 75% of everolimus is partitioned in erythrocytes and 25% is partitioned in plasma. In plasma, 75% of everolimus is bound to plasma proteins.

to free fraction 1 week earlier [5]. However, in another report, the author observed no additional benefit of monitoring free cyclosporine compared to total cyclosporine level monitored in plasma in renal transplant recipients. For example, 1 week before rejection, mean total plasma cyclosporine was 100 ng/mL, and at rejection it was reduced to 58 ng/mL. Similarly, free cyclosporine concentration was also reduced from 1.79 ng/mL 1 week prior to rejection to 0.73 ng/mL at rejection. However, 1 week after the rejection episode, both total and free plasma cycloserine values were increased to 95 and 1.45 ng/mL, respectively. Similarly for acute nephrotoxic episode, both total and free cyclosporine values were increased proportionally. The authors employed membrane dialysis using stainless-steel equipment for separating bound cyclosporine from free cyclosporine in plasma, and concentrations were determined using high-performance liquid chromatography (HPLC) [6].

Falck et al. reported that intracellular T lymphocyte cyclosporine levels declined prior to acute rejection in kidney transplant recipients. In a prospective single-center study, 20 kidney transplant recipients (mean age, 54 years) receiving cyclosporine were recruited within 2 weeks of post-transplant and followed up for 3 months. The authors isolated T lymphocytes from 7 mL of whole blood using Prepacyte (cell separating reagent) and determined intracellular cyclosporine concentration using a validated liquid chromatography combined with tandem mass spectrometry (LC–MS/MS). The authors reported that 7 patients who experienced biopsy verified acute rejection within 3 months of post-transplantation showed decreased intracellular cyclosporine concentration 1 week prior to rejection. The decline was more significant (average 27.1% decline) 3 days prior to clinically recognizable signs of rejection. Moreover, intracellular cyclosporine area under the curve 0–12h (AUC_{0-12h}) measured during stable phase was 182% higher in rejection-free patients, but no difference was observed between C2 cyclosporine levels in patients experiencing rejection versus stable patients. The authors concluded that intracellular T lymphocyte concentration tends to decline 1 week prior to rejection but more significantly 3 days prior to rejection episode [7].

In general, ultrafiltration is considered the most suitable method for analysis of free drug concentration. In this method, serum is centrifuged with an ultrafiltration device, and then free drug concentration is measured in the protein-free ultrafiltrate. The Centrifee Micropartition ultrafiltration device is widely used, and the cutoff concentration of the filter used in the device is 30,000 (other cutoff concentrations are also available, but this cutoff is most commonly used for determination of free drug concentration). Oellerich and Muller-Vahl demonstrated that the ultrafiltration method is suitable for routine measurement of free phenytoin in clinical laboratories because results compared well with the equilibrium dialysis method, which is considered the gold standard [8]. However, cyclosporine is monitored in whole blood, and the ultrafiltration technique cannot be used for determination of the free cyclosporine level.

Several methods, including ultracentrifugation, erythrocyte partitioning, equilibrium dialysis using stainless-steel chambers, and microdialysis, have been used for measuring unbound cyclosporine concentration. Measurement of free (unbound) cyclosporine is difficult due to binding of cyclosporine to devices used for separating bound cyclosporine from free cyclosporine. However, using stainless-steel equilibrium apparatus, free (unbound) cyclosporine concentration can be accurately measured. Akhlagi et al. showed that free cyclosporine fraction in plasma is highly variable, ranging from 0.52 to 3.94% with an overall mean of 1.53% in specimens collected from heart, lung, and heart–lung transplant recipients. Free fraction of cyclosporine was also negatively correlated with age of the patient but did not vary with transplant type or etiology of organ failure. The free fractions were significantly lower in hypercholesterolemic transplant recipients compared to normocholesterolemic transplant recipients. Administration of the cholesterol-lowering drug simvastatin resulted in a significant increase in mean free fraction of cyclosporine due to lipid reduction. In addition, variation in free fraction could be significantly affected by serum lipoproteins levels. Therefore, the lipidemic status of patients should be considered during therapeutic drug monitoring of cyclosporine [9]. In another study, the authors showed that following simvastatin therapy, the mean plasma unbound fraction of cyclosporine increased from 1.4 to 1.82% in heart transplant recipients. Clearance of cyclosporine was also increased. The authors used the equilibrium dialysis method for analysis of free cyclosporine [10]. Moreover, heart transplant recipients with a lower level of unbound cyclosporine are more prone to cardiac rejection [11].

Due to the inherent difficulty of monitoring free cyclosporine, alternative specimens such as saliva have been investigated as an appropriate matrix for free cyclosporine. Mendonza et al. described an LC–MS/MS technique for determination of cyclosporine concentrations in saliva. For a highly protein-bound drug such as cyclosporine, saliva offered a simple way to determine free cyclosporine concentration. The authors used an Aqua Perfect C_{18} column maintained at 65°C for their analysis, and cyclosporine C was used as the internal standard. Electrospray tandem mass spectrometry was used for quantification of cyclosporine [12]. Another approach is to use mathematical equation to calculate the free cyclosporine level from the total cyclosporine level and concentrations of serum LDL cholesterol, HDL cholesterol, and albumin [13].

4.4 MONITORING FREE (UNBOUND) FRACTION OF TACROLIMUS AND SIROLIMUS

Therapeutic drug monitoring is useful for solid organ transplant recipients who are receiving tacrolimus for immunosuppressant therapy. The consensus report on tacrolimus monitoring recommended use of analytic methods with a lower limit of quantitation of 1 ng/mL. The target whole blood tacrolimus concentration should be 8–12 ng/mL for early exposure. Moreover, careful validation of the analytic method for determination of whole blood tacrolimus level is essential, as is participation in an external proficiency testing program. Moreover, certified calibrator materials must be used for chromatographic methods such as LC–MS/MS). In addition, intermethod bias should be accounted for when comparing clinical trial outcomes [14].

Approximately 14.3% of tacrolimus is found in plasma, and the rest is distributed in cellular components of blood (mostly erythrocytes but a very small fraction is associated with lymphocytes). In plasma, tacrolimus is associated mostly with soluble proteins (average, 61.2%), followed by HDL (28.1%), LDL (7.8%), and VLDL (1.4%). The in vitro fraction of unbound tacrolimus in plasma of healthy subjects was estimated to be 1.2 ± 0.12% [15]. Zahir et al. reported that the association of tacrolimus with erythrocytes varies significantly from day 1 of transplant (average, 74.4%) to day 60 of transplant (average, 80.4%) among liver transplant recipients. In patients experiencing tacrolimus-related side effects, unbound tacrolimus levels measured in whole blood were significantly elevated compared to those of patients not experiencing toxicity (average unbound tacrolimus was 0.85 ng/L in patients experiencing side effects vs. 0.53 ng/L in stable patients). However, total whole blood tacrolimus levels were comparable between stable patients and patients experiencing tacrolimus-related side effects (8.1 ng/mL in stable patients vs. 9.3 ng/mL in patients experiencing side effects). In addition, unbound tacrolimus concentrations were significantly lower in patients experiencing rejection (average unbound tacrolimus of 0.28 ng/L in patients experiencing rejection vs. 0.70 ng/L in stable patients). Moreover, the percentage of tacrolimus associated with leukocytes was also lower during rejection episodes. However, the total tacrolimus level was 8.6 ng/mL (mean) in stable patients and 7.6 ng/mL in patients experiencing rejection, both of which were within therapeutic range. The authors employed equilibrium dialysis using stainless-steel apparatus for measurement of free fraction [16].

Sirolimus (rapamycin) is approximately 94.5% distributed to erythrocytes, 3.1% in plasma, 1.01% in lymphocytes, and 1.0% in granulocytes. In plasma, approximately 2% of sirolimus is unbound (free), and the rest is bound to plasma proteins. Lipoproteins are not the major plasma binding protein of sirolimus. There is a slight variation of free fraction of sirolimus in plasma over a sirolimus concentration range of 5–100 ng/mL. Because only a small fraction of sirolimus is distributed in plasma, only 0.1% of sirolimus in whole blood concentration is found in free form [17,18]. In general, sirolimus is monitored in whole blood, and the unbound concentration of sirolimus is not determined. In humans, more than 75% of everolimus is partitioned in erythrocytes, and approximately 25% is found in plasma. In plasma, 75% of everolimus is bound to plasma proteins and 25% is free [19] (Table 4.1).

4.5 MYCOPHENOLIC ACID: A BRIEF INTRODUCTION

Mycophenolate mofetil is a prodrug of mycophenolic acid that after oral administration is rapidly hydrolyzed to mycophenolic acid. Another formulation of mycophenolic acid is mycophenolate sodium, which can also be administered orally. Mycophenolic acid is a potent selective and reversible inhibitor of inosine monophosphate dehydrogenase, which is a key enzyme involved in de novo synthesis of guanine nucleotides. Currently for renal transplant recipients, mycophenolate mofetil is administered at a dosage of 1 g twice daily or, for mycophenolate sodium, the dosage is 720 mg twice daily (bioequivalent of 1 g mycophenolate mofetil). However, dosage may vary widely between route of administration (oral vs. intravenous) and transplant type. After oral administration, bioavailability is approximately 94%, but in one report oral bioavailability in renal transplant patients was 80.7% [20]. Mycophenolic acid is strongly protein bound (97–99%), and only a small fraction of mycophenolic acid is circulated in the free form, which is the pharmacologically active form. The 12-h dose interval of mycophenolic acid plasma concentration versus time profile shows a rapid absorption where peak concentration is achieved approximately 1 h after administration followed by distribution and decreasing plasma concentration reaching a plateau within 3 or 4 h. In whole blood, 99.9% of mycophenolic acid is found in plasma fraction, whereas only 0.01% is found in cellular components of blood, justifying therapeutic drug monitoring using serum or plasma [21].

The main metabolite of mycophenolic acid is formed via activity of liver enzyme uridine diphosphate glucuronyl transferase, where mycophenolic acid phenolic glucuronide is formed (7-O-mycophenolic acid β-glucuronide or MPAG). Glucuronidation also produces mycophenolic acid acyl glucuronide, which is a minor metabolite. Whereas MPAG has no pharmacological activity, the minor metabolite mycophenolic acid acyl glucuronide does has pharmacological activity. MPAG is present in plasma at 20- to 100-fold higher concentration than mycophenolic acid [22]. Most of the dosage of mycophenolic acid is excreted in urine as MPAG. A small amount is recovered in feces. However, MPAG is also excreted in bile, which may be deconjugated by glucuronidase shed by bacteria present in the gastrointestinal tract. As a result, this enterohepatic recirculation of mycophenolic acid may account for approximately 40% (range, 10–60%) of mycophenolic acid exposure in a patient receiving this drug [23]. Therefore, due to enterohepatic recirculation, a secondary peak concentration of mycophenolic acid is usually observed 4–8 h after ingestion of a dose. A significant portion of between-occasion variability of mycophenolic acid trough concentration in an individual patient is due to day to day fluctuations in enterohepatic recirculation. Many factors influence elimination of mycophenolic acid, including significant renal or liver disease, drug–drug interactions, genetic factors, diarrhea, and patient compliance [24].

Myfortic is an enteric formulation of mycophenolate sodium that is formulated as a delayed-release tablet. Enteric-coded mycophenolate sodium 720 mg twice a day has been found to be equivalent to mycophenolate mofetil 1000 mg twice a day. Enteric-coded mycophenolate sodium may have fewer gastrointestinal side effects and other side effects compared to mycophenolate mofetil [25]. Although mycophenolic acid area under the curve, maximum serum concentration, and trough serum concentration did not differ significantly between heart transplant recipients receiving enteric-coated mycophenolate sodium and those receiving mycophenolate mofetil, the peak serum concentration was observed approximately 1 h later with enteric-coated mycophenolate sodium (Myfortic) compared to mycophenolate mofetil [26].

4.6 RATIONALE FOR THERAPEUTIC DRUG MONITORING OF MYCOPHENOLIC ACID

With the increasing use of mycophenolate mofetil or mycophenolate sodium in solid organ transplant, the need for more accurate dosing has become evident. However, few studies have investigated the clinical usefulness of therapeutic drug monitoring of mycophenolic acid, the active drug, in solid organ transplantation in a prospective way, and such studies have produced conflicting results. According to the consensus report on therapeutic drug monitoring of mycophenolic acid in solid organ transplantation, limited sampling strategies (LSSs) monitoring (several specific timed points after dosing) is preferred compared to a single mycophenolic acid trough concentration (pre-dose) measurement for dosing of mycophenolic acid in solid organ transplant recipients. Use of LSSs can improve early graft outcome in terms of acute rejection, although avoidance of drug-related adverse effects has not been demonstrated. Moreover, whether therapeutic drug monitoring of mycophenolic acid will be required for maintenance immunosuppression therapy is not clear. Therefore, general routine use of therapeutic drug monitoring of mycophenolic acid cannot be recommended, although specific patient populations may benefit from prolonged concentration controlled mycophenolic acid dosing. These patient populations include patients who are at increased immunological risk; patients undergoing minimization or withdrawal of immunosuppressive therapy; and patients experiencing altered renal, hepatic, or bowl function. Drug–drug interactions and noncompliance can also be determined from therapeutic drug monitoring [27].

Although rationale for routine therapeutic drug monitoring in maintenance immunosuppressive therapy is unclear, pre-dose levels of mycophenolic acid vary widely even in stable transplant recipients receiving this drug. In addition, AUC_{0-12h} is also monitored and probably provides a better assessment of exposure of mycophenolic acid. Limited sampling approach and use of Bayesian estimation of mycophenolic acid AUC have been described for therapeutic drug monitoring. Usually, three blood specimens collected 2 or 3h after dosing are sufficient to estimate AUC_{0-12h} for mycophenolic acid [28]. It has been usually accepted that clinical efficacy as well as avoidance of rejection and hematological toxicities of mycophenolic acid can be achieved by therapeutic drug monitoring. Individual dosing is recommended due to large interindividual variability in pharmacokinetic and pharmacodynamics of mycophenolic acid. In general, in the presence of cyclosporine, the recommended pre-dose mycophenolic acid concentration in serum or plasma is 1.0–3.5 mg/L, although AUC_{0-12h} for mycophenolic acid is also used for therapeutic drug monitoring with suggested reference range (Table 4.2). Borrows et al., using 5600 trough mycophenolic acid samples (12h after dose) from 121 renal transplant patients receiving mycophenolate mofetil and tacrolimus in a steroid sparing protocol (steroids for 7 days only), observed that a mycophenolic acid trough level of 1.60 mg/L during the early transplant phase best discriminated patients who experienced rejection versus those who did not. Similarly, in the post-transplant phase, the mycophenolic level of

Table 4.2 Therapeutic Range of Mycophenolic Acid*

Parameter	Comedication	Therapeutic Range
Trough (predose) concentration	Cyclosporine	1.0–3.5 mg/L (1.0–3.5 µg/mL)
AUC_{0-12h}	Cyclosporine	30–60 mg × h/L (30–60 µg × h/mL)
Trough (predose) concentration	Tacrolimus	1.9–4.0 mg/L (1.9–4.0 µg/mL)
AUC_{0-12h}	Tacrolimus	30–60 mg × h/L (30–60 µg × h/mL)

Patients receiving mycophenolic acid and co-medication.

2.75 mg/L best discriminated patients with and without rejection. However, higher mycophenolic acid levels were also associated with anemia, lower hemoglobin, lower white cell count, as well as incidence of leukopenia [29].

4.6.1 SERUM PROTEIN BINDING OF MYCOPHENOLIC ACID

Mycophenolic acid is strongly bound to serum protein (97–99%), mostly albumin, in patients with normal renal and liver function. Binding of mycophenolic acid to α_1 acid glycoprotein in serum is minimal. Nowak and Shaw reported various parameters of reversible binding of mycophenolic acid with human serum albumin [30]. The authors also studied the distribution of mycophenolic acid in whole blood using [14C] mycophenolic acid and observed that 99.99% radioactivity was found in plasma, indicating that distribution of mycophenolic acid in erythrocytes or other cellular components of blood was negligible. Mycophenolic acid is reversibly bound to human serum albumin with a dissociation constant (K_d) of 13.56 µmol/L. One mole of albumin is capable of binding 1.8 mol of mycophenolic acid. As albumin concentration was increased from 0.07 to 6.9 g/dL, the free fraction of mycophenolic acid decreased from an average of 53.3 to 0.92%. Mycophenolic acid did not bind significantly to α_1 acid glycoprotein. Mycophenolic acid serum protein binding was not significantly affected by warfarin, digoxin, phenytoin, cyclosporine A, or prednisone even at high concentrations, but sodium salicylate concentrations from 10 to 500 mg/L increased free mycophenolic acid fraction in normal human serum from 1.36 to 8.26%. The authors further demonstrated that the free fraction of mycophenolic acid has pharmacological activity as evidenced by the observation that 50% of inhibition (IC_{50}) of inosine monophosphate dehydrogenase isoform II was increased by 5.4-fold as the concentration of human serum albumin added to the enzyme reaction mixture was increased from 0 to 5.0 g/dL. Furthermore, the IC_{50} mycophenolic acid concentration for phytohemagglutinin A-stimulated human peripheral blood mononuclear cells increased 4.8-fold when incubation was performed in the presence of 1 g/dL human serum albumin versus no serum albumin added. The authors further demonstrated that free mycophenolic acid levels determined by reference equilibrium dialysis method and ultrafiltration method produced comparable result. The authors performed the ultrafiltration procedure using the Centrifree Micropartition

Table 4.3 Various Characteristics of Plasma Protein Binding of Mycophenolic Acid

- Mycophenolic acid is mostly found in plasma (99.9%), and protein binding of mycophenolic acid in plasma is 97–99% in patients with normal renal and liver function.
- Only free mycophenolic acid (1–3% of total mycophenolic acid level) is pharmacologically active in patients with normal renal and liver function.
- Mycophenolic acid is reversibly bound to albumin in plasma with a dissociation constant (K_d) of 13.56 µmol/L.
- One mole of albumin is capable of binding 1.8 mol of mycophenolic acid. In another report, the K_d value was 13.24 µmol/L and 1 mol of human albumin was capable of binding 1.72 mol of mycophenolic acid.
- Free mycophenolic acid concentration is significantly affected by plasma albumin concentration. When albumin concentration was increased from 0.07 g/dL to 6.9 g/dL, the free fraction of mycophenolic acid decreased from average 53.3% to 0.92%.
- In general, it is assumed that if plasma albumin concentration is less than 3.1 g/dL (30 g/L), significantly elevated free mycophenolic acid may be observed in these patients compared to patients with albumin level >3.1 g/dL. For these hypoalbuminemic patients (albumin <3.1 g/dL), monitoring free mycophenolic acid level is desirable.
- Sodium salicylate concentration from 10 to 500 mg/L increased free mycophenolic acid fraction in normal human serum from 1.36 to 8.26%.

system (Amicon, Beverly, MA), which is commonly used for monitoring free drug concentration in clinical laboratories [30]. Vial et al. reported that the K_d value for mycophenolic acid was 13.24 µmol/L, and 1 mol of human albumin is capable of binding 1.72 mol of mycophenolic acid [31]. Interestingly, 7-*O*-mycophenolic acid glucuronide, the major metabolite of mycophenolic acid, is 82% bound to plasma proteins [32]. Various characteristics of protein binding of mycophenolic acid are summarized in Table 4.3.

4.6.2 CONDITIONS THAT INCREASE FREE MYCOPHENOLIC ACID LEVEL

Because mycophenolic acid is strongly protein bound, pharmacological activities of mycophenolic acid are due to its free fraction only. It has been demonstrated that only free mycophenolic acid is capable of inhibiting inosine monophosphate dehydrogenase [33]. Moreover, only free mycophenolic acid can be metabolized to inactive MPAG (major metabolite) and active mycophenolic acid acyl glucuronide (minor metabolite). Traditionally, total mycophenolic acid level is monitored with an assumption that approximately 97–99% would be protein bound. In general, in transplant recipients with normal albumin concentration as well as normal renal and liver function, the free fraction of mycophenolic acid is 2 or 3%, and free mycophenolic acid concentration can be predicted from total mycophenolic acid concentration. Ensom et al. reported that the average free fraction of mycophenolic acid in stable lung transplant recipients was 2.9% (range, 2.0–3.4%). Mean albumin concentration in these patients was 3.7 g/dL [34]. Beckebaum et al. observed a median free mycophenolic acid fraction of 1.16% (range, 0.85–2.16%) in stable liver transplant patients also receiving cyclosporine, and they reported a median free fraction of 0.98% (range, 0.72–1.7%) in stable liver transplant patients also receiving tacrolimus. None of the patients studied were hypoalbuminemic (albumin range, 3.5–5.1 g/dL). Serum creatinine varied from 1.1 to 2.3 mg/dL (median, 1.5 mg/dL) [35]. Jiao et al. reported that in Chinese renal transplant recipients on day 10 of transplant, mean fraction of free mycophenolic acid was 3.5%, whereas the mean fraction of mycophenolic acid metabolite (MPAG) was 34.6%. The mean total and free AUC_{0-12h} of mycophenolic acid were 20.2 and 0.7 mg × h/L, respectively [36]. However, many conditions may lead to significantly increased free mycophenolic acid concentrations, and for these patients, monitoring only total mycophenolic acid concentration may provide misleading information regarding exposure of mycophenolic acid. Major causes of decreased protein binding of mycophenolic acid include the following:

- Hypoalbuminemia
- Uremia
- Liver disease (hypoalbuminemia is a common feature of liver disease)
- Elevated mycophenolic acid glucuronide
- Hyperbilirubinemia

Various conditions that may increase free mycophenolic acid are summarized in Table 4.4.

Hypoalbuminemia is the major cause of elevated free mycophenolic acid because albumin is the major mycophenolic acid binding protein in plasma. Many pathological conditions, such as uremia and liver disease, may also cause hypoalbuminemia. For these patients, traditionally monitored total mycophenolic acid concentration may be within the therapeutic window, but the free mycophenolic acid level may be elevated,

Table 4.4 Various Clinical Conditions That May Increase Free Mycophenolic Acid Concentrations After Transplantation

- Significant hypoalbuminemia (albumin below 3.1 g/dL) may cause increased concentration of free mycophenolic acid.
- Time of transplant (usually free fraction is higher immediately after transplantation and then free fraction is reduced with time, probably due to improved graft function and improved albumin concentration).
- Increased concentration of mycophenolic acid glucuronide metabolite may increase free mycophenolic acid concentration due to displacement of mycophenolic acid from albumin binding.
- Significant renal dysfunction may increase free mycophenolic acid concentration due to hypoalbuminemia as well as accumulation of mycophenolic acid glucuronide metabolite.
- Liver disease may also increase free mycophenolic acid concentration.
- One strongly protein-bound drug can displace mycophenolic acid from protein binding site causing increased free mycophenolic acid concentration.

causing toxicity. For these patients, monitoring free mycophenolic acid should be more beneficial. In a study of 42 renal transplant recipients, Atcheson et al. observed a significant relationship between low plasma albumin concentrations and elevated free mycophenolic acid fraction (>3%) using Spearman correlation. Receiver operating characteristic curve analysis showed that the cutoff value for albumin was 3.1 g/dL. In general, patients with albumin concentration less than 3.1 g/dL showed elevated percentage of free mycophenolic acid (>3%). At that cutoff, albumin was found to be a good predictor of elevated free mycophenolic acid concentration, with sensitivity and specificity of 0.75 and 0.80, respectively. The authors concluded that clinicians should consider monitoring free mycophenolic acid concentrations in hypoalbuminemic patients with plasma albumin levels less than 3.1 g/dL [37].

In uremic patients, the free fraction of mycophenolic acid may be elevated due to hypoalbuminemia as well as accumulation of MPAG in plasma. MPAG is capable of displacing mycophenolic acid from protein binding sites because MPAG is also strongly bound to protein (~82%). It is assumed that both hypoalbuminemia and accumulation of MPAG are responsible for the increased free fraction of mycophenolic acid in patients with renal insufficiency. Elevated free fraction in these patients leads to higher clearance and lower AUC for total mycophenolic acid. In patients with chronic renal failure, both total and free mycophenolic acid should be measured in order to avoid mycophenolic acid toxicity induced by increased free mycophenolic acid concentration. Kaplan et al. studied 8 renal transplant recipients (1 patient had both kidney and pancreas transplant) with chronic renal insufficiency and 15 renal transplant patients with preserved renal function and observed that average free mycophenolic acid fractions were more than double those of patients with normal renal function (5.8 ± 2.7 vs. 2.5 ± 0.4). Such differences were both clinically and statistically significant. The authors concluded that mycophenolic acid protein binding is decreased and free mycophenolic acid concentrations are increased in chronic renal failure patients [38]. Weber et al. observed that renal impairment had no effect on total mycophenolic acid AUC_{0-12h} values, but free fraction in children (median, 1.65%; range, 0.4–13.8%) who received renal transplantation was significantly modulated by renal function and serum albumin concentration because patients with renal insufficiency or low serum albumin showed higher free fraction of mycophenolic acid as well as free mycophenolic acid AUC_{0-12h}. In addition, patients with renal insufficiency showed significantly higher MPAG AUC_{0-12h} because mycophenolic acid glucuronide is cleared by the kidney [39].

CASE REPORT

A 58-year-old man with end stage renal failure secondary to polycystic kidney disease received renal transplant and subsequently developed highly elevated free mycophenolic acid fraction associated with severe toxicity over a period of 5 days. During this time, although his serum creatinine was reduced from 0.85 mmol/L (0.96 mg/dL) to 0.5 mmol/L (0.56 mg/dL), he became markedly jaundiced as bilirubin increased from 17 μmol/L (1.0 mg/dL) to 161 μmol/L (9.4 mg/dL). His serum albumin level was also reduced from 3.6 to less than 2 g/dL. Although his liver enzymes were normal before transplant, they were elevated after transplant (alkaline phosphatase, 137 U/L; γ-glutamyltransferase, 301 U/L). On day 5, his 2-h cyclosporine level (837 ng/mL) and total mycophenolic acid AUC_{0-6h} (12.6 mg × h/L) were low, but total MPAG AUC_{0-6h} was elevated (1317 mg × h/L). Mycophenolic acid dose was not changed, but cyclosporine was substituted with tacrolimus. The patient subsequently experienced severe nausea, vomiting, hematemesis, and pancytopenia (nadir white cell count $1.6 × 10^9$/L, platelet count $32 × 10^9$/L, and hemoglobin 7.3 mg/dL). This severe toxicity was resolved after cessation of therapy with mycophenolic acid mofetil. Retrospective analysis revealed that free mycophenolic acid AUC_{0-6h} was significantly elevated (2.3 mg × h/L), as was the free fraction, which was highly elevated to 18.3%, thus explaining the observed toxicity despite the fact that the total mycophenolic acid level was relatively low. This case illustrates severe mycophenolic acid toxicity caused by increased free fraction despite total mycophenolic acid level being relatively low. Moreover, high free mycophenolic acid concentration may be associated with hypoalbuminemia and hyperbilirubinemia [40].

CASE REPORT

A 34-year-old Caucasian female patient presented to the clinic with a 1-day history of fever and myalgia. The patient had undergone a pancreas–kidney transplant 2 years ago. The patient was initially maintained on cyclosporine and prednisone. However, 3 months before admission, her serum creatinine was increased to 5 mg/dL with calculated creatinine clearance of 9 mL/min. At that time, renal biopsy showed grade III chronic rejection along with grade II acute rejection, and the patient was prescribed mycophenolate mofetil at 750 mg twice daily as a prophylaxis against rejection. The next morning after her presentation to the clinic, a full pharmacokinetic profile of mycophenolic acid, free mycophenolic acid, as well as MPAG was assessed along with cyclosporine. Her trough cyclosporine level of 240 ng/mL and cyclosporine 12 h AUC (4900 ng × h/mL) were within therapeutic range. Her total mycophenolic acid 12 h AUC was 36.8 µg × h/mL, which was again within therapeutic range. However, her free mycophenolic acid fraction was 13.8% (normal, ≤ 3%), and her free mycophenolic acid 12 h AUC was 5.07 µg × h/mL (normal, 0.08–1.95 µg × h/mL). Therefore, the patient was experiencing mycophenolic acid-induced toxicity due to significantly elevated free fraction, which was probably related to multiple factors, including hypoalbuminemia (albumin in this patient was 2.7 g/dL), chronic renal failure (serum creatinine during episode was 6.7 mg/dL), and highly elevated 12 h AUC of MPAG (5899 µg × h/mL; normal in stable renal transplant patients, <750 µg × h/mL). Therapy with mycophenolate mofetil was discontinued, and her symptoms improved within 1 week (at admission, hemoglobin was 5.4 g/dL, whereas 1 week after discontinuation of therapy, it was 10 g/dL). The patient's infection was also resolved because early antigen as well as culture of cytomegalovirus were negative [41].

In general, the free fraction of mycophenolic acid is elevated immediately after transplantation and then reduces as the graft becomes more stable. Weber et al. reported that median total mycophenolic acid AUC_{0-12h} value increased twofold from 32.4 mg × h/L (range, 13.9–57.0 mg × h/L) at 3 weeks post-transplant to 65.1 mg × h/L (range, 32.6–114 mg × h/L) at 3 months post-transplant in pediatric renal transplant recipients. However, median AUC_{0-12h} for free mycophenolic acid did not change during this period because mycophenolic acid free fraction declined more than 35% from 3 weeks post-transplant to 3 months post-transplant (1.4% free in the initial phase of post-transplant to 0.9% in the stable phase) [42].

Reine et al. reported that albumin levels correlated with free fraction of mycophenolic acid in liver transplant recipients. Moreover, the authors observed that both total and free mycophenolic acid levels were equally good predictors of the immunosuppressive effect of mycophenolic acid as estimated by inosine monophosphate dehydrogenase activity [43]. Interestingly, Shen et al. observed that fraction of free mycophenolic acid as well as free mycophenolic acid AUC_{0-12h} were higher in liver transplant recipients who received transplant from a living donor compared to liver transplant recipients who received transplant from a deceased donor [44].

Kim et al. investigated the population pharmacokinetics of free mycophenolic acid in pediatric patients ($n = 31$) and young adults ($n = 5$) undergoing allogenic hematopoietic cell transplantation. The pharmacokinetics of unbound mycophenolic acid could be well described by using a two-compartmental model with linear elimination and first-order absorption. The important clinical covariates affecting unbound mycophenolic acid pharmacokinetics were weight, estimated creatinine clearance, and total bilirubin. In individuals with hepatic dysfunction (total bilirubin >10 mg/dL), unbound mycophenolic acid clearance was approximately threefold lower compared to that in patients with normal liver function or mild hepatic impairment [45]. Kiang et al. used multiple regression analysis of various factors in order to predict free mycophenolic acid fraction (MPAf). Various factors that the authors considered were weight, age, height, total daily mycophenolic acid dosage, albumin, and serum creatinine. The authors used data from 91 patients for the regression analysis and derived the following equation:

$$MPAf = 1.865 + (0.0357 \times age\ in\ years) + (0.0125 \times weight\ in\ Kg)$$
$$- (0.0202 \times height\ in\ cm) - (0.000323 \times total\ daily\ dosage\ in\ mg)$$
$$+ (0.0122 \times albumin\ in\ gm/L) + (0.0160 \times creatinine\ in\ \mu mol/L).$$

Nevertheless, none of these variables were significant predictors of MPAf [46].

Van Hest studied pharmacokinetic modeling of the plasma protein binding of mycophenolic acid in renal transplant patients in an attempt to describe the relationship between renal function and albumin concentration and MPAG concentration with unbound fraction of mycophenolic acid. The hypothesis for the underlying mechanism is that low plasma albumin concentration and accumulation of MPAG metabolite result in decreased protein binding of mycophenolic acid. Subsequent increase in unbound fraction of mycophenolic acid leads to an increased clearance of total mycophenolic acid. The authors observed that the time profile of unbound fraction of mycophenolic acid and total MPAG metabolite concentration could be adequately described by a two-compartment pharmacokinetic model with a link between the central compartments representing the glucuronidation of free mycophenolic acid to form MPAG. A reduction of creatinine clearance from 60 to 25 mL/min correlated with an increase in free fraction from 2.7 to 3.5%. Moreover, accumulation of MPAG concentration from 50 to 150 mg/L correlated with an increase in free fraction from 2.8 to 3.7%. In addition, a decrease in albumin concentration from 40 to 30 g/L correlated with an increase in free fraction from 2.6 to 3.5% [47].

> ### CASE REPORT
>
> A 36-year-old woman presented for hematopoietic cell transplantation due to severe myelodysplastic syndrome. On day 4, the patient developed septic shock and oliguric acute renal failure. She was intubated, and continuous venovenous dialysis was initiated. All nephrotoxic drugs including immunosuppressants were stopped. On day 6 and on day 8, mycophenolate mofetil and cyclosporine were restarted at reduced dosages to promote engraftment. On day 8, her total mycophenolic acid trough level was 2.4 mg/L, and mycophenolic acid AUC_{0-12h} was 58.33 mg × h/L, both of which were within therapeutic range. However, unbound trough mycophenolic acid was 0.05 mg/L and unbound mycophenolic acid AUC_{0-12h} was 1.67 mg × h/L—both in the toxic range. In organ transplant, unbound mycophenolic acid AUC_{0-12h} greater than 0.4 mg × h/L is associated with increased risk of neutropenia and infection. Serum creatinine for the patient was 2.97 mg/dL, total bilirubin was 19.8 mg/dL, and liver enzymes were highly elevated (aspartate aminotransferase, 1931 U/L; alanine aminotransferase, 2383 U/L). Despite all efforts, the patient was removed from life support on day 29 [48].

Kaplan et al. assessed free mycophenolic acid, total mycophenolic acid, and MPAG kinetics in a patient with renal failure receiving mycophenolate mofetil for a pancreas transplant because the patient presented with signs of mycophenolate mofetil toxicity. The authors observed that mycophenolic acid glucuronide AUC in the patient was extremely high (5899 µm × h/mL), but total mycophenolic acid AUC (36.8 µm × h/mL) was within the expected range. The free fraction of the mycophenolic acid was 13.8%, which was significantly elevated. The patient also had leukopenia. The authors concluded that patients with severe renal insufficiency may have markedly increased free mycophenolic acid concentration that may not be reflected in total mycophenolic acid concentration [49].

Although most authors measure free mycophenolic acid concentrations directly in serum or plasma collected from patients, Huang et al. developed a mathematic equation to predict free mycophenolic acid fraction from serum creatinine and total bilirubin concentration in serum. The equation proposed by the authors is as follows:

Unbound mycophenolic acid fraction = [0.928 + (serum creatinine mg/dL) × 0.392] (× 1.48 if total bilirubin 3 mg/dL or higher)

Unbound free mycophenolic acid concentration can then be estimated by multiplying total mycophenolic acid concentration with the unbound mycophenolic acid fraction. Interestingly, serum albumin was not significant in the regression model. The model showed low bias but poor precision, and the authors commented that direct measurement of free mycophenolic acid is superior to this mathematical modeling approach of estimating free mycophenolic acid concentration [50].

4.6.3 CLINICAL UTILITY OF MONITORING FREE MYCOPHENOLIC ACID

As mentioned previously, hypoalbuminemia, hyperbilirubinemia, uremia, and elevated concentration of mycophenolic acid glucuronide can all contribute to significantly elevate free mycophenolic acid concentration without affecting total mycophenolic acid concentration. Therefore, for these patients, monitoring free mycophenolic acid level instead of traditionally monitored total mycophenolic acid level should be more useful. Free mycophenolic acid AUC in addition to total mycophenolic acid AUC are useful in renal transplant patients with poor graft function early after transplantation, patients with chronic renal failure, liver transplant patients in the early post-transplantation period, and any patient with low serum albumin. Based on a study of 54 pediatric renal transplant recipients (aged 2.2–17.8 years), Weber et al. observed an association between total mycophenolic acid AUC_{0-12h} and acute rejection. Using receiver operator curve characteristics, the authors commented that AUC_{0-12h} of 33.8 mg × h/L in the initial phase of post-transplant had a diagnostic sensitivity of 75% and specificity of 64%. The respective pre-dose concentration was 1.2 mg/L, with a sensitivity of 83% and a specificity of 64%. In contrast, high free mycophenolic acid but not total mycophenolic acid AUC_{0-12h} values were associated with increased risk of mycophenolate mofetil-related side effects, such as leukopenia and infection. Low protein binding of mycophenolic acid favors its access from circulation to bone marrow, thus causing leukopenia by inhibiting leukocyte maturation from precursor cells. The authors concluded that for the assessment of the toxic effect of mycophenolate mofetil regarding leukopenia and infection, measurement of free mycophenolic acid is more appropriate [51].

4.6.4 DRUG–MYCOPHENOLIC ACID INTERACTION

Few clinically significant drug–mycophenolic acid interactions that lead to elevated free mycophenolic acid level have been described. Nowak and Shaw described displacement of mycophenolic acid from protein binding site by salicylate [30]. Fenofibrate, which is strongly protein bound, may displace mycophenolic acid from the protein binding site, causing toxicity from elevated free fraction.

CASE REPORT

A 57-year-old man was admitted to the hospital for febrile neutropenia. He had undergone kidney transplantation 17 years ago. The patient's immunosuppressive medications were mycophenolate mofetil (500 mg three times a day) and meprednisone 4 mg daily. His hypertension was treated with losartan 50 mg daily and dyslipidemia was treated with ezetimibe 10 mg/simvastatin 20 mg daily over a period of 4 years until 2 weeks before admission, when fenofibrate 200 mg per day was started due to persistently elevated triglyceride levels. On admission, his white blood cell count was 3130/μL with neutropenia (absolute neutrophile count, 313/μL), indicating mycophenolic acid toxicity. Both mycophenolate mofetil and fenofibrate were discontinued while therapy with piperacillin tazobactam 4.5 g three times per day and granulocyte stimulation factor 300 μg per day was initiated. Three days after admission, his white blood cell count was increased to 7280/μL with 22% neutrophils. Mycophenolate mofetil was restarted and granulocyte stimulation factor was discontinued, and 1 month after discharge his white blood cell count was 4480/μL and absolute neutrophil count was 1296/μL. The initiation of fenofibrate in this patient may have precipitated mycophenolic acid-induced neutropenia because fenofibrate is approximately 99% bound to serum albumin and may have displaced mycophenolic acid from protein binding, causing elevated free fraction of mycophenolic acid. In addition, competition of fenofibrate with liver enzyme with uridine diphosphate glucuronyl transferase that also conjugated mycophenolic acid may have reduced metabolism of mycophenolic acid to inactive MPAG metabolite. Both factors may be responsible for mycophenolic acid-induced neutropenia in this patient [52].

Mycophenolate mofetil or mycophenolate sodium is usually used along with another immunosuppressant, such as cyclosporine, tacrolimus, or sirolimus. In general, exposure to mycophenolic acid is 30–40% lower when it is given in combination with cyclosporine than when it is given in combination with tacrolimus or sirolimus. In general, a higher dose of mycophenolate mofetil or sodium may be needed when it is administered in combination with cyclosporine because cyclosporine inhibits biliary secretion of MPAG metabolite due to inhibition of multidrug resistance-associated protein 2. Therefore, enterohepatic recirculation of MPAG back to mycophenolic acid is impaired [53]. However, another complication of cyclosporine-induced inhibition of enterohepatic circulation of mycophenolic acid is the accumulation of MPAG metabolite in plasma, which is capable of displacing mycophenolic acid from the protein binding site, leading to an increased concentration of pharmacologically active free mycophenolic acid. Transiently higher free mycophenolic acid may then accelerate metabolism of mycophenolic acid to MPAG, thus lowering total mycophenolic acid AUC. However, these patients still may have adequate immunosuppression because only free mycophenolic acid is pharmacologically active [54].

Sevelamer may decrease exposure of mycophenolic acid by up to 25% due to reduced gastrointestinal absorption. Cholestyramine may influence mycophenolic acid exposure due to binding or interference with enterohepatic recirculation. Reduced bioavailability of mycophenolic acid if co-administered with antacids is possibly due to chelation. Co-administration of sustained-release ferrous sulfate and mycophenolate mofetil resulted in a 90% decrease in mycophenolic acid exposure due to chelation. Polycarbophil also reduces exposure of mycophenolic acid due to chelation between mycophenolic acid and calcium ion [55].

Several antibiotics have clinically significant interaction with mycophenolic acid. Rifampin significantly reduces total mycophenolic acid AUC_{0-12h} (17.5% decrease) mainly due to reduction in enterohepatic recirculation of mycophenolic acid. Total MPAG AUC_{0-12h} also increased by 34.4% with increased urinary recovery of MPAG as well as mycophenolic acid acyl glucuronide. Rifampin may also induce glucuronidation of mycophenolic acid, thus reducing exposure of mycophenolic acid [56]. Kodawara et al. observed a reduction in serum mycophenolic acid concentration when ciprofloxacin was co-administered with mycophenolic acid, partly due to inhibition of deconjugation of MPAG by β-glucuronidase in the intestine. Therefore, ciprofloxicin blocks eneterohepatic recirculation of mycophenolic acid. In addition, enoxacin showed similar inhibitory effect, but the antibiotics levofloxacin and ofloxacin showed no inhibitory effect [57]. Norfloxicin and metronidazole alone or in combination can reduce AUC of mycophenolic acid, most likely due to reduced enterohepatic recirculation. Naderer et al. reported that compared to therapy with mycophenolate mofetil alone, the area under the plasma concentartion curves of mycophenolic acid (1-g single dose, study period 48 h) were reduced by 10, 19, and 33% when mycophenolate mofetil was administered with norfloxacin, metronidazole, and norfloxacin and metronidazole, respectively [58]. Although St. John's wort, an herbal antidepressant, can significantly reduce the whole blood concentartions of cyclosporine and tracrolimus, causing potential treatment failure, it has no

Table 4.5 Interaction of Various Drugs with Mycophenolic Acid

Interacting Drug with Mycophenolic Acid	Comments
Other immunosuppressants: Cyclosporine, tacrolimus, and Sirolimus	Higher mycophenolic acid level in patients also receiving tacrolimus or sirolimus compared to patients receiving mycophenolic acid with cyclosporine because cyclosporine inhibits biliary secretion of mycophenolic acid glucuronide.
Resins and binders	Sevelamer may decrease exposure of mycophenolic acid by up to 25% due to reduced gastrointestinal absorption. Cholestyramine may influence mycophenolic acid exposure due to binding or interference with enterohepatic recirculation.
Antacids	Reduced bioavailability of mycophenolic acid possibly due to chelation.
Metal ions	Co-administration of sustained-release ferrous sulfate and mycophenolate mofetil resulted in 90% decrease in mycophenolic acid exposure due to chelation. Polycarbophil also reduces exposure of mycophenolic acid due to chelation between mycophenolic acid and calcium ion.
Antibiotics	Norfloxacin, metronidazole, and a combination of norfloxacin and metronidazole reduce AUC of mycophenolic acid. Ciprofloxacin and enoxacin also reduce serum concentration of mycophenolic acid by inhibiting enterohepatic recirculation of mycophenolic acid. Rifampicin may also reduce exposure to mycophenolic acid.
St. John's wort	No significant interaction.
Salicylate	Displaces mycophenolic acid from protein binding site.
Fenofibrate	Fenofibrate, which is strongly protein bound, may displace mycophenolic acid from protein binding site, causing toxicity from elevated free fraction of mycophenolic acid.

interaction with mycophenolic acid. This may be due to the fact that mycophenolic acid is not metabolized by cytochrome P450 mixed function oxidase enzymes in the liver, which is induced by components of St. John's wort [59] (Table 4.5).

4.6.5 ANALYTICAL METHODS FOR DETERMINATION OF FREE MYCOPHENOLIC ACID

The standard method for determination of mycophenolic acid in serum or plasma is HPLC combined with a suitable detector. Although ultraviolet detector (UV) could be used for determination of mycophenolic acid, LC–MS and LC–MS/MS are superior analytical techniques compared to HPLC-UV. Immunoassays are commercially available for determination of mycophenolic acid in serum or plasma, but such methods suffer from metabolite cross-reactivity, especially mycophenolic acid acyl glucuronide (the minor metabolite). Usually, free mycophenolic acid is determined in protein-free ultrafiltrate, which can be prepared using a suitable filtration device. The Centrifree Micropartition system with a molecular weight cutoff of 30,000 is a filtration device commonly used for preparing protein-free ultrafiltrate for determination of free phenytoin, free valproic acid, and free carbamazepine. Such filtration device is also commonly used by many investigators for determination of free mycophenolic acid concentration. Another approach to measure free mycophenolic acid is to use saliva as the biological matrix.

Many methods using chromatographic techniques have been described in the literature for measurement of total and free mycophenolic acid. Streit et al. described an LC–MS/MS method for analysis of free and total mycophenolic acid in human plasma in which free mycophenolic acid was isolated from plasma using ultrafiltration. The authors used an online extraction cartridge with a column switching technique, chromatography using C-18 column, and electrospray tandem mass spectrometry for quantification of free and total mycophenolic acid. The chromatography analysis time was only 4 min, and the lower limit of quantification of free mycophenolic acid was 0.5 µg/L. The method was linear up to 1000 µg/L [60].

Zeng et al. described an HPLC-UV method for determination of total and free mycophenolic acid in human plasma. The authors measured total mycophenolic acid after protein precipitation using supernatant (20 µL) and free mycophenolic acid in the protein-free ultrafiltrate, where 100 µL ultrafiltrate was directly injected into the C-18 HPLC column. The mobile phase composition was 0.05 mol/L sodium phosphate buffer (pH 2.31)–acetonitrile (50:50 by volume for free mycophenolic acid analysis but 55:45 by volume for total mycophenolic acid analysis). Elution of peaks was monitored at 254 nm. In specimens collected from five pediatric bone marrow transplant recipients receiving intravenous mycophenolic acid mofetil, total mycophenolic acid concentrations in serum varied from 70 to 7800 µg/L, whereas free mycophenolic acid concentrations ranged from 2.1 to 107.5 µg/L [61]. Willis et al. measured free mycophenolic acid in protein-free ultrafiltrate (200-µL sample size) using HPLC combined with atmospheric pressure chemical ionization tandem mass spectrometry. Mycophenolic acid was extracted from the ultrafiltrate using a C-18 solid phase extraction column, and detection was achieved using selected reactant monitoring mode (for mycophenolic acid, m/z 318.9 → 190.9; for internal standard, indomethacin, m/z 356.0 → 297.1). The chromatographic run time was 12 min [62]. Heinig et al. used LC–MS for determination of mycophenolic acid and its glucuronide metabolite in plasma and ultrafiltrate, as well as dried blood spot and dried plasma spot [63]. Wiesen et al. used LC–MS/MS for determination of mycophenolic acid and its glucuronide metabolite in saliva and plasma [64]. Mendonza et al. also used LC–MS/MS for determination of mycophenolic acid concentration in saliva. In 11 kidney transplant recipients, mean salivary mycophenolic acid concentration was 31.4 µg/L (range, 2.6–220.4 µg/L), which correlated well with unbound mycophenolic acid levels in plasma, indicating that saliva can be used for determination of free mycophenolic acid [65].

Rebollo et al. modified the EMIT immunoassay (Siemens Diagnostics, Deerfield, IL) for application on the Viva-E analyzer for determination of free mycophenolic acid. The authors used the Centrifree Micropartition system for preparation of protein-free ultrafiltrate and then determined free mycophenolic acid concentration in the ultrafiltrate. However, the analyzer was programmed so that for determination of mycophenolic acid concentration in the ultrafiltrate, 30 μL of the specimen was used (for determination of total mycophenolic acid using EMIT, only 3 μL of the specimen is needed). Appropriate adjustments of reagent volumes were also made. The limit of quantitation for free mycophenolic acid was 5 ng/mL, which was comparable to the limit of quantitation achieved by LC–MS/MS [66].

4.7 CONCLUSION

Therapeutic drug monitoring of mycophenolic acid using serum or plasma is useful for avoiding rejection as well as toxicity such as neutropenia. In general, pre-dose concentration is measured, but better correlation exists between mycophenolic acid AUC_{0-12h} and clinical efficacy as well as toxicity. Interindividual pharmacokinetics of mycophenolic acid, however, is highly variable, and there are overlapping concentrations between therapeutic range and toxicity. Mycophenolic acid is strongly protein bound (97–99%), mostly to serum albumin. Whereas for solid organ transplant recipients with normal renal and liver function, therapeutic drug monitoring of total mycophenolic acid is sufficient, for transplant recipients with renal insufficiency, hypoalbuminemia, and liver disease, the free fraction of mycophenolic acid may be significantly elevated, so monitoring free mycophenolic acid along with traditionally monitored total mycophenolic acid is strongly recommended.

REFERENCES

[1] Watson I, Potter J, Yatscoff R, Fraser A, et al. Ther Drug Monit [Editorial] 1997;19:125.
[2] Dasgupta A. Usefulness of monitoring free (unbound) concentrations of therapeutic drugs in patient management. Clin Chim Acta 2007;377:1–13.
[3] Levy RH, Moreland TA. Rationale for monitoring free drug levels. Clin Pharmacokinet 1984;9(Suppl. 1):1–9.
[4] Musteata FM, Pawliszyn J, Qian MG, Wu JT, et al. Determination of drug plasma protein binding by solid phase microextraction. J Pharm Sci 2006;95:1712–22.
[5] Lindholm A, Henricsson S. Intra and interindividual varaiability in free fraction of cyclosporine in plasma in recipients of renal transplants. Ther Drug Monit 1989;11:623–30.
[6] Lindholm A. Monitoring of the free concentartion of cyclosporine in plasma in man. Eur J Clin Pharmacol 1991;40:571–5.
[7] Falck P, Asberg A, Guldseth H, Bremer S, et al. Declining intracellular T-lymphocyte concentration of cyclosporine A preceds acute rejection in kidney transplant recipients. Transplantation 2008;85:179–84.

[8] Oellerich M, Muller-Vahl H. The EMIT free level ultrafiltration technique compared with equilibrium dialysis and ultracentifugation to determine protein binding of free phenytoin. Clin Pharmacokinet 1984;9(Suppl. 1):61–70.

[9] Akhlaghi F, Ashley J, Keogh A, Brown K. Cyclosporine plasma unbound fraction in heart and lung transplantion recipients. Ther Drug Monit 1999;21:8–16.

[10] Akhlaghi F, McLachlan A, Keogh AM, Brown KF. Effect of simvastatin on cyclosporine unbound fraction and apparent blood clearance in heart transplant recipients. Br J Clin Pharmacol 1997;44:537–42.

[11] Akhlaghi F, Keogh AM, Brown KF. Unbound cyclosporine and allograft rejection after heart transplanatation. Transplantation 1999;67:54–9.

[12] Mendonza A, Gohh R, Akhlaghi F. Determination of cyclosporine in saliva using liquid chromatography-tandem mass spectrometry. Ther Drug Monit 2004;26:569–75.

[13] Akhlaghi F, Ashley JJ, Keogh AM, Brown KF. Indirect estimation of the unbound fraction of cyclosporine in plasma. Ther Drug Monit 1998;20:301–8.

[14] Wallemacq P, Armstrong VW, Brunet M, Haufroid V, et al. Opportunities to optimize tacrolimus therapy in solid organ transplanttaion: report of the European consensus conference. Ther Drug Monit 2009;31:139–52.

[15] Zahir H, Nand RA, Brown KF, Tattam BN, et al. Validation of methods to study the distribution and protein binding of tacrolimus in human blood. J Pharmacol Toxicol Methods 2001;46:27–35.

[16] Zahir H, McCaughan G, Gleeson M, Nada RA, et al. Changes in tacrolimus distribution in blood and plasma protein binding following liver transplant. Ther Drug Monit 2004;26:506–15.

[17] Trepainer D, Gallant H, Legatt DF, Yatscoff RW. Rapamycin: distribution, pharmacokinetics and therapeutic range investigation: an update. Clin Biochem 1998;31: 345–51.

[18] Yatscoff R, LeGatt D, Keenan R, Chackowsky P. Blood distribution of rapamycin. Transplantation 1993;56:1202–6.

[19] Kirchner GI, Meier-Wiedenbach I, Manns MP. Clinical pharmacokinetics of everolimus. Clin Pharmacokinet 2004;43:83–95.

[20] Pescovitz MD, Conti DE, Dunn J, Gonwa T, et al. Intravenous mycophenolate mofetil: safety, tolerability and pharmacokinetics. Clin Transplant 2000;14:179–88.

[21] Langman LJ, LeGatt DF, Yatscoff RW. Blood distribution of mycophenolic acid. Ther Drug Monit 1994;16:602–7.

[22] Schutz E, Shipkova M, Armstrong VW, Wieland E, et al. Identification of a pharmacologically active metabolite of mycophenolic acid in plasma of transplant recipients treated with mycophenolate mofetil. Clin Chem 1999;45:419–22.

[23] Bullingham RE, Nicholls A, Hale M. Phramacokinetics of mycophenolate mofetil (RS61443): a short review. Transplant Proc 1996;28:925–9.

[24] Shaw LM, Figurski M, Milone MC, Trofe J, et al. Therapeutic drug monitoring of mycophenolic acid. Clin J Am Soc Nephrol 2007;2:1062–72.

[25] Qureshi A, Scheinfeld N. Myfortic (mycophenolate sodium) delayed released tablets. Dermatol Online J 2008;14(8):4.

[26] Hummel M, Yonan N, Ross H, Miller LW, et al. Pharmacokinetics and variability of mycophenolic acid from enteric coated mycophenolate sodium compared with mycophenolate mofetil in de novo heart transplant recipients. Clin Transplant 2007;21:18–23.

[27] Kuypers DR, Le Meur Y, Cantarovich M, Tredger MJ, et al. Consensus report on theraputic drug monitoring of mycophenolic acid in solid organ transplantation. Clin J Am Soc Nephrol 2010;5:341–58.

[28] Musuamba FT, Rousseau A, Bosmans JL, Senessael JJ, et al. Limited sampling models and Bayesian estimation for mycophenolic acid area under the curve prediction in stable renal transplant patients co-medicated with ciclosporin or sirolimus. Clin Pharmacokinet 2009;48:745–58.

[29] Borrows R, Chusney G, Loucaidou M, James A, et al. Mycophenolic acid 12 h trough level monitoring in renal transplantion: association with acute rejection and toxicity. Am J Transplant 2006;6:121–8.

[30] Nowak I, Shaw LM. Mycophenolic acid binding to human serum albumin: characterization and relation to pharamcodynamics. Clin Chem 1995;41:1011–7.

[31] Vial Y, Tod M, Hornecker M, Urien S, et al. In vitro influence of fatty acids and bilirubin on binding of mycophenolic acid to human serum albumin. J Pharm Biomed Anal 2011;54:607–9.

[32] de Winter BC, vam Gelder T, Sombogaard F, Shaw LM, et al. Pharamacokinetic role of protein binding of mycophenolic acid and its glucuronide metabolite in renal transplant recipients. J Pharmacokinet Pharmacodyn 2009;36:541–64.

[33] Nowak I, Shaw LM. Effect of mycophenolic acid glucuronide on inosine monophaosphate dehydrogenase activity. Ther Drug Monit 1997;19:358–60.

[34] Ensom MH, Partovi N, Decarie D, Dumont RJ, et al. Pharmacokinetics and protein binding of mycophenolic acid in stable lung transplant recipients. Ther Drug Monit 2002;24:310–4.

[35] Beckebaum S, Armstrong VW, Cicinnati VR, Streit F, et al. Pharmacokinetics of mycophenolic acid and its glucuronide metabolites in stable adult liver transplant recipients with renal dysfunction on a low dose calcineurin inhibitor regimen and mycophenolate mofetil. Ther Drug Monit 2009;31:205–10.

[36] Jiao Z, Zhong JY, Zhang M, Shi XJ, et al. Total and free mycophenolic acid and its 7-O-glucuronide metabolite in Chinese adult renal transplant patients: pharamcokinetics and applications of limited sampling strategies. Eur J Clin Pharmacol 2007;63:23–37.

[37] Atcheson BA, Taylor PJ, Kirkpatrick CM, Duffull SB, et al. Free mycophenolic acid should be monitored in renal transplant recipients with hypoalbuminemia. Ther Drug Monit 2004;26:284–6.

[38] Kaplan B, Meier-Kriesche HU, Friedman G, Mulgaonkar S, et al. The effect of renal insufficiency on mycophenolic acid protein binding. J Clin Pharmacol 1999;39:715–20.

[39] Weber LT, Shipkova M, Lamersdorf T, Niedmann PD, et al. Pharamcokinetics of mycophenolic acid (MPA) and determination of MPA free fraction in pediatric and adult renal transplant recipients: German study group on mycophenolate mofetil therapy in pediatric renal transplant recipients. J Am Soc Nephrol 1998;9:1511–20.

[40] Mudge DW, Atcheson BA, Taylor PJ, Pillans PI, et al. Severe toxicity associated with a markedly elevated mycophenolic acid free fraction in a renal transplant recipient. Ther Drug Monit 2004;26:453–5.

[41] Bruce K, Scott G, Ratnaj N, Stephen M, et al. Decreased protein binding of mycophenolic acid associated with leukopenia in a pancreas transplant patient with renal failure. Transplantation 1998;65:1127–9.

[42] Weber LT, Lamersdorf T, Shipkova M, Niedmann PD, et al. Area under the plasma concentration time curve for total but not free mycophenolic acid increases in the stable phase after renal transplantation: a longitudinal study in perdiatric patients: German study group on mycophenolate mofetil therapy in pediatric renal transplant recipients. Ther Drug Monit 1999;21:498–506.

[43] Reine PA, Vethe NT, Kongsgaard UE, Andersen AM, et al. Mycophenolate pharmacokinetics and inosine monophosphate dehydrogenase activity in liver transplant recipients with an emphasis on therapeutic drug monitoring. Scand J Clin Lab Invest 2013;73:117–24.

[44] Shen B, Chen B, Zhang W, Mao H. Comparison of pharmacokinetics of mycophenolic acid and its metabolites between living donor liver trasnplant recipients and deceased donor liver transplant recipients. Liver Transpl 2009;15:1473–80.

[45] Kim H, Long-Boyle J, Rydholm N, Orchard PJ, et al. Population pharmacokinetics of unbound mycophenolic acid in pediatric and young adult patients undergoing allogenic hematopoietic cell transplant. J Clin Pharmacol 2012;52:1665–75.

[46] Kiang TK, Ng K, Ensom MH. Multiple regression analysis of factors predicting mycophenolic acid free fraction in 91 adult organ transplant recipients. Ther Drug Monit 2013;35:867–71.

[47] van Hest RM, van Gelder T, Vulto AG, Shaw LM, et al. Pharmacokinetic modelling of the plasma protein binding of mycophenolic acid in renal transplant recipients. Clin Pharmacokinet 2009;48:463–76.

[48] Jacobson P, Long J, Rogosheske J, Brunstein C, et al. High unbound mycophenolic acid concentration in a hematopoietic cell transplantation pateint with sepsis and renal and hepatic failure. Biol Blood Marrow Transplant 2005;11:977–8.

[49] Kaplan B, Gruber SA, Nallamathou R, Katz SM, et al. Decreased protein binding of mycophenolic acid associated with leukopenia in a pancreas transplant recipient with renal failure. Transplantataion 1998;65:1127–9.

[50] Huang J, Jacobson P, Brundage R. Prediction of unbound mycophenolic caid concentartions in patients after hematopoietic cell transplantation. Ther Drug Monit 2007;29:385–90.

[51] Weber LT, Shipkova M, Armstraong VW, Wagner N, et al. The pharmacokinetic pharmacodynamic relatiopnship for total and free mycophenolic acid in pediatric renal transplant recipients: a report of the German study group on mycophenolate mofetil therapy. J Am Soc Nephrol 2002;13:759–68.

[52] Alvarez PA, Egozcue J, Sleiman J, Moretti L, et al. Severe neutropenia in a renal transplant patient suggesting an interaction between mycophenolic acid and fenofibrate. Curr Drug Saf 2012;7:24–9.

[53] Hessenlink DA, van Hest RM, Mathot RA, Bonthuis F, et al. Cyclosporine interacts with mycophenolic acid by inhibiting the multidrug resistance associated protein 2. Am J Transplant 2005;5:987–94.

[54] Kiberd BA, Puthenparumpil JJ, Fraser A, Tell SE, et al. Impact of mycophenolate mofetil loading on drug exposure in the early posttransplant period. Transplant Proc 2005;37:2320–3.

[55] Staatz C, Tett SE. Clinical pharamcokinetics and pharmacodynamics of mycophenolate in solid organ transplant recipients. Clin Pharmacokinet 2007;46:13–58.

[56] Naesens M, Kuypers DR, Streit F, Armstrong WV, et al. Rifampin induces alterations in mycophenolic acid glucuronidation and elimination: implications for drug exposure in renal allograft recipients. Clin Pharmacol Ther 2006;80:509–21.

[57] Kodawara T, Masuda S, Yano Y, Matsubara K, et al. Inhibitory effect of ciprofloxacin on β-glucuronidase mediated deconjugation of mycophenolic acid glucuronide. Biopharm Drug Dispos 2014 Feb 24 [e-pub ahead of print].

[58] Naderer OJ, Dupuis RE, Heinzen EL, Wiwattanawongsa K, et al. The influence of norfloxacin and metronidazole on the disposition of mycophenolate mofetil. J Clin Pharmacol 2005;45:219–26.

[59] Dasgupta A. Herabal supplements and therapeutic drug monitoring: focus on digoxin immunoassays and interaction with St. John's wort. Ther Drug Monit 2008;30:212–7.

[60] Streit F, Shipkova M, Armstrong VW, Oellerich M. Validation of a rapid liquid chromatography-tandem mass spectrometry method for free and total mycophenolic acid. Clin Chem 2004;50:152–9.

[61] Zeng L, Nath CE, Shaw PJ, Earl JW, et al. HPLC-UV assay for monitoring total and unbound mycophenolic acid concentrations in children. Biomed Chromatogr 2009;23:92–100.

[62] Willis C, Taylor PJ, Salm P, Tett SE, et al. Quantification of free mycophenolic acid by high performance liquid chromatography-atmospheric pressure chemical ionization tandem mass spectrometry. J Chromatogr B Biomed Sci Appl 2000;748:151–6.

[63] Heinig K, Bucheli F, Hartenbach R, Gajate-Perez A. Determination of mycophenolic acid and its phenyl glucuronide in human plasma, ultrafiltrate, blood, DBS and dried plasma spot. Bioanalysis 2010;2:1423–35.

[64] Wiesen MH, Farowski F, Feldkotter M, Hoppe B, et al. Liquid chromatography-tandem mass spectrometry method for the quantification of mycophenolic acid and its phenolic glucuronide in saliva and plasma using a standardized saliva collection devise. J Chromatogr A 2012;1241:52–9.

[65] Mendobza AE, Gohh RY, Akhlaghi F. Analysis of mycophenolic acid in saliva using liquid chromatography tandem mass spectrometry. Ther Drug Monit 2006;28:402–6.

[66] Rebollo N, Calvo MV, Martin-Suarez A, Dominguez-Gil A. Modification of the EMIT immunoassay for the measurement of unbound mycophenolic acid in plasma. Clin Biochem 2011;44:260–3.

Pharmacogenomics aspect of immunosuppressant therapy

5

Loralie Langman[1], Teun van Gelder[2], and Ron H.N. van Schaik[3]

[1]*Department of Laboratory Medicine and Pathology, Mayo Clinic College of Medicine, Rochester, MN, USA;* [2]*Departments of Internal Medicine and Hospital Pharmacy, Erasmus University Medical Center, Rotterdam, Netherlands;* [3]*European Specialist Laboratory Medicine, Department of Clinical Chemistry, Erasmus University Medical Center, Rotterdam, Netherlands*

5.1 INTRODUCTION

Pharmacogenetics is the discipline that translates information on genetic variability into prediction of the pharmacokinetics (PK) and pharmacodynamics effects of drugs and was assumed to revolutionize pharmacotherapy. Patients would no longer be treated with standard drugs in a typical dose but, rather, the best drug in the correct dose would be selected for each individual based on a genetic test. In addition, individuals who were likely to experience adverse events would be identified before drug treatment. Unfortunately, this prediction has not materialized [1].

Although variations in the DNA, often single nucleotide polymorphisms (SNPs), have found correlations between pharmacokinetic and pharmacogenetic parameters for a large number of drugs, very few physicians have ordered pharmacogenetic tests for their patients outside clinical trials. Very few transplant programs have adopted the practice of preemptively genotyping transplant recipients and making selection of the optimal drug regimen and starting dose based on one or more of these polymorphisms. One of the main reasons for the reserved attitude toward implementation of genotype-based dosing is the lack of studies that show a clinical benefit over currently used approaches. A significant effect of genotype on dose-corrected drug concentrations does not necessarily imply an improved clinical outcome following implementation of genotyping. However, some novel and promising leads have been reported.

5.2 INDIVIDUAL GENES

Various enzymes are responsible for metabolism of immunosuppressant drugs, and polymorphisms of genes coding such enzymes play an important role in metabolism and disposition of immunosuppressants. However, isoforms of the cytochrome P450 enzymes play a very important role in metabolism of various immunosuppressants

M. Oellerich & A. Dasgupta (Eds): Personalized Immunosuppression in Transplantation.
DOI: http://dx.doi.org/10.1016/B978-0-12-800885-0.00005-9

by the liver, and genes encoding such enzymes have been widely studied to understand interindividual differences in metabolism of immunosuppressants.

5.2.1 CYTOCHROME P450

The cytochrome P450 enzymes (CYPs) are a superfamily of enzymes, all of which contain one molecule of heme that is noncovalently bound to the polypeptide chain. The enzymes require reduced nicotinamide adenine dinucleotide phosphate (NADPH) as a cofactor to carry out the oxidation of substrates. The hydrogen ion (H^+) is supplied through the enzyme NADPH–cytochrome P450 oxidoreductase (POR) [2]. More than 50 individual CYPs have been identified in humans [2], but only a few are known to be important for metabolism of xenobiotics. The liver expresses the greatest abundance of the proteins, thus ensuring efficient first-pass metabolism of drugs. CYPs are also expressed throughout the gastrointestinal tract and in lower amounts in lung, kidney, and even in the central nervous system [2]. The expression of the different CYPs can differ markedly as a result of dietary and environmental exposure to inducers or through interindividual changes resulting from heritable polymorphic differences in gene structure; tissue-specific expression patterns can affect overall drug metabolism and clearance [2].

5.2.1.1 CYP3A5

CYP3A5 is part of a cluster of cytochrome P450 genes on chromosome 7q21.1. CYP3A5 is expressed as a 52.5-kDa protein. The deduced 502-amino acid CYP3A5 protein shares 85% sequence similarity with CYP3A4. Analysis of enzymatic activity established that CYP3A4 and CYP3A5 have overlapping substrate specificity [3].

CYP3A5 is an enzyme that is not expressed in most Caucasians, due to a genetic polymorphism described in 2001 [4,5]. The 6986A > G SNP causes a splicing defect. This *CYP3A5*3* variant has an allele frequency of 90%; thus, most Caucasians are CYP3A5 non-expressers (*CYP3A5*3/*3*) [6]. In contrast, 70% of the African population are CYP3A5 expressers because they are carriers of one or two *CYP3A5*1* alleles [4,5].

The importance of the *CYP3A5*3* allele first became apparent for its effect on tacrolimus metabolism, in which *CYP3A5*3/*3* individuals showed significantly higher dose-corrected trough concentrations [7]. These initial findings have been confirmed by several groups so that the effect of this polymorphism for tacrolimus PK is virtually undisputed [8,9]. Also, the effects of *CYP3A4*1B* are thought to be caused by linkage of the variant to the active *CYP3A5*1* allele rather than caused by increased CYP3A4 activity. In a prospective study, Thervet et al. [10] showed that dosing based on CYP3A5 genotype, with 0.15 mg/kg b.i.d. for expressers and 0.075 mg/kg b.i.d. for non-expressers, resulted in a significantly higher proportion of patients ending up in the tacrolimus therapeutic window compared with a non-genotyping approach. However, a difference in clinical endpoint—reduced acute rejections—has thus far never been shown. Possibly, this is due to the cotreatment with mycophenolate mofetil and steroids, or it may be the result of extensive therapeutic drug monitoring, which causes tacrolimus concentrations to correct very soon during therapy, thereby correcting for any genotyping effect.

In patients who are homozygous for the *CYP3A5*3* allele (CYP3A5 non-express-ers), sirolimus clearance was found to be low, and obviously this would allow for a reduced starting dose [11–13]. In contrast, in a study of 113 kidney transplant recipients, no significant association was found between *CYP3A4*, *CYP3A5*, or *PPARA* geno-types (the *PPARA* gene encodes peroxisome proliferator activated receptor α) and the sirolimus concentration:dose ratio [14]; thus, this association is still uncertain.

CYP3A5 genotyping might be useful to guide tacrolimus and sirolimus dosing, but a preliminary study did not support a clinically relevant role for CYP3A5 geno-typing in predicting everolimus dose requirement [15]. In the same study, this clini-cal finding was supported by an in vitro study with liver microsomes that showed that CYP3A4 is a better catalyst of everolimus metabolism than CYP3A5, whereas the opposite was observed for tacrolimus. Also in both heart and lung transplant recipients, a minor role for CYP3A5 in explaining everolimus variability was found, although not all studies have reported similar findings [16,17]. Moes et al. performed a population pharmacokinetic study in 53 renal transplant patients [18]. They found that genetic polymorphisms in genes coding for *ABCB1*, *CYP3A5*, *CYP2C8*, and *PXR* had no clinically relevant effect on everolimus PK. They also concluded that everolimus pre-dose plus C2 in a limited sampling model better estimated everoli-mus systemic exposure compared to the widely used pre-dose-only concentration monitoring strategy, which is currently routinely applied.

5.2.1.2 CYP3A4

On the protein level, as well as because of its involvement in the metabolism of 35–50% of all drugs, the CYP3A subfamily is of major importance. The human P450 3A sub-family contains three members: P450s 3A4, 3A5, and 3A7 [19]. P450 3A4 probably has the broadest catalytic selectivity and is the most abundant P450 expressed in human liver and small intestine. P450 contributes to the metabolism of approximately half the drugs in use today [20]. The CYP3A4 is a 52-kDa protein that localizes to the endo-plasmic reticulum, primarily located in hepatocytes and the biliary epithelial cells of the liver and the villous columnar epithelial of the jejunum [3].

In humans, the CYP3A4 protein is encoded by the *CYP3A4* gene [21]. This gene is part of a cluster of cytochrome P450 genes on chromosome 7q21.1 [22]. The P450 3A4 gene has been sequenced and is 27 kb long with 13 exons. The promoter motif contains a basal transcription element (−35 to −50). Also present in the 5'-untrans-lated region are putative AP-3, p53, hepatocyte nuclear factor-4 and -5 elements, a glucocorticoid response element, and estrogen receptor element sequences [20].

CYP3A4 was long thought to be the most important enzyme in the metabolism of cyclosporine and tacrolimus. However, not many clinically relevant polymor-phisms were known, either because of low frequency (<1%: *CYP3A4*2, 4, 5, 6, 7, 8, 9, 11, 12, 13, 14, 15, 16, 17, 18, 19, 20, 21*) or because of unclear or no effect on enzyme activity (*CYP3A4*1B, *3, *10*). The first potentially relevant CYP3A4 SNP investigated with respect to immunosuppressants was *CYP3A4-V*, later renamed

*CYP3A4*1B* (−392A > G; www.cypalleles.ki.se), first described by Rebbeck et al. [23]. This polymorphism has an allele frequency of approximately 5–10% in the Caucasian population [23,24] and 35–67% in African Americans [25,26], but the clinical effect is controversial. Originally, it was thought to encode increased enzymatic activity, as established in vitro [27], but subsequent studies raised doubt on this finding [28]. Later, it was found that this polymorphism was in linkage with the active *CYP3A5*1* allele, present in 15–20% of the Caucasian population. It is now assumed that the increase in CYP3A4 activity was not due to the *CYP3A4-V* polymorphism but, rather, was caused by the contribution of CYP3A5 expression, as encoded by the *CYP3A5*1* allele [29].

However, the most important contribution comes from the recently discovered CYP3A4 intron 6 C > T SNP (rs35599367) [30], defining the *CYP3A4*22* variant allele (www.cypalleles.ki.se). This polymorphism affects hepatic expression of CYP3A4 and has an allele frequency of 5% in the Caucasian population [31], and it was shown to be significantly associated with a decreased CYP3A4 activity in vivo, as shown by the metabolism of the CYP3A4 phenotype probes midazolam and erythromycin in cancer patients [32]. The metabolism of tacrolimus was also significantly affected by this variant, and combination of *CYP3A5* and *CYP3A4* genotype status, thus forming CYP3A combined predicted phenotype, could explain more than 60% of tacrolimus pharmacokinetic variability [31,33,34].

For cyclosporine, some studies indeed showed a higher dose requirement for reaching target concentrations for *CYP3A4*1B* carriers, a higher oral cyclosporine clearance, or a lower dose-adjusted area under the concentration time curve (AUC) in healthy volunteers [35,36]. However, in other studies, including 554 kidney transplant patients, no significant association between *CYP3A4*1B* and cyclosporine PK could be shown [37]. In a population pharmacokinetic model, a significant effect of this variant allele on cyclosporine PK was still demonstrated [38], however, making any firm conclusions on the contribution of this variant to cyclosporine PK unclear.

Also, cyclosporine PK proved to be affected by the *CYP3A4*22* variant allele, resulting in a 1.6-fold higher dose-adjusted concentration in 99 Caucasian renal transplant recipients [39], whereas a 15% decreased cyclosporine clearance was demonstrated in 298 adult renal transplant patients carrying a *CYP3A4*22* allele, compared to *CYP3A4*1/*1* individuals [40]. Also, a decreased renal function was shown in cyclosporine-treated renal transplant patients when they were carrying a *CYP3A4*22* allele, thus putting these patients at increased risk of cyclosporine-induced nephrotoxicity [41].

For sirolimus, the average concentration corrected for dose was found to be significantly lower in *CYP3A4*1B* renal transplant carriers ($n = 69$) [13], consistent with an increased activity, either directly on CYP3A4 or by linkage to CYP3A5, because the *CYP3A5*1* allele required significantly more sirolimus to reach adequate blood trough concentrations. A study on *CYP3A4*22* demonstrated a 20% lower metabolic rate of sirolimus ($p = 0.04$), but no significant association could be demonstrated between this genotype and sirolimus dose or dose-corrected trough concentrations in kidney transplant recipients [14].

5.2.2 *POR*

Cytochrome P450 oxidoreductase (EC 1.6.2.4 NADPH-ferrihemoprotein oxidoreductase, POR) has a major role in metabolism. POR is a diflavin reductase that contains both flavin mononucleotide and flavin adenine dinucleotide (FAD) as cofactors and uses NADPH as an electron donor [42]. All cytochrome P450s depend on POR for their supply of electrons for their catalytic activities to metabolize drugs, xenobiotics, and steroid hormones. POR also supplies electrons to many other proteins and small molecules, including heme oxygenase, squalene monooxygenase, and cytochrome b5 [42–45]. As early as the 1960s, POR was shown to be localized in the endoplasmic reticulum near the cytochrome P450 proteins [46–49].

Human POR is a 78-kDa membrane-bound protein with 680 amino acids and is encoded by a gene located on chromosome 7q11.23 (GenBank: NM_000941) that contains 16 exons—15 coding exons and 1 untranslated exon (NT007933) [42,45]. POR is bound to the membranes of endoplasmic reticulum by an N-terminal hydrophobic anchor that is approximately 55 amino acids long [42]. Because all microsomal P450s depend on POR for the supply of electrons, alterations of POR may affect P450 enzyme activities [42]. Therefore, because oxidative metabolism of calcineurin inhibitors (CNIs) is essentially mediated by the cytochrome P450 subfamily 3A (CYP3A) isoenzymes, alterations in POR could have significant consequences to levels of CNIs.

POR is highly polymorphic, and more than 40 variant alleles have been described, with 1508C > T (rs1057868; *POR*28*) being the most common SNP [50,51]. *POR*28* encodes the amino acid variant p.A503V, which lies in the FAD binding domain [51]. *POR*28* has been found to be present in approximately 25% of all alleles, with minor differences among different population groups [51,52].

This variant has been associated with differential enzyme activity of CYP1A2, CYP2C19, CYP2D6, and CYP3A [45,50,51,53–56], with the nature and the magnitude of the effect depending on the CYP isoform investigated [50]. Several studies have shown that CYP3A4 and -3A5 activity is affected by *POR*28* [56,57]. However, others have suggested that the impact of the *POR*28* variant is substrate specific [53], making it difficult to predict what effect this SNP may have on the metabolism of drugs for which the activity has not previously been characterized. The effect of p.A503V on metabolism of immunosuppressive drugs used in organ transplantation has been extensively studied.

For cyclosporine, it has been shown that there was a decrease in the dose-adjusted drug concentrations for *POR*28/*28* homozygous individuals compared with patients carrying a *POR*1* allele. This was in patients not carrying the *CYP3A4*22* (decrease-of-function allele). CYP3A5 non-expressers were also excluded from the analysis because if cyclosporine is preferentially metabolized by CYP3A4, the effect of CYP3A5 in cyclosporine oxidation is contradictory. For this reason, one cannot rule out potential confounding effects of CYP3A5 expression on cyclosporine PK [45].

A study measuring the impact of the p.A503V allele of POR on metabolism of tacrolimus was carried out in healthy Chinese men [58]. It found no significant differences in tacrolimus PK between the *POR*28* CC and the *POR*28* T allele in all subjects. Further analysis showed no significant differences in tacrolimus PK between the *POR*28* CC homozygotes and *POR*28* T heterozygotes in CYP3A5 non-expressers (*CYP3A5*3/*3*). However, the mean tacrolimus exposure for the *POR*28* CC homozygotes in CYP3A5 expressers (*CYP3A5*1/*1* or *1/*3*) was much higher than that for the *POR*28* CT heterozygotes. Of 298 renal allograft recipients who were subcategorized according to CYP3A5 expression, which is known to have a significant impact on tacrolimus metabolism, among the CYP3A4 expressers, lower levels of tacrolimus were detected in carriers of the p.A503V allele of POR and these expressers required higher dosages throughout the treatment. In CYP3A5 non-expressers (*CYP3A5*3/*3*), the p.A503V allele of POR had no impact [57]. These studies suggest a role for p.A503V allele of POR in the variability of tacrolimus exposure levels. Further in vitro studies of CYP3A5 activities comparing normal and p.A503V POR are required to test this hypothesis [42].

Several studies have shown that CYP3A5 activity is affected by *POR*28* in tacrolimus-treated kidney transplant recipients. A gain of CYP3A5 activity has been linked to the *POR*28* genotype in kidney transplant recipients expressing CYP3A5 and carrying at least one POR*28 variant allele, and they showed significantly lower tacrolimus exposure early post-transplantation [45]. These patients required significantly higher daily tacrolimus doses to maintain similar trough concentrations during the first year after transplantation compared with *POR*1/*1* patients expressing CYP3A5 [45]. This is consistent with previous observations that *POR*28* is associated with increased early tacrolimus dose requirements in patients carrying a *CYP3A5*1* allele [57]. In the latter study, CYP3A5 expressers also carrying the *POR*28* allele had significantly lower tacrolimus AUC and C_{max} compared with those expressing *POR*1/*1*, supporting the hypothesis that the *POR*28* allele might be associated with an increased CYP3A5 metabolic activity and, as a consequence, a higher tacrolimus dose requirement. Because this effect was only observed in patients expressing CYP3A5, it suggests that *POR*28* may have a more significant effect on CYP3A5 activity with respect to tacrolimus metabolism.

5.2.3 *ABCB1*

ABCB1 (adenosine triphosphate-binding cassette subfamily B member 1), also known as P-glycoprotein (P-gp) or multidrug-resistance protein 1 (MDR1) or cluster of differentiation 243 (CD243), acts as a transmembrane efflux pump involved in energy-dependent export of xenobiotics from inside the cell [59,60]. ABCB1 is extensively distributed and expressed in the intestinal epithelium, where it pumps xenobiotics (e.g., toxins and drugs) back into the intestinal lumen; in liver cells, where it pumps them into bile ducts; in the cells of the proximal tubular of the kidney, where it pumps them into urine-conducting ducts; and in the capillary endothelial cells comprising the blood–brain barrier and blood–testis barrier, where it pumps them back into the capillaries [61]. The specific tissue expression of ABCB1 suggests that it functions as a protective barrier that ultimately affects drug absorption from the gut and distribution among body compartments as well as metabolism and excretion [60,62,63].

P-gp is a 170-kDa transmembrane glycoprotein that includes 10–15 kDa of N-terminal glycosylation. The N-terminal half of the molecule contains six transmembrane domains, followed by a large cytoplasmic domain with an ATP binding site, and then a second section with six transmembrane domains and an ATP binding site that shows more than 65% of amino acid similarity with the first half of the polypeptide [64].

ABCB1 has a broad substrate specificity [65], including immunosuppressant drugs. As the old MDR1 name implies, ABCB1 removes drugs from the intracellular compartment of lymphocytes, their main therapeutic target. For this reason, the activity of ABCB1 may affect intracellular concentrations and may influence the immunosuppressive effect. In addition, P-gp has a higher expression on CD8$^+$ T cells than on CD4$^+$ T cells and therefore could potentially influence the intralymphocytic drug concentrations more so for CD8$^+$ T cells than for CD4$^+$ T cells [60].

ABCB1 lies on chromosome 7q21.12 and contains 29 exons in a genomic region spanning 209.6 kb [66]. The two most 5′ exons are untranslated. The *ABCB1* promoter region contains a few low-frequency polymorphisms, but they do have varying effects on the promoter [67]. Several SNPs have been identified in *ABCB1* that may affect protein expression and function. To date, the most studied polymorphism that affects P-gp expression in human tissues is the C to T transition at position 3435 (*3435T > C*, Ile1145Ile) within exon 26 (rs1045642). This SNP does not produce altered amino acid sequences (synonymous mutation) and consequently is not expected to change the function of the protein [68]. However, messenger RNA (mRNA) expression of the *3435C* allele has been shown to be higher than that of the *3435T* allele. The *3435C > T* substitution has been associated with reduced mRNA expression [69] and effects on mRNA secondary structure, altering its stability [68] and affecting the timing of cotranslational folding and insertion of P-gp into the membrane, thereby altering substrate specificity [70].

Predictably, the *ABCB1 3435CC* genotype is associated with a higher ABCB1 function compared with the *3435CT* and *3435TT* genotypes [70–72], suggesting that the *3435TT* genotype is less efficient in removing CNIs from cells. Thus, ideally they need lesser amounts of a given drug to reach the same concentrations [73]. This is supported by the fact that in cyclosporine-treated patients, *3435TT* carriers had 1.7-fold increased intracellular drug concentrations [71]. Interestingly, cyclosporine is a known potent competitive inhibitor of ABCB1 and consequently negatively affects its own transport. As a result of the inhibition of the ABCB1 by cyclosporine, the effect of genotypic variability may be dampened.

In addition, in studies using tacrolimus, it has been shown that in patients with the *3435CC* genotype, patients' tacrolimus is more effectively pumped out of the cells, which may lead to lower tacrolimus concentrations at the site of action. Pharmacodynamic studies have supported this by showing that *3435CC* genotype patients needed higher tacrolimus concentrations to achieve the same interleukin-2 (IL-2) inhibition compared with the *TT* genotype [60,69]. Because ABCB1 may affect intrarenal (either native kidney or transplanted kidney) tacrolimus concentrations, due to its expression in renal tubular cells, some investigators have attempted to correlate expression of ABCB1 to development of chronic histologic kidney damage. Naesens et al. found that this type of damage was correlated with low ABCB1 expression [74]. Moore et al. showed that patients with the non-CC genotype of *ABCB1* had an increased risk for long-term graft failure (hazard ratio, 1.69; 95% confidence interval, 1.20–2.40; $P = 0.003$) [75]. A French group found that the presence of ABCB1 polymorphisms in donors influenced long-term graft outcome adversely, with a decrease in renal function and graft loss in transplant recipients receiving cyclosporine [76].

In contrast to cyclosporine, there is no inhibition of ABCB1 activity as a result of the presence of sirolimus [77]. The implication is that it is more likely that polymorphisms in the *ABCB1* gene will affect sirolimus PK. In one study, mean sirolimus concentration/dose ratio was 48% higher in patients with the *ABCB1 3435CT/TT* genotype than those with the *3435CC* genotype, and it was 24% higher in *IL-10-1082GG* homozygotes compared with *-1082AG/AA* [78]. Also, hyperlipidemia was found to be related to *ABCB1* genotype in a study from the same group that reported higher triglyceride and low-density lipoprotein cholesterol levels in *ABCB1 3435T* carriers than in 3435CC homozygotes [79]. In a pharmacodynamic study, Woillard et al. found that an mTOR gene variant haplotype was significantly associated with a decrease in hemoglobin levels in sirolimus-treated patients [80].

As previously mentioned, *ABCB1 3435C > T* is a silent polymorphism, which means that it does not cause an amino acid change, but it has been suggested that it results in mRNA instability or altered transfer RNA functioning [68,81]. It is in strong linkage disequilibrium with two other coding SNPs (*1236C > T* and *2677G > T*), forming two abundant haplotypes (*ABCB1*1* and *ABCB1*13*) [68]. An effect of these haplotypes has been described for tacrolimus [82] and for cyclosporine [83] in a small number ($N = 9$) of Asian heart transplant recipients. However, in a larger study ($N = 98$) in renal transplant recipients [84], the latter finding could not be confirmed, suggesting that genetic variability in MDR1 is unlikely to contribute much to interindividual differences in cyclosporine PK. Haplotype analysis may therefore be a superior method to analyze the effects of genetic variability in this gene on drug PK.

5.2.4 UGT1A9

Enzymes of the UDP glycosyltransferase (UGT; EC 2.4.1.17) superfamily covalently link glycosyl groups to lipophilic substrates, making them more water soluble and therefore more readily excreted [3]. Several UGT1A enzymes are encoded by the *UGT1A* gene complex on chromosome 2q37. Within this complex, nine viable first exons are independently spliced to four common exons to generate nine *UGT1A* transcripts with unique 5′ ends and identical 3′ ends. UGT1A9, like each first exon within the *UGT1A* gene complex, is considered a unique gene linked to the four common exons [85,86]. The protein is a 56-kDa protein and highly expressed in kidney, jejunum, ileum, colon, and rectum, with lower expression in liver [3].

The UGT1A9 plays an important role in the metabolism of mycophenolic acid, in which it inactivates mycophenolic acid by glucuronidation to mycophenolic acid glucuronide, with a minor contribution of UGT1A8 [87]. The inactive UGT allelic variant *UGT1A9*3* (98T > C), with a minor allele frequency of 3% [88], was associated with a significant 50% increase in mycophenolic acid concentration in both tacrolimus and cyclosporine cotreated patients, indicating that indeed UGT1A9 plays an essential role in mycophenolic acid metabolism. However, the clinically important point is mycophenolic acid underexposure, giving rise to an increased risk of transplant rejection. For this, the effects of the *-275T > A* and *-2152C > T* polymorphisms are of importance because these linked SNPs encode a 1.4–1.6 increased UGT1A9 hepatic expression and activity [89]. Carriers of this promoter polymorphism, comprising 10–12% of the population, indeed showed a 20% lower mycophenolic acid exposure ($p = 0.012$) compared to noncarriers in 163 tacrolimus cotreated patients in the Fixed Dose versus Concentration Controlled mycophenolate mofetil study [88]. Surprisingly, this effect was not seen in the 175 mycophenolate mofetil/cyclosporine cotreated individuals; the reason for this difference is not clear. This observation was confirmed by other studies [90] that showed a 27% lower AUC. Most important, however, was the significantly increased odds ratio of 13.3 ($p < 0.05$) for acute rejection for this promoter polymorphism in fixed-dose mycophenolate mofetil-treated patients receiving tacrolimus [88], making this particular polymorphism thus far the only molecular marker in drug-metabolizing enzymes that is predictive of the clinical outcome of acute rejection. Its implementation in current clinical practice, however, has thus far not been realized. The UGT1A9 gene polymorphism may be especially clinically relevant in a setting in which no therapeutic drug monitoring is performed for mycophenolic acid.

5.2.5 OTHER GENETIC FACTORS

The mechanism of action of mycophenolic acid is the inhibition of the target enzyme inosine-5′-monophosphate dehydrogenase (IMPDH). Two isoforms of IMPDH exist, derived from different genes [32]. In activated lymphocytes, IMPDH type II predominates over type I. It has been described that the IMPDH type II *3757T > C* polymorphism is associated with increased IMPDH activity in mycophenolate mofetil-treated renal transplant recipients. However, this explains only 8% of the interpatient variability in IMPDH activity, and it is therefore unlikely to have an important impact on clinical outcome [91,92].

The CNIs are well-known for their nephrotoxic effects. In daily practice, this may become manifest as an acute oligoanuria, but more often there is a more subtle rise in serum creatinine without other clear cause. Constriction of the afferent vessel to the glomerulus and direct renal tubular toxicity are considered to be the main mechanisms responsible for the nephrotoxic effects. The acute nephrotoxic effects, observed mostly in the immediate post-transplant period, are due to a reduction in blood flow. High local tacrolimus concentrations are assumed to be related to this adverse effect of tacrolimus, which is rapidly reversible upon dose reduction. In the DeKAF (Long-Term Deterioration of Kidney Allograft Function) study, several SNPs in the *XPC, CYP2C9, PAX4, MTRR*, and *GAN* genes were investigated for their association with nephrotoxicity [93]. Remarkably, for acute cyclosporine nephrotoxicity, several associations with genetic variants could be demonstrated, whereas for acute tacrolimus-induced nephrotoxicity this was not the case. One could envision that in order to prevent chronic nephrotoxicity due to cyclosporine, genotyping would be performed, but this has not yet reached daily practice.

5.3 CONCLUSIONS

In patients receiving a transplant, drug concentration measurements are performed routinely at every outpatient visit and during hospital admission. Target concentrations have been defined depending on the type of organ transplanted, the perceived risk of rejection, time post-transplantation, co-medication, and adverse events. However, the evidence that therapeutic drug monitoring does improve outcome is weak at best, and yet the monitoring of drug concentrations is widely accepted. Pharmacogenetic tests to further individualize drug therapy are rarely used, despite reported associations between drug dose requirement and genotype. Evidence that implementation of a pharmacogenetic test will improve clinical outcome is thus far lacking. The only applicable outcome is a doubling of the starting tacrolimus dose in patients who express CYP3A5, and even for this intervention little evidence exists to demonstrate improved clinical outcome. Moreover, with efficient therapeutic drug monitoring, it is possible to rapidly correct for the effect of genotypic deviations in PK, thus decreasing the utility of a genotyping approach [91].

The future of pharmacogenetics will be in treatment models in which patient characteristics are combined with polymorphisms in multiple genes. These models should focus on pharmacodynamic parameters, drug transporter proteins, and predictors of toxicity. Such models will provide more information than the relatively small candidate gene studies performed so far. For implementation of these findings into clinical practice, linkage of genotype data to medication prescription systems within electronic health records will be crucial.

REFERENCES

[1] Elens L, Hesselink DA, van Schaik RH, van Gelder T. Pharmacogenetics in kidney transplantation: recent updates and potential clinical applications. Mol Diagn Ther 2012;16:331–45.

[2] Gonzalez FJ, Coughtrie M, Tukey RH. Chapter 6. Drug metabolism. In: Brunton L, Chabner B, Knollmann B, editors. Goodman & Gilman's the pharmacological basis of therapeutics (12th ed.). New York, NY: McGraw-Hill; 2011.

[3] Hamosh A. Omim®—online Mendelian inheritance in man®. Baltimore, MD: McKusick-Nathans Institute of Genetic Medicine, Johns Hopkins University School of Medicine; 2014.

[4] Hustert E, Haberl M, Burk O, Wolbold R, et al. The genetic determinants of the *CYP3A5* polymorphism. Pharmacogenetics 2001;11:773–9.

[5] Kuehl P, Zhang J, Lin Y, Lamba J, et al. Sequence diversity in *CYP3A* promoters and characterization of the genetic basis of polymorphic CYP3A5 expression. Nat Genet 2001;27:383–91.

[6] van Schaik RH, van der Heiden IP, van den Anker JN, Lindemans J. *CYP3A5* variant allele frequencies in Dutch Caucasians. Clin Chem 2002;48:1668–71.

[7] Hesselink DA, van Schaik RH, van der Heiden IP, van der Werf M, et al. Genetic polymorphisms of the *CYP3A4*, *CYP3A5*, and *MDR-1* genes and pharmacokinetics of the calcineurin inhibitors cyclosporine and tacrolimus. Clin Pharmacol Ther 2003;74:245–54.

[8] Hesselink DA, Bouamar R, Elens L, van Schaik RH, et al. The role of pharmacogenetics in the disposition of and response to tacrolimus in solid organ transplantation. Clin Pharmacokinet 2014;53:123–39.

[9] Buendia JA, Bramuglia G, Staatz CE. Effects of combinational *CYP3A5 6986A > G* polymorphism in graft liver and native intestine on the pharmacokinetics of tacrolimus in liver transplant patients: a meta-analysis. Ther Drug Monit 2014;36:442–7.

[10] Thervet E, Loriot MA, Barbier S, Buchler M, et al. Optimization of initial tacrolimus dose using pharmacogenetic testing. Clin Pharmacol Ther 2010;87:721–6.

[11] Le Meur Y, Djebli N, Szelag JC, Hoizey G, et al. *CYP3A5*3* influences sirolimus oral clearance in *de novo* and stable renal transplant recipients. Clin Pharmacol Ther 2006;80:51–60.

[12] Miao LY, Huang CR, Hou JQ, Qian MY. Association study of *ABCB1* and *CYP3A5* gene polymorphisms with sirolimus trough concentration and dose requirements in Chinese renal transplant recipients. Biopharm Drug Dispos 2008;29:1–5.

[13] Anglicheau D, Le Corre D, Lechaton S, Laurent-Puig P, et al. Consequences of genetic polymorphisms for sirolimus requirements after renal transplant in patients on primary sirolimus therapy. Am J Transplant 2005;5:595–603.

[14] Woillard JB, Kamar N, Coste S, Rostaing L, et al. Effect of *CYP3A4*22, POR*28*, and *PPARA rs4253728* on sirolimus *in vitro* metabolism and trough concentrations in kidney transplant recipients. Clin Chem 2013;59:1761–9.

[15] Picard N, Rouguieg-Malki K, Kamar N, Rostaing L, et al. *CYP3A5* genotype does not influence everolimus *in vitro* metabolism and clinical pharmacokinetics in renal transplant recipients. Transplantation 2011;91:652–6.

[16] Kniepeiss D, Renner W, Trummer O, Wagner D, et al. The role of *CYP3A5* genotypes in dose requirements of tacrolimus and everolimus after heart transplantation. Clin Transplant 2011;25:146–50.

[17] Schoeppler KE, Aquilante CL, Kiser TH, Fish DN, et al. The impact of genetic polymorphisms, diltiazem, and demographic variables on everolimus trough concentrations in lung transplant recipients. Clin Transplant 2014;28:590–7.

[18] Moes DJ, Press RR, den Hartigh J, van der Straaten T, et al. Population pharmacokinetics and pharmacogenetics of everolimus in renal transplant patients. Clin Pharmacokinet 2012;51:467–80.

[19] Nelson DR, Koymans L, Kamataki T, Stegeman JJ, et al. P450 superfamily: update on new sequences, gene mapping, accession numbers and nomenclature. Pharmacogenetics 1996;6:1–42.

[20] Guengerich FP. Cytochrome P-450 3A4: regulation and role in drug metabolism. Annu Rev Pharmacol Toxicol 1999;39:1–17.

[21] Hashimoto H, Toide K, Kitamura R, Fujita M, et al. Gene structure of *CYP3A4*, an adult-specific form of cytochrome P450 in human livers, and its transcriptional control. Eur J Biochem 1993;218:585–95.

[22] Inoue K, Inazawa J, Nakagawa H, Shimada T, et al. Assignment of the human cytochrome P-450 nifedipine oxidase gene (*CYP3A4*) to chromosome 7 at band q22.1 by fluorescence *in situ* hybridization. Jpn J Hum Genet 1992;37:133–8.

[23] Rebbeck TR, Jaffe JM, Walker AH, Wein AJ, et al. Modification of clinical presentation of prostate tumors by a novel genetic variant in *CYP3A4*. J Natl Cancer Inst 1998;90:1225–9.

[24] van Schaik RH, de Wildt SN, van Iperen NM, Uitterlinden AG, et al. *CYP3A4*-V polymorphism detection by PCR-restriction fragment length polymorphism analysis and its allelic frequency among 199 Dutch Caucasians. Clin Chem 2000;46:1834–6.

[25] Lamba JK, Lin YS, Thummel K, Daly A, et al. Common allelic variants of cytochrome P4503A4 and their prevalence in different populations. Pharmacogenetics 2002;12:121–32.

[26] Walker AH, Jaffe JM, Gunasegaram S, Cummings SA, et al. Characterization of an allelic variant in the nifedipine-specific element of *CYP3A4*: ethnic distribution and implications for prostate cancer risk. Mutations in brief no. 191. Online. Hum Mutat 1998;12:289.

[27] Amirimani B, Ning B, Deitz AC, Weber BL, et al. Increased transcriptional activity of the *CYP3A4**1B promoter variant. Environ Mol Mutagen 2003;42:299–305.

[28] Spurdle AB, Goodwin B, Hodgson E, Hopper JL, et al. The *CYP3A4**1B polymorphism has no functional significance and is not associated with risk of breast or ovarian cancer. Pharmacogenetics 2002;12:355–66.

[29] Lamba JK, Lin YS, Schuetz EG, Thummel KE. Genetic contribution to variable human CYP3A-mediated metabolism. Adv Drug Deliv Rev 2002;54:1271–94.

[30] Wang D, Guo Y, Wrighton SA, Cooke GE, et al. Intronic polymorphism in *CYP3A4* affects hepatic expression and response to statin drugs. Pharmacogenomics J 2011;11:274–86.

[31] Elens L, Bouamar R, Hesselink DA, Haufroid V, et al. A new functional *CYP3A4* intron 6 polymorphism significantly affects tacrolimus pharmacokinetics in kidney transplant recipients. Clin Chem 2011;57:1574–83.

[32] Elens L, Nieuweboer A, Clarke SJ, Charles KA, et al. *CYP3A4* intron 6 C > T SNP (*CYP3A4**22) encodes lower CYP3A4 activity in cancer patients, as measured with probes midazolam and erythromycin. Pharmacogenomics 2013;14:137–49.

[33] Elens L, Capron A, van Schaik RH, De Meyer M, et al. Impact of *CYP3A4**22 allele on tacrolimus pharmacokinetics in early period after renal transplantation: toward updated genotype-based dosage guidelines. Ther Drug Monit 2013;35:608–16.

[34] Elens L, Hesselink DA, van Schaik RH, van Gelder T. The *CYP3A4**22 allele affects the predictive value of a pharmacogenetic algorithm predicting tacrolimus predose concentrations. Br J Clin Pharmacol 2013;75:1545–7.

[35] Elens L, Bouamar R, Shuker N, Hesselink DA, et al. Clinical implementation of pharmacogenetics in kidney transplantation: calcineurin inhibitors in the starting blocks. Br J Clin Pharmacol 2014;77:715–28.

[36] Wang J. *CYP3A* polymorphisms and immunosuppressive drugs in solid-organ transplantation. Expert Rev Mol Diagn 2009;9:383–90.

[37] Kuypers DR, de Jonge H, Naesens M, Lerut E, et al. *CYP3A5* and *CYP3A4* but not *MDR1* single-nucleotide polymorphisms determine long-term tacrolimus disposition and drug-related nephrotoxicity in renal recipients. Clin Pharmacol Ther 2007;82:711–25.

[38] Hesselink DA, van Gelder T, van Schaik RH, Balk AH, et al. Population pharmacokinetics of cyclosporine in kidney and heart transplant recipients and the influence of

ethnicity and genetic polymorphisms in the *MDR-1*, *CYP3A4*, and *CYP3A5* genes. Clin Pharmacol Ther 2004;76:545–56.

[39] Elens L, van Schaik RH, Panin N, de Meyer M, et al. Effect of a new functional *CYP3A4* polymorphism on calcineurin inhibitors' dose requirements and trough blood levels in stable renal transplant patients. Pharmacogenomics 2011;12:1383–96.

[40] Moes DJ, Swen JJ, den Hartigh J, van der Straaten T, et al. Effect of CYP3A4*22, *CYP3A5*3*, and *CYP3A* combined genotypes on cyclosporine, everolimus, and tacrolimus pharmacokinetics in renal transplantation. CPT Pharmacometrics Syst Pharmacol 2014;3:e100.

[41] Elens L, Bouamar R, Hesselink DA, Haufroid V, et al. The new *CYP3A4* intron 6 C > T polymorphism (*CYP3A4*22*) is associated with an increased risk of delayed graft function and worse renal function in cyclosporine-treated kidney transplant patients. Pharmacogenet Genomics 2012;22:373–80.

[42] Pandey AV, Fluck CE. NADPH P450 oxidoreductase: structure, function, and pathology of diseases. Pharmacol Ther 2013;138:229–54.

[43] Hubbard PA, Shen AL, Paschke R, Kasper CB, et al. NADPH-cytochrome P450 oxidoreductase. Structural basis for hydride and electron transfer. J Biol Chem 2001;276:29163–70.

[44] Masters BS. The journey from NADPH-cytochrome P450 oxidoreductase to nitric oxide synthases. Biochem Biophys Res Commun 2005;338:507–19.

[45] Elens L, Hesselink DA, Bouamar R, Budde K, et al. Impact of *POR*28* on the pharmacokinetics of tacrolimus and cyclosporine a in renal transplant patients. Ther Drug Monit 2014;36:71–9.

[46] Lu AY, Coon MJ. Role of hemoprotein P-450 in fatty acid omega-hydroxylation in a soluble enzyme system from liver microsomes. J Biol Chem 1968;243:1331–2.

[47] Lu AY, Junk KW, Coon MJ. Resolution of the cytochrome P-450-containing omega-hydroxylation system of liver microsomes into three components. J Biol Chem 1969;244:3714–21.

[48] Williams Jr. CH, Kamin H. Microsomal triphosphopyridine nucleotide-cytochrome C reductase of liver. J Biol Chem 1962;237:587–95.

[49] Phillips AH, Langdon RG. Hepatic triphosphopyridine nucleotide-cytochrome C reductase: isolation, characterization, and kinetic studies. J Biol Chem 1962;237:2652–60.

[50] Agrawal V, Huang N, Miller WL. Pharmacogenetics of P450 oxidoreductase: effect of sequence variants on activities of CYP1A2 and CYP2C19. Pharmacogenet Genomics 2008;18:569–76.

[51] Huang N, Agrawal V, Giacomini KM, Miller WL. Genetics of P450 oxidoreductase: sequence variation in 842 individuals of four ethnicities and activities of 15 missense mutations. Proc Natl Acad Sci USA 2008;105:1733–8.

[52] Huang N, Pandey AV, Agrawal V, Reardon W, et al. Diversity and function of mutations in P450 oxidoreductase in patients with Antley-Bixler syndrome and disordered steroidogenesis. Am J Hum Genet 2005;76:729–49.

[53] Agrawal V, Choi JH, Giacomini KM, Miller WL. Substrate-specific modulation of CYP3A4 activity by genetic variants of cytochrome P450 oxidoreductase. Pharmacogenet Genomics 2010;20:611–8.

[54] Gomes AM, Winter S, Klein K, Turpeinen M, et al. Pharmacogenomics of human liver cytochrome P450 oxidoreductase: multifactorial analysis and impact on microsomal drug oxidation. Pharmacogenomics 2009;10:579–99.

[55] Gomes LG, Huang N, Agrawal V, Mendonca BB, et al. The common P450 oxidoreductase variant A503V is not a modifier gene for 21-hydroxylase deficiency. J Clin Endocrinol Metab 2008;93:2913–6.

[56] Oneda B, Crettol S, Jaquenoud Sirot E, Bochud M, et al. The P450 oxidoreductase genotype is associated with CYP3A activity *in vivo* as measured by the midazolam phenotyping test. Pharmacogenet Genomics 2009;19:877–83.

[57] de Jonge H, Metalidis C, Naesens M, Lambrechts D, et al. The P450 oxidoreductase *28 SNP is associated with low initial tacrolimus exposure and increased dose requirements in CYP3A5-expressing renal recipients. Pharmacogenomics 2011;12:1281–91.

[58] Zhang JJ, Zhang H, Ding XL, Ma S, et al. Effect of the P450 oxidoreductase 28 polymorphism on the pharmacokinetics of tacrolimus in Chinese healthy male volunteers. Eur J Clin Pharmacol 2013;69:807–12.

[59] Ueda K, Clark DP, Chen CJ, Roninson IB, et al. The human multidrug resistance (*MDR1*) gene. cDNA cloning and transcription initiation. J Biol Chem 1987;262:505–8.

[60] Vafadari R, Bouamar R, Hesselink DA, Kraaijeveld R, et al. Genetic polymorphisms in ABCB1 influence the pharmacodynamics of tacrolimus. Ther Drug Monit 2013;35:459–65.

[61] Thiebaut F, Tsuruo T, Hamada H, Gottesman MM, et al. Cellular localization of the multidrug-resistance gene product P-glycoprotein in normal human tissues. Proc Natl Acad Sci 1987;84:7735–8.

[62] Ayrton A, Morgan P. Role of transport proteins in drug absorption, distribution and excretion. Xenobiotica 2001;31:469–97.

[63] Rong G, Jing L, Deng-Qing L, Hong-Shan Z, et al. Influence of *CYP3A5* and *MDR1* (*ABCB1*) polymorphisms on the pharmacokinetics of tacrolimus in Chinese renal transplant recipients. Transplant Proc 2010;42:3455–8.

[64] Viguié F. ABCB1 ATP-binding cassette, sub-family B (MDR/TAP), member 1. Atlas Genet Cytogenet Oncol Haematol 1998;2:45–6.

[65] Dean M. The human ATP-binding cassette (ABC) transporter superfamily. Bethesda, MD: National Center for Biotechnology Information (US); 2002.

[66] Bodor M, Kelly EJ, Ho RJ. Characterization of the human *MDR1* gene. AAPS J 2005;7:E1–E5.

[67] Wang B, Ngoi S, Wang J, Chong SS, et al. The promoter region of the *MDR1* gene is largely invariant, but different single nucleotide polymorphism haplotypes affect MDR1 promoter activity differently in different cell lines. Mol Pharmacol 2006;70:267–76.

[68] Wang D, Johnson AD, Papp AC, Kroetz DL, et al. Multidrug resistance polypeptide 1 (*MDR1, ABCB1*) variant *3435C > T* affects mRNA stability. Pharmacogenet Genomics 2005;15:693–704.

[69] Hoffmeyer S, Burk O, von Richter O, Arnold HP, et al. Functional polymorphisms of the human multidrug-resistance gene: multiple sequence variations and correlation of one allele with P-glycoprotein expression and activity *in vivo*. Proc Natl Acad Sci USA 2000;97:3473–8.

[70] Kimchi-Sarfaty C, Oh JM, Kim IW, Sauna ZE, et al. A "silent" polymorphism in the MDR1 gene changes substrate specificity. Science 2007;315:525–8.

[71] Crettol S, Venetz JP, Fontana M, Aubert JD, et al. Influence of *ABCB1* genetic polymorphisms on cyclosporine intracellular concentration in transplant recipients. Pharmacogenet Genomics 2008;18:307–15.

[72] Hitzl M, Drescher S, van der Kuip H, Schaffeler E, et al. The *C3435T* mutation in the human *MDR1* gene is associated with altered efflux of the P-glycoprotein substrate rhodamine 123 from CD56+ natural killer cells. Pharmacogenetics 2001;11:293–8.

[73] Mendes J, Martinho A, Simoes O, Mota A, et al. Genetic polymorphisms in *CYP3A5* and *MDR1* genes and their correlations with plasma levels of tacrolimus and cyclosporine in renal transplant recipients. Transpl Proc 2009;41:840–2.

[74] Naesens M, Lerut E, de Jonge H, Van Damme B, et al. Donor age and renal P-glycoprotein expression associate with chronic histological damage in renal allografts. J Am Soc Nephrol 2009;20:2468–80.

[75] Moore J, McKnight AJ, Dohler B, Simmonds MJ, et al. Donor *ABCB1* variant associates with increased risk for kidney allograft failure. J Am Soc Nephrol 2012;23:1891–9.

[76] Woillard JB, Rerolle JP, Picard N, Rousseau A, et al. Donor P-gp polymorphisms strongly influence renal function and graft loss in a cohort of renal transplant recipients on cyclosporine therapy in a long-term follow-up. Clin Pharmacol Ther 2010;88:95–100.

[77] Llaudo I, Colom H, Gimenez-Bonafe P, Torras J, et al. Do drug transporter (*ABCB1*) SNPs and P-glycoprotein function influence cyclosporine and macrolides exposure in renal transplant patients? Results of the pharmacogenomic substudy within the symphony study. Transpl Int 2013;26:177–86.

[78] Sam WJ, Chamberlain CE, Lee SJ, Goldstein JA, et al. Associations of *ABCB1 3435C > T* and *IL-10-1082g > A* polymorphisms with long-term sirolimus dose requirements in renal transplant patients. Transplantation 2011;92:1342–7.

[79] Sam WJ, Chamberlain CE, Lee SJ, Goldstein JA, et al. Associations of *ABCB1* and *IL-10* genetic polymorphisms with sirolimus-induced dyslipidemia in renal transplant recipients. Transplantation 2012;94:971–7.

[80] Woillard JB, Kamar N, Rousseau A, Rostaing L, et al. Association of sirolimus adverse effects with m-TOR, p70s6k or Raptor polymorphisms in kidney transplant recipients. Pharmacogenet Genomics 2012;22:725–32.

[81] Fung KL, Gottesman MM. A synonymous polymorphism in a common *MDR1* (*ABCB1*) haplotype shapes protein function. Biochim Biophys Acta 2009;1794:860–71.

[82] Anglicheau D, Verstuyft C, Laurent-Puig P, Becquemont L, et al. Association of the multidrug resistance-1 gene single-nucleotide polymorphisms with the tacrolimus dose requirements in renal transplant recipients. J Am Soc Nephrol 2003;14:1889–96.

[83] Chowbay B, Cumaraswamy S, Cheung YB, Zhou Q, et al. Genetic polymorphisms in MDR1 and CYP3A4 genes in Asians and the influence of *MDR1* haplotypes on cyclosporin disposition in heart transplant recipients. Pharmacogenetics 2003;13:89–95.

[84] Mai I, Stormer E, Goldammer M, Johne A, et al. *MDR1* haplotypes do not affect the steady-state pharmacokinetics of cyclosporine in renal transplant patients. J Clin Pharmacol 2003;43:1101–7.

[85] Gong QH, Cho JW, Huang T, Potter C, et al. Thirteen UDPglucuronosyltransferase genes are encoded at the human *UGT1* gene complex locus. Pharmacogenetics 2001;11:357–68.

[86] Mackenzie PI, Bock KW, Burchell B, Guillemette C, et al. Nomenclature update for the mammalian UDP glycosyltransferase (*UGT*) gene superfamily. Pharmacogenet Genomics 2005;15:677–85.

[87] Bernard O, Guillemette C. The main role of *UGT1A9* in the hepatic metabolism of mycophenolic acid and the effects of naturally occurring variants. Drug Metab Dispos 2004;32:775–8.

[88] van Schaik RH, van Agteren M, de Fijter JW, Hartmann A, et al. *UGT1A9-275T > A/-2152C > T* polymorphisms correlate with low MPA exposure and acute rejection in MMF/tacrolimus-treated kidney transplant patients. Clin Pharmacol Ther 2009;86:319–27.

[89] Girard H, Court MH, Bernard O, Fortier LC, et al. Identification of common polymorphisms in the promoter of the *UGT1A9* gene: evidence that UGT1A9 protein and activity levels are strongly genetically controlled in the liver. Pharmacogenetics 2004;14:501–15.

[90] Sanchez-Fructuoso AI, Maestro ML, Calvo N, Viudarreta M, et al. The prevalence of uridine diphosphate-glucuronosyltransferase 1A9 (*UGT1A9*) gene promoter region single-nucleotide polymorphisms *T-275A* and *C-2152T* and its influence on mycophenolic acid pharmacokinetics in stable renal transplant patients. Transplant Proc 2009;41:2313–6.

[91] van Gelder T, van Schaik RH, Hesselink DA. Pharmacogenetics and immunosuppressive drugs in solid organ transplantation. Nat Rev Nephrol 2014;10:725–31.

[92] Shah S, Harwood SM, Dohler B, Opelz G, et al. Inosine monophosphate dehydrogenase polymorphisms and renal allograft outcome. Transplantation 2012;94:486–91.

[93] Jacobson PA, Schladt D, Israni A, Oetting WS, et al. Genetic and clinical determinants of early, acute calcineurin inhibitor-related nephrotoxicity: results from a kidney transplant consortium. Transplantation 2012;93:624–31.

Biomarker monitoring in immunosuppressant therapy: an overview

Maria Shipkova

Head Laboratory for Therapeutic Drug Monitoring and Clinical Toxicology, Central Institute for Clinical Chemistry and Laboratory Medicine, Klinikum Stuttgart, Germany

6.1 INTRODUCTION

Although remarkable achievements in organ transplantation have occurred during the past two decades, some key challenges remain open and new ways must be found to master them. These include the prolongation of the survival of the transplanted organs as well as the reduction of comorbidities and mortality that are related to the side effects of anti-rejection therapy, such as nephrotoxicity, cardiovascular disease, diabetes, infections, and malignancy. A key issue for these two obstacles is a suboptimal guidance of immunosuppressive therapy for an individual donor and recipient combination. Both the risk of rejection and allograft loss, on the one hand, and the development of therapy-related complications, on the other hand, depend on a broad variety of patient-specific factors, such as genetically determined susceptibility, sensitization by preexisting alloantibodies, previous transplantations, preexisting morbidity, time on dialysis, age, and polymorphisms of genes involved in pharmacokinetics and pharmacodynamics. The risk for acute rejection and graft loss is highest early after the transplantation; therefore, the most powerful immunosuppression is applied in this period. To counteract the occurrence of side effects, it is essential to taper immunosuppression to an appropriate maintenance level thereafter. The optimal rate of decrease as well as the optimal level to target are not well established, and it can be assumed that they will be quite different in patients with different risk factor profiles [1].

Dose minimization is often performed empirically by clinicians. Therapeutic drug monitoring (TDM), biochemical markers for organ injury, clinical events, and biopsies are the most frequently used tools to guide immunosuppressive therapy. TDM is a well-established approach that has been used in recent years for some immunosuppressive drugs, such as calcineurin inhibitors (CNIs), mTOR inhibitors, and, in limited use, mycophenolate. It is certainly an important instrument for determining pharmacokinetic inter- and intrapatient variability to improve patient compliance to therapy and particularly to avoid several side effects related to overdosing [2].

M. Oellerich & A. Dasgupta (Eds): Personalized Immunosuppression in Transplantation.
DOI: http://dx.doi.org/10.1016/B978-0-12-800885-0.00006-0

125

However, clinical experience clearly shows that despite the fact that drug concentrations are adjusted according to guidelines for therapeutic range, outcomes differ among patients. Both over- and under-immunosuppression occur, and multiple factors, such as individual sensitivity to immunosuppression or additive, synergistic, or antagonistic pharmacological effects of coadministered drugs, may be important in these cases. Moreover, TDM does not support guidance of therapy minimization/weaning, does not help to identify tolerant transplant recipients [3,4], and is not applied to important components of current immunosuppressive regimens such as corticosteroids or biologicals.

Classical biochemical markers, such creatinine, proteinuria, enzyme activities, bilirubin, and troponins, are very popular because most of them are highly sensitive and easily accessible. However, they possess low specificity for rejection, do not reflect early responsiveness of the immune system, and represent only a crude approach to monitoring therapy with drug side effects and clinical complications remaining common [5]. Most frequently, if abnormality is noted, histological evaluation by biopsy is considered. Biopsies are the gold standard for determining sensitivity and specificity in order to diagnose the status of the transplanted organ and indirectly provide information on the immune reaction against it. However, biopsies are invasive, and there is a delay between histological changes and the first occurrence of clinical or biochemical signs of rejection. Results are imprecise and depend on the experience of the evaluating pathologist. Implementation of protocol biopsies in some centers has demonstrated the occurrence of subclinical rejections. These rejections may have a potentially negative impact on organ survival. Although it may be suggested that therapy optimization would benefit from protocol biopsies, they are risky and the need for serial use over a long time period is a major limitation for their more global clinical adoption [6,7].

Considering all these important issues, it is a common consensus that there is an urgent need for more sophisticated and less invasive biomarkers to complement current clinical practices that allow further optimization and individualization of the immunosuppressive therapy. Such new biomarkers in combination with the respective analytical methods have to satisfy high analytical and diagnostic requirements. They should be noninvasive, easily available, not very laborious, and analytically accurate. They should also be suitable for standardization and ensure reproducibility of results across laboratories. Furthermore, such biomarkers should be cost-effective. Further requirements are an adequate diagnostic specificity and sensitivity as well as a rapid turnaround time to allow the timely adjustment of immunosuppressive therapy to prevent both under- and over-immunosuppression. They should also indicate drug toxicity and signs of specific unresponsiveness to donor alloantigens. To become clinically useful, they should be prospectively validated in an independent multicenter patient cohort, should be approved by the regulatory authorities, and must be commercialized. Finally, external quality assurance tools should be established [4,8]. This chapter provides an overview of different biomarkers that are currently under investigation and considers their reliability and appropriateness to meet the requirements needed for use in transplantation medicine.

6.2 CURRENT IMMUNOSUPPRESSIVE AGENTS AND THEIR EFFECTS ON IMMUNE RESPONSIVENESS

Effective immunosuppression in transplantation relies on preventing a response of the transplant recipient's immune system that would cause rejection of the allograft and at the same time preserving immunologic control of infections and malignancy. Current immunosuppressive regimens mostly include combinations of steroids, CNIs, antiproliferative agents (mycophenolate or mTOR inhibitors), and antibody-based therapies. These drugs primarily target different pathways of T-cell activation (signals 1–3), thereby inhibiting T-cell activation or proliferation, or lead to T-cell depletion. Multiple immune mediators, such as cytokines, chemokines, and cytotoxic molecules, are affected. Combining drugs with different sites of action allows for dosage adjustments to minimize toxicities and side effects [9]. Recent progress in molecular and cellular immunology has further elucidated the interactions between antigen-presenting cells (APCs) and T and B cells. Also, the triggers of B-cell activation and antibody synthesis have been widely unraveled, opening new perspectives for development of B-cell-specific immunosuppression [10,11]. In addition, novel regulatory cells (regulatory T and B cells as well as suppressive APCs) have been identified and have become the focus of intensive research, similar to the complex interplay between innate and adaptive immunity in allograft recognition. Better understanding of rejection processes together with the prospect of avoiding side effects related to classical immunosuppressants such as CNIs and steroids fostered the development and adoption of biologics for organ transplantations, offering promising new therapeutic alternatives. Table 6.1 summarizes the most well-established immunosuppressant agents and their mechanisms of action. Potential promising biomarkers to complement current clinical practices for the guidance of immunosuppressive therapy can be derived from these mechanisms of action.

6.3 BIOMARKERS TO GUIDE IMMUNOSUPPRESSANT THERAPY

According to the definition given by the Biomarkers Definitions Working Group, a biological biomarker is "a characteristic that is objectively measured and evaluated as an indicator of normal biological processes, pathogenic processes, or pharmacological responses to therapeutic intervention" [12]. In general, biomarkers applied as a tool for management of immunosuppression in transplantation can be divided into two groups: biomarkers associated directly with the pharmacological effect of an immunosuppressive agent (drug specific) and biomarkers that are non-drug specific and reflect the net effect of immunosuppression by combined therapies and individual responsiveness of the patient's immune system (Figure 6.1).

Drug-specific biomarkers include those related to drug pharmacodynamics and pharmacogenetics. They complement pharmacokinetic parameters such as single

Table 6.1 Immunsuppressive Drugs and their Mechanisms of Action

Agents	Main Mechanisms of Action
Pharmacological	
• Corticosteroids (Methylprednisolone, Prednisolone)	Broad range of effects on various phases of the immune responses such as inhibition of cytokine transcription by Antigen presenting cells (APCs), reduction of adhesion molecule expression, induction of apoptosis of immunocompetent cells as well as suppression of inflammatory cell activation.
• Calcineurininhibitors (Ciclosporin A, Tacrolimus)	Prevention of T-cell activation by inhibition of signal 2 (transduction of the costimulatory signal). Cyclosporine A and Tacrolimus bind to the intracellular proteins cyclophilin and FK-binding protein (FKBP) respectively to create active drug complexes. These complexes inactivate calcineurin, a pivotal enzyme in the T cell receptor-signaling pathway resulting in inhibition of the dephosphorylation of nuclear factor of activated T lymphocytes (NFAT) followed bysuppression of the transcription of pro-inflammatory cytokine genes (e.g. interleukin-2, interferon-γ).
• Thiopurine (Azathioprine)	The active metabolites 6-thioguanine nucleotides are purine analogues. They interfere with the normal purine synthesis thus inhibiting the DNA synthesis and cell proliferation of both T- and B-lymphocytes.
• Mycophenolates (Mycophenolat mofetil, Mycophenolat sodium)	Suppression of purine synthesis, DNA synthesis and finally cell proliferation (primarily T cells but also B cells) by potent inhibition of inosine monophosphate dehydrogenase (IMPDH), a key enzyme in the de novo purine synthesis.
• mTOR-Inhibitors (Sirolimus, Everolimus)	Inhibition of signal 3 transduction (cytokine release) and cell proliferation (primarily T cells). To become active the two drugs bind to the same immunophilin as tacrolimus (FKBP), but without an effect on the calcineurin activity. The active complex is a highly specific inhibitor of mammalian target of rapamycin complex 1 (mTORC1) and suppresses cell cycle progression and T cell proliferation.
Biological	
• Depleting agents (e.g. Alemtuzumab, Antithymocyte globuline, Rituximab)	Interference with signals 1–3 and depletion of immunocompetent cells. The CD52 molecule on mononuclear cells is the target of Alemtuzumab, whereas the CD20 molecule on B cells is the target of Rituximab. The immunosuppressive effect of Antithymocyte globuline, a polyclonal agent, is mediated mainly through interacting with a variety of surface markers e.g. CD45, CD3, CD4 on the lymphocytes.
• Non- depleting agents e.g. Basiliximab,	Inhibition of signal 3 transduction (cytokine release) and T-cell proliferation. Basiliximab binds to a chain of the interleukin-2 receptor on activated T lymphocytes, renders them unresponsive to interleukin-2, and prevents their interleukin-2 induced clonal expansion.
Eculizumab	Inhibition of complement activation by blockade of the cleavage of the complement protein C5 and interference with the formation of the membrane attack complex.
Belatacept	Blockade of costimulation (signal 2) by competition with CD28 for CD80/CD86 binding

signal 1: T-Cell receptor engagement, signal 2: costimulation, signal 3: inflammatory stimulus via cytokines.

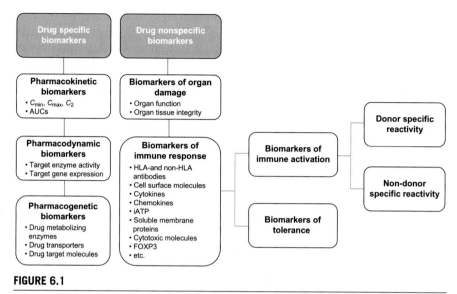

FIGURE 6.1

Biomarkers supporting management of immunosuppression in transplantation.

drug concentrations measured in plasma or whole blood representing the classical TDM approach. There are also some new directions of investigation aiming at elucidation of the putative role of free drug concentrations and particularly of intracellular and/or tissue drug concentrations to improve validity of TDM results for clinical practice. Based on the results of two single-center studies of liver and kidney transplant recipients, it has been suggested that tacrolimus concentration determined in liver biopsies or isolated mononuclear blood cells is beneficial for the prediction of risk for acute rejection compared to whole-drug concentrations [13,14]. However, the need for biopsy-gained tissue material and laborious isolation of peripheral blood cells are currently the main limitations to this new approach. Currently, with the availability of liquid chromatography combined with tandem mass spectrometry (LC–MS/MS) instruments in clinical laboratories, it is possible to accurately measure very low drug concentrations in biological matrix. Further technical developments may support the applicability of intracellular drug concentrations. In fact, the available evidence is still very limited, and much more work must be done (see Chapter 9).

Specific pharmacodynamic biomarkers include target enzyme activity and target gene expression. Research during recent years has focused on calcineurin phosphatase activity and nuclear factor of activated T lymphocytes (NFAT) regulated gene expression to identify pharmacological action of CNIs, inosine monophosphate dehydrogenase (IMPDH) activity and gene expression to monitor therapy with mycophenolate, and P70S6 kinase activity to follow therapy with mTOR inhibitors. Currently, several biomarkers complement the traditional TDM approach in the management of immunosuppressive therapy.

6.4 CALCINEURIN PHOSPHATE

Many investigators have examined the pharmacodynamic action of CNIs on the enzyme calcineurin phosphatase in isolated peripheral blood mononuclear cells, with more studies having been performed with cyclosporine (CsA) compared to tacrolimus. Patient populations included kidney, liver, and lung solid transplant recipients [15]. Most studies, but not all, suggested that calcineurin activity is closely related to CNI concentrations and particularly to C_2 (2 h after dosage) drug concentrations [16,17]. Both Fukudo et al. [18] and Koefoed-Nielsen et al. [19] observed greater inhibition of the enzyme with CsA compared to tacrolimus. With both drugs, a broad interindividual variation of this biomarker has been observed. In a group consisting of 107 lung transplant patients receiving CsA, azathioprine, and steroids, Sanquer et al. reported that calcineurin activity was linked to both acute and chronic rejection [20]. Moreover, the occurrence of malignancies and viral infections was significantly increased in patients showing very low levels of enzyme activity. The authors suggested an optimal range for the activity between 12 and 102 pmol/mg/min in their patient population. Fukudo et al. [18,21] described a transient increase of calcineurin phosphatase activity in living-donor kidney transplant recipients with acute rejection as well as an association between high enzyme activity and acute rejection in liver transplant patients on therapy with either CsA or tacrolimus. In addition, in liver transplant recipients with tacrolimus therapy, a link between low activity and nephrotoxicity was demonstrated. An interesting observation reported by Blanchet et al. was that candidates for liver transplantation with alcoholic cirrhosis or hepatocellular carcinoma showed a deficiency in pre-transplant calcineurin activity compared with other liver diseases [22]. The authors speculated that this fact may lower the risk of acute rejection in these patients after transplantation but also may increase the risk of cancer. This fact may serve as a basis for therapy optimization.

The results suggest that monitoring of pre- and post-transplantation calcineurin activity may represent a promising tool to complement TDM of CNIs. However, all studies published were single-center investigations and include limited number of patients. An important obstacle for the broader distribution of these assays is their laborious and time-consuming workup, including the need for cell isolation, incubation, and analytics. Regarding analytics, an advantageous step compared to older methods using radioisotope, spectrophotometric, or fluorometric detection is the development of the first LC–MS/MS-based method for measurement of calcineurin activity by Carr et al. [23].

6.5 NUCLEAR FACTOR OF ACTIVATED T LYMPHOCYTES REGULATED GENE EXPRESSION

Another approach to investigate the specific pharmacodynamic effects of CNIs is based on monitoring the inhibition of the dephosphorylation of NFATs that is directly related to calcineurin inhibition (Table 6.1). The inhibited dephosphorylation prevents nuclear translocation of NFAT and subsequent transcriptional activation of the NFAT regulated expression of a variety of genes required for T-cell activation, including interleukin-2 (IL-2), interferon-γ (IFN-γ), and granulocyte macrophage colony-stimulating factor. During recent years, the research group of Zeier has extensively investigated the residual expression of these genes as a tool for pharmacodynamic monitoring of treatment with CsA and tacrolimus [24]. A combination of three genes is used to adjust for random variations in expression of individual genes. The percentage inhibition of this expression at specific time points after a drug dose compared to pre-dose expression as a reference is determined and used to guide therapy. The method relies on *ex vivo* stimulation of whole blood by phorbol 12-myristate 13-acetate and ionomycin (3 h, 37°C), avoiding artifacts associated with cell isolation [24]. Gene expression is quantified using the reverse-transcription polymerase chain reaction (RT-PCR) technique with a commercially available LightCycler "Cyclosporine Monitoring" amplification kit and can be performed semiautomatically. These characteristics seem to be a promising basis for method standardization; however, until recently, no cross-validation experience with this procedure had been reported. The reduction of gene transcripts was found to be inversely correlated with the individual CsA or tacrolimus concentration. Low residual expression (<15%) of the three genes was associated with signs of probable over-immunosuppression, such as increased frequency of recurrent infections and malignancies in stable patients treated with CsA [25]. In addition, in a small biopsy-controlled pilot study, the group investigated the utility of this pharmacodynamic approach to monitor tailoring of CsA dose in stable renal transplant recipients [26]. The dose reduction was free from adverse events, such as acute rejections, when the residual expression remained below 30%. Almost complete clinical evidence with this method has been generated by the same group and demonstrated more promising results with CsA than with tacrolimus, probably due to a higher variability of the time to reach adequate levels of suppression after tacrolimus intake. Moreover, a very high inhibition of residual gene expression in nearly all patients early post-transplantation complicates the use of the biomarker in this phase [27]. As a next step, confirmation of the first results in larger randomized prospective and particularly multicenter studies is required to validate the value of this approach for clinical routine.

A comprehensive review of this topic is given in Chapter 11.

6.6 INOSINE MONOPHOSPHATE DEHYDROGENASE

IMPDH types I and II are inhibited in peripheral blood mononuclear cells by mycophenolic acid (MPA). Therefore, determination of the enzyme activity in samples of patients treated with mycophenolate represents a promising approach to monitor pharmacodynamic effects of this therapy. Both radiometric and nonradiometric methods have been described for this purpose [28]. The publication of a highly reproducible and well-validated IMPDH assay, based on the chromatographic determination of newly generated xanthosine-5′-monophosphate in mononuclear cell lysates by Glander et al. contributed significantly to progress in research involving this biomarker [29,30]. Interlaboratory transfer was successful, and the assay was used in several clinical trials, including pediatric and adult kidney transplant recipients [31–34]. Vethe et al. established a modified procedure based on the determination of IMPDH activity in $CD4^+$ cells, which are more directly involved in immunological processes [35]. In clinical trials, substantial interindividual variations in IMPDH activity was reported [30–34,36]. This variability was more than 10-fold, even when determined pre-transplantation and before initiation of therapy with mycophenolate, indicating the potential importance of the basic IMPDH activity for the individual therapeutic response. In a retrospective study with kidney transplant recipients, patients with low IMPDH activity in the pre-transplantation phase had more complications related to the mycophenolate therapy requiring dose reductions early after transplantation, whereas patients with high IMPDH activity had more rejections, especially in the case of additional dose reductions [33]. A significant association between inhibition of IMPDH activity and the occurrence of acute rejection has been confirmed in three independent clinical studies [37–39]. The pharmacodynamic biomarkers investigated were the area under the time curve of IMPDH enzyme activity (IMPDH-AUC)$_{0–12h}$, IMPDH-AUC$_{0–4h}$, and pre-dose IMPDH activity, respectively. Although two of the studies were focused on IMPDH activity immediately after transplantation, Chiarelli et al. investigated stable patients on long-term mycophenolate mofetil therapy [38]. Furthermore, Molinaro et al. described significantly higher pre-transplant IMPDH gene expression (both isoenzyme 1 and isoenzyme 2) in patients who experienced acute rejections compared to non-rejectors [40]. Pre-transplant messenger RNA (mRNA) expression was also associated with hematological side effects. The significant associations disappeared after transplantation, and the authors suggested a role of the cotherapy with steroids. An interesting new finding was reported by Dostalek et al., who observed significantly lower IMPDH gene expression, protein level, and enzyme activity in kidney transplant recipients with diabetes mellitus compared to those without [41]. Based on this finding, the authors suggested a possible need to optimize dosing of mycophenolate in patients with diabetes according to their IMPDH expression/activity. This finding must be proven in larger studies. However, based on review of all studies, it could be suggested that MPA plasma concentrations interpreted in the context of the individual IMPDH activity could provide a more straightforward approach to guide the therapy than classical TDM alone.

In general, mycophenolate administration was proven to result in strong inhibition of IMPDH activity, which was better related to peak drug concentrations (within 2 h after drug intake) than to pre-dose concentrations [3,42]. Changes in IMPDH activity after transplantation reflected inversely the progress of the respective mycophenolic concentration [38,42]. In addition, significant correlation between IMPDH inhibition and free mycophenolic concentration as well as the concentration of the pharmacologically active acyl glucuronide metabolite has been reported [43]. Although associated with promising initial results, wide application of IMPDH activity measurement is limited in clinical practice due to the need for cell separation, incubation, and long analytical run times. Sample instability precludes transfer of whole blood samples to central laboratories where the analyses are established; therefore, cell isolation has to be performed locally. Two LC–MS/MS-based procedures to support monitoring of IMPDH activity have been published [44,45].

6.7 PHOSPHORYLATION OF mTOR DOWNSTREAM EFFECTORS

Compared to CNIs and mycophenolate, there are very few studies targeting pharmacodynamic monitoring of therapy with the mTOR inhibitors everolimus and sirolimus. Drug effects on mTOR activity have been investigated by measurement of the phosphorylation of mTOR downstream effectors p70S6 kinase and S6 protein [46]. Most studies applied a Western blot analysis in lysates of isolated peripheral mononuclear cells. Using this technique, Hartmann et al. studied the phosphorylation status of p70S6 kinase in peripheral blood mononuclear cells in 36 renal transplant patients on combined therapy with sirolimus and either CNIs or mycophenolate mofetil. Although no correlation between the p70S6 kinase phosphorylation and sirolimus trough concentrations was found, p70S6 kinase phosphorylation was significantly inhibited when sirolimus trough concentrations were greater than or equal to 6 ng/mL. Some patients exhibited a strong reduction in phospho-p70S6 kinase despite low trough concentrations of sirolimus, indicating individual enzyme susceptibility. A high degree of phosphorylation was observed in all patients who experienced a rejection event independently of the sirolimus trough concentrations. In contrast, non-rejecters showed significant inhibition of phosphorylation [47]. The results of a study of kidney transplant patients suggested that comedication with tacrolimus limits the inhibitory effect of sirolimus on the activation of the p70S6 kinase [48]. Again, the potency of inhibition of p70s6 kinase phosphorylation varied among patients and failed to correlate with drug trough concentrations. Although these results suggest that the phosphorylation status of p70S6 kinase appeared to provide relevant information on the pharmacodynamic effect of sirolimus, the use of this assay is hampered by its very laborious analytical procedure and the semiquantitative readout. There are two reports on the development of enzyme-linked immunosorbent assay (ELISA) methods to follow the phosphorylation of the p70S6 kinase [49,50] and another one on the use of a phospho-flow cytometry (using FACSDiva 6.1.3 software) to measure the level of phosphorylated S6 ribosomal protein (p-S6RP) [51]. Whereas an acceptable correlation between Western blot analysis and ELISA was registered, no reports on the comparability with the phospho-flow cytometry method are available. An advantage of the two newer analytical approaches is that they allow quantitative evaluation. In addition, the phospho-flow cytometry works by using whole blood, avoiding the laborious cell isolation step. Whether these analytical alternatives will help to foster the research on pharmacodynamic monitoring of the therapy with mTOR inhibitors, which is still in its very preliminary phase, remains to be determined. Therefore, drug-specific pharmacodynamic biomarkers appear to have a promising potential to improve the management of immunosuppressive therapy when combined with classical TDM. However, currently available methods are not practical for routine use, they do not allow timely reporting of results to support therapeutic decisions, they are not standardized, and profound validation data are not available for most of them. In addition, their diagnostic potential has been investigated only in small single-center clinical trials.

6.8 PHARMACOGENETIC BIOMARKERS

Studies during approximately the past decade have investigated genetic variations of drug-metabolizing enzymes and drug transporters [52–54]. Genetic background is thought to considerably account for the variability in drug disposition and therapeutic effects. For *CYP3A5* expressors who carry at least one wild-type *CYP3A5*1* allele, it has been shown that a one and a half to two times higher tacrolimus dose is required to achieve target blood concentrations. Approximately 85% of people with a sub-Saharan genetic origin are *CYP3A5* expressors, whereas approximately 85% of Caucasians do not express the enzyme because they are homozygous for a mutant allele, the most common being *CYP3A5*3* (6986A > G, rs776746) [52,55]. Passey et al. proposed a dosing algorithm that allows predicting tacrolimus clearance and dose based on *CYP3A5* genotype and clinical and ethnic information [56]. However, although this genetic variation obviously has an impact on tacrolimus pharmacokinetics, it remains open whether it is also clinically relevant in tacrolimus-treated transplant patients and can improve clinical outcome. Recently, other genes (e.g., *P450 oxidoreductase *28* or the nuclear receptor pregnane X) have also been discussed as having an impact on the interindividual response to therapy. There also may be value in using *CYP3A5* genotyping to predict the optimal dose for sirolimus, but this must first be investigated in clinical trials. Polymorphisms in the ATP-binding cassette transporters *ABC1* (P-glycoprotein) and *ABCC2* (multidrug resistance-associated protein 2) have not been clearly proven to be associated with either toxicity or efficacy in patients treated with CNIs, mTOR inhibitors, or MPA. However, more studies are needed, and it is not unlikely that ABCB1 transporter polymorphisms have some impact on CNI-mediated toxicity and intralymphocyte drug concentrations. Although UDP-glucuronosyltransferase plays an important role in the metabolism of MPA, according to current experience, the polymorphisms of this enzyme family do not seem to be clinically relevant to individualize MPA dosing and to improve outcome.

Genetic polymorphisms influencing the pharmacodynamics of immunosuppressants, such as mTOR and mycophenolate, have been reported. Woillard et al. described a significant association between an mTOR valiant haplotype (AGAAA (rs1770345/rs2300095/rs2076655/rs1883965/rs12732063) (frequency = 0.055)) and decreased hemoglobin concentrations under sirolimus treatment [57]. In a recent study, *IMPDH1* and *IMPDH2* were resequenced using DNA from 288 individuals from three ethnic groups [58]. In IMPDH1, 73 SNPs (59 novel) and in IMPDH2, 25

SNPs (24 novel) were identified. Two alloenzymes, IMPDH1 Leu275 and IMPDH2 Phe263, displayed a strong decrease in cytosolic IMPDH activity. The polymorphisms in type 1 and type 2 *IMPDH* genes and the association with clinical outcome were investigated in 456 renal transplant patients on mycophenolate mofetil who were part of the Apomygre or FDCC clinical trials [59]. It was demonstrated that the *IMPDH1* rs2278294 SNP was associated with a lower risk of acute rejection and a higher risk of leukopenia during the first year post-transplantation. These results provide insight that variation in MPA response may result, in part, from genetic variation in IMPDH and that IMPDH1 genotyping together with MPA and CNI TDM could improve MPA treatment outcome during the first year post-transplantation.

Although genotyping has become a standard technique in many laboratories and many genetic variants have been discovered, particularly in drug-metabolizing enzymes, none has the potential to meaningfully complement the standard practices for guidance of immunosuppressive therapy. However, it has become increasingly apparent that immunosuppressive drug response phenotypes seem to be more complex and the result of combined effects of genetic variation at multiple gene loci and environmental factors. More research in this field is needed. Chapter 5 elucidates the role of pharmacogenetic biomarkers in-depth.

6.9 BIOMARKERS NONSPECIFIC FOR SINGLE DRUG ACTION

Biomarkers nonspecific for the action of a particular immunosuppressive drug can be divided into those reflecting the damage of the transplanted organ and biomarkers revealing the reactivity status of the graft recipient's immune system (Figure 6.1).

6.9.1 BIOMARKERS OF ORGAN DAMAGE

Altered levels of biomarkers of organ damage may be associated with changes in the function of the transplanted organ or its tissue integrity. Under-immunosuppression, over-immunosuppression, or drug side effects may contribute to organ damage. Commonly used biochemical parameters in this category include creatinine, various enzymes (AST, ALT, LDH, etc.), neutrophil gelatinase-associated lipocalin (a marker of kidney injury), kidney injury molecule-1, serum and urine protein, bilirubin, and troponins. Their broad use is the result of the availability of reliable commercial tests that can be run on consolidated automated analytical systems with short turnaround time. However, as previously mentioned, they are unspecific for a particular disease or tissue damage, and change is an indicator of an already advanced graft injury. Many experimental studies during recent years have targeted the discovery of new, more specific, and noninvasive biomarkers allowing detection of ongoing injury to the donor organ in its early stage. There are reports on potential mRNA and protein biomarkers that could be monitored in the blood or urine as surrogate for the detection of transplant injury. For example, Ling et al. identified a panel of 40 peptides in urine of kidney transplant recipients specific for acute rejection. Transcriptional signals for the corresponding genes from paired renal transplant biopsies matched with the urine samples. A six-gene biomarker panel (*COL1A2*, *COL3A1*, *UMOD*, *MMP-7*, *SERPING1*, and *TIMP1*) classified acute rejection with high specificity and sensitivity (area under receiver operating characteristic curve = 0.98) and suggested the important role of collagen remodeling for this process. The authors concluded that detection of the corresponding proteolytic degradation products in urine could provide a noninvasive diagnostic approach [60]. Kurian et al. applied DNA microarrays, tandem mass spectroscopy proteomics, and bioinformatics to identify genomic and proteomic markers of mild and moderate/severe chronic allograft nephropathy in peripheral blood of two distinct cohorts of kidney transplant patients with biopsy-documented histology ($N = 77$ in total) [61]. A consensus analysis revealed 393 (mild) and 63 (moderate/severe) final candidate biomarkers with predictive accuracy for chronic allograft nephropathy of 80 and 92%, respectively. Proteomic profiles show more than 500 candidates each for both stages of chronic allograft nephropathy, including 302 proteins unique to mild and 509 unique to moderate/severe diseases. In 2009, Garcia Moreira et al. reported on the use of cell-free DNA both in plasma and in urine as a noninvasive acute rejection marker in renal transplantation [62]. Cell-free DNAs are small DNA fragments spilled into the blood or urine from dead cells and cells undergoing apoptosis. Total cell-free DNA (t-cfDNA) and donor-derived cell-free DNA (dd-cfDNA) for the *HBB* (hemoglobin, β) and the *TSPY1* (testis-specific protein, Y-linked 1) genes were analyzed by quantitative PCR in samples obtained from 100 renal transplant recipients during the first 3 months after transplantation. Plasma t-cfDNA concentrations increased markedly during episodes of acute rejection, often before clinical diagnosis, and returned to reference values after treatment. However, the authors observed similar increases during severe post-transplantation infections and therefore proposed the use of the combination of plasma t-cfDNA and procalcitonin, a specific marker of bacterial infections, to improve the diagnostic specificity. Although it appears promising in regard to a higher sensitivity and earlier detection of damage compared to classical biochemical markers, it cannot be expected that these two candidate molecules will provide a better specificity regarding the allograft tissue integrity because the allograft is not definitively the source of their generation. More advanced application of the circulating cell-free DNA analysis is feasible because modern genomic techniques offer the required sensitivity to distinguish recipient- from donor-specific cell DNA released into the body fluids and allow reliable estimation of the proportion of the donor-specific molecules derived from the allograft. First promising results with this new approach have been published, and a comprehensive discussion on the advantages and difficulties of this biomarker is provided in Chapter 7. Further research is needed to assess to what degree this approach can distinguish between different causes of graft injury or information on the level of injury. It can be expected that the combination with other biomarkers will be needed to improve specificity for detection of acute or chronic rejection [63,64]. Oellerich et al. provide data showing that graft-derived cell-free DNA may also be helpful to individualize immunosuppressive regimens [65].

6.9.2 BIOMARKERS OF IMMUNE RESPONSE

The importance of considering the effective immune responsiveness of a transplant recipient when making decisions regarding personalized therapeutic schemes is well recognized, and many experimental and clinical studies have attempted to identify the most appropriate biomarkers with a goal to achieve personalized therapy. Scientific and clinical interests focus not only on options for immune monitoring that support the diagnosis of an ongoing clinical event but also on options that make it possible to predict the risk of clinical complications. Biomarkers of immune response can be divided into biomarkers of immune activation and biomarkers of tolerance (Figure 6.1). Biomarkers of immune activation are directly related to the effective level of immunosuppression and should possess high validity for early identification of inappropriate drug combinations or dosing associated with either under- or over-immunosuppression. They should allow for tailoring immunosuppression in a controlled manner and for identifying patients who may develop operational tolerance. Both biomarkers that reflect the donor-specific immune reactivity and those that are not donor specific are of importance. Whereas the first group provides information on immune cell reactivity directed specifically toward the allograft and is a cornerstone to uncovering under-immunosuppression that may promote rejection and shorten organ survival, the second group makes it possible to determine a patient's general immune status and is particularly helpful for detecting over-immunosuppression. Biomarkers of functional immunity that are currently under investigation include a broad variety of molecules, such as donor-specific and non-donor-specific antibodies, cell surface molecules, intracellular and circulating cytokines, chemokines, cytotoxic molecules, soluble proteins shed from the cell membranes, and mediators such as intracellular ATP (iATP).

The analysis of anti-human leukocyte antigen (anti-HLA) antibodies, including donor-specific antibodies, by ELISA and flow cytometry-based and LUMINEX-based assessment is a well-established systematic method of monitoring transplant recipients. Evidence from large studies with kidney transplant recipients has indicated that patients with serum anti-HLA antibodies and particularly those with anti-donor HLA antibodies have significantly worse outcomes [66,67]. Therefore, pre-transplant antibody specificities (virtual cross-matching) are currently routinely determined. Furthermore, newer evidence that de novo post-transplant anti-donor class II antibodies are associated with graft injury resulted in implementation of post-transplant antibody monitoring [68–70]. In addition, there is growing evidence that measurement of some non-HLA antibodies, such as the anti-endothelial cell antibodies or antibodies to the major histocompatibility complex class I-related chain A (anti-MICA), may be beneficial as a tool to estimate donor-reactive immunity and improve risk stratification both pre- and post-transplant [71–74]. However, confirmation of these finding in large prospective studies is needed before monitoring with these antibodies can be implemented routinely. In addition, more work on obtaining an advanced assay standardization and appropriate cutoffs to sort positive test results is required. One important expectation for donor-specific antibodies is that they may be used as an exclusion criterion when patients are being selected for weaning of immunosuppression or to reintroduce stronger immunosuppression if they appear during a weaning procedure [7].

The upregulation of cytokine synthesis and the activation of surface receptors/ costimulatory molecules of T cells lead to T-cell proliferation, a key step during acute rejection episodes. Both of these biomarker groups are affected by treatment with immunosuppressive drugs (Table 6.1). Therefore, some of them, such as the cytokines INF-γ, IL-2, IL-10, and transforming growth factor-β or the surface markers of lymphocyte activation CD25, CD71, CD26, CD27, CD28, CD30, CD154, etc., have been identified as candidate biomarkers associated with clinical outcome and response to the immunosuppressive therapy [75,76]. A considerable number of studies evaluating these markers are experimental studies in which the direct effect of different immunosuppressants has been investigated. Some of these studies have also provided useful information on possible synergistic and antagonistic interactions between immunosuppressive drugs used in combined therapy [75,77]. However, the number of clinical studies in which the diagnostic/predictive value of these biomarkers has been investigated is limited, and the patient cohorts included are small. Early studies demonstrated that the percentage of IL-2 producing $CD8^+$ T cells was associated with inhibited IL-2 secretion during treatment with CsA [78]. Also, an association between the percentage of IL-2 producing $CD8^+$ T cells and graft stability in liver or kidney transplant recipients was suggested [79]. In a study of 24 liver transplant patients that aimed to evaluate whether specific biomarkers reflect immune response reactivity and predict rejection associated with withdrawal of immunosuppression, Millan et al. observed that the frequency of $CD4^+$ and $CD8^+$ T cells producing INF-γ as well as $CD8^+$ cells producing IL-2 was significantly higher in organ rejecters versus non-rejecters [80]. Furthermore, organ rejecters showed increased percentage of INF-γ producing $CD8^+$ cells before transplantation. The results suggested that this biomarker could be used to estimate risk of rejection and to set an appropriate initial therapy. In another study of the same group, a pre-transplantation cutoff value of 55.8% for $\%CD8^+/IFN-\gamma^+$ and a percentage inhibition for soluble IFN-γ, $\%CD8^+/IFN-\gamma^+$, and $\%CD8^+/IL-2^+$ lower than 40% during the first week post-transplantation were associated with a high risk of acute rejection [81]. There were no differences in drug concentrations between rejecters and non-rejecters. The authors suggested a low susceptibility to immunosuppressive drugs for the patients with low percentage inhibition.

Clinical studies aiming at the association of surface molecule expression as a marker of T-cell activation under immunosuppression are limited and often report conflicting results. Ashokkumar et al. reported on an association between high expression of CD154 on $CD19^+$ cells and CD154 on $CD4^-$ and increased risk of rejection in pediatric populations with intestinal [82] and liver transplantation [83], respectively. Boleslawski et al. found an association between high CD28 expression on $CD3^+$ cells and risk of rejection as well as low expression of the same marker on $CD8^+$ cells and risk of malignancies [84,85]. The two studies were performed on liver transplant recipients. Wieland et al. reported a significant association between low

CD26 expression on T cells and freedom from rejection early after kidney transplantation [86]. The group was able to confirm this finding in an independent and larger population and extended this result with the observation that CD26 expression on effector T cells ($CD3^+$ $CD8^+$) is a more specific biomarker for rejection than the expression on all $CD3^+$ lymphocytes (E. Wieland et al., unpublished data).

Although analytical techniques to perform analysis on cytokines and cell surface molecules are widely available (e.g., ELISA and flow cytometry), these biomarkers are not frequently used in clinical trials. This is probably due to two very important limitations of most of these procedures: They are laborious (sometimes requiring cell isolation from whole blood) and include mitogenic stimulation that can take up to 72h for some protocols. Exceptions are the expression on CD28 and CD26 that can both be performed directly in whole blood and do not need a stimulation step. Such analysis can be completed within 2 or 3h after receipt of the patient sample. Other important limitations with this group of markers include the lack of standardization and limited data on method validation, which are prerequisite for performing large multicenter studies or comparing results generated at different analytical sites. The same limitations are responsible for the low frequency of application of assays for the assessment of lymphocyte proliferation, such as proliferating cell nuclear antigen/DNA expression, carboxy-fluorescein succinimidyl ester (a fluorescent cell stain dye) dilution assay, and DNA incorporation of ^{3}H-thymidine or its analog BrdU (bromodeoxyuridine). In the few small studies that have been published, an association of proliferation biomarkers with both risks of under-immunosuppression (acute rejection) and over-immunosuppression (leukopenia and viral infections) has been suggested [75].

Another nonspecific approach to follow T-cell activation is the use of the enzyme-linked immunospot (ELISPOT) assay. In this assay, cytokine-secreting T cells are counted after in vitro stimulation of recipient peripheral blood mononuclear cells by donor-specific or -nonspecific antigens for 18–48h. This assay is commercially available as a ready-to-use kit, and the readout can be automated by video imaging. It can be used for detecting T cells secreting cytokines such as IL-2, INF-γ, or IL-10. In particular, the application with INF-γ is under extensive investigation, and the main topic of interest is the use of the INF-γ ELISPOT to determine the donor-specific memory T-cell reactivity. Recent research in transplantation immunology indicated that especially the memory cell pool may have a deleterious role on graft outcome, even a long time after transplantation, and highlighted the need for biomarkers to measure memory alloreactivity [8]. Studies from single centers indicate that heightened T-cell alloreactivity measured with the ELISPOT assay correlates with acute and chronic rejection and with poor long-term allograft function [87]. In a retrospective study of 130 kidney transplant recipients, Augustine et al. suggested that antibody induction therapy preferentially benefits transplant candidates with strong pre-transplant donor-reactive cellular immunity and that if confirmed prospectively, pre-transplant ELISPOT assessments could permit individualized use of induction therapy in patients [88]. Bestard et al. [89] reported the first results of the successful use of the donor-specific INF-γ ELISPOT response to make decisions on both CNI-free and CNI-based initial therapy after transplantation and on therapy optimization, including mycophenolate and corticosteroids weaning and CNI minimization 6–12 months thereafter. This prospective study included 120 de novo renal transplant patients. These promising results, however, require validation in large-scale prospective randomized trials. The distinctiveness of the INF-γ ELISPOT assay compared to most other biomarkers in research is the fact that international consortia both in Europe and in the United States (RISET, CTOT) have implemented a rigorous approach to validate this assay, enabling its highly standardized use in multiple laboratories [90,91]. Drawbacks for the introduction of this technique in the clinic are its complexity, labor and time intensity, as well as high costs.

As a result of increasing evidence, increasing attention has been focused on chemokines such as CXCL9 and CXCL10. These small molecules are downstream of INF-γ signaling and attract CXCR3$^+$ T cells into the graft. The chemokines are secreted by several cell types and can also be measured in urine samples. Chemokine concentrations have been associated with both rejection and graft dysfunction pre- and post-transplantation [92–94]. A possible problem with the clinical usefulness of pretransplant concentrations is a depletion or inactivation of the CXCR3$^+$ responder cells due to the use of induction therapies [6]. Again, the evidence is derived from small single-center studies and must be confirmed in larger and independent cohorts.

One way to investigate the overall function of lymphocytes is to determine their ability to produce iATP after stimulation with phytohemagglutinin. Based on this principle, Cylex, Inc., introduced an immune function assay that is commercially available under the trade name ImmuKnow. This assay has also been approved by the US Food and Drug Administration (FDA). In 2013, this company was acquired by Viracor-IBT Laboratories, Inc. Studies using the ImmuKnow assay showed that high CD4$^+$ T-cell iATP concentrations were associated with risk of acute rejection in recipients of kidney, liver, heart, and small bowel transplants, whereas low CD4$^+$ T-cell iATP concentrations were linked to higher risk of infections [95–99]. From meta-analysis, a target immunological response zone could be determined, allowing the assessment of the relative risk of infection and rejection. However, not all studies were able to confirm these associations [100]. Possible reasons for the inconsistent results are the use of only single time point measurements and lack of information on the individual baseline values in some trials, the uncertainty regarding the advantage of using different target ranges for different organs and patient populations, as well as the limited power of the studies in some cases. A potential explanation for the inconclusive findings regarding the prediction of acute rejection is the fact that the assay reflects the general immune status but not the specific reactivity directed toward the allograft. However, this feature is beneficial to detect over-immunosuppression, and this is in accordance with the published literature, with the vast majority of studies reporting on a significant relationship between ImmuKnow test results and the occurrence of infections [100–102]. Interesting preliminary data from liver transplant recipients indicated that titrating immunosuppressive therapy according the iATP concentrations reduced the risk of infections compared to standard monitoring practice [103]. In general, serial longitudinal use of this assay appears to provide a diagnostically conclusive tool for identifying over-immunosuppression and to indicate an increased risk of short-term mortality, but more evidence must be generated to support appropriate interpretation of the test results. Disadvantages from an analytical standpoint are the laborious and time-intensive procedure, the need of cell isolation and incubation, the requirement of very fast processing of the material after sampling, and the high cost.

Several studies have demonstrated that the technically simple sCD30 measurement in serum allows prediction of the incidence of acute allograft rejection and may differentiate graft deterioration from chronic allograft nephropathy [104]. sCD30 is the soluble form of CD30, a member of the TNF receptor family expressed on CD4[+] and CD8[+] T lymphocytes, B and natural killer cells, as well as some nonlymphoid cells that represents a costimulatory molecule with an important role in T- and B-cell growth, differentiation, and function. Upon activation of CD30[+] T cells, CD30 is enzymatically cleaved, leaving the soluble protein molecule in the plasma, which can be then used as a measure of this cell activation. Its release after allogenic stimulation has been shown to be mediated by memory T cells and regulated by INF-γ and IL-2 [105]. Most results with this biomarker have been reported with kidney transplant recipients by Opelz et al. High pre-transplant concentrations (>100 U/mL) were significantly related to the incidence of acute allograft rejection, need of anti-rejection treatment in the first year post-transplantation, as well as risk of graft loss during the 5-year follow-up [106]. High plasma sCD30 concentrations early after transplantation (3–5 days) were an additional prognostic marker for acute rejection [107]. In general, sCD30 values greater than 40 U/mL at 1 month post-transplantation were associated with a significantly lower 3-year graft survival rate, irrespective of the pre-transplant concentrations [108]. One-year sCD30 concentrations were reported to differentiate graft deterioration from chronic allograft nephropathy [109]. High sCD30 concentrations, both pre- and post-transplantation, were shown to be a risk factor for low graft survival independent of antibody sensitization and HLA mismatch [106,108,110], with a particularly poor prognosis for patients with simultaneously high levels of these markers.

However, these promising results were not confirmed in some studies by other groups [111–113]. One possible explanation is the lower number of patients included in these studies or a shorter follow-up, as well as a high biological variability of sCD30 levels with time and with variable therapeutic regimens, particularly regarding induction therapy [6,114]. An association between increased serum creatinine and sCD30 concentrations has been reported that may complicate interpretation of results close to the proposed cutoffs [115]. Similar to the ImmuKnow assay, a possible benefit of longitudinal serial evaluations has been suggested [116]. Data with non-renal transplant recipients are very limited and inconsistent. Finally, data on using this biomarker to guide therapeutic decisions are still lacking. Therefore, further clinical trials are required to validate the diagnostic value of sCD30 in transplantation. However, advantages of this biomarker are the availability of commercial assays based on the ELISA technology that can be easily performed, it does not require ex vivo stimulation of immune cells, and it offers a certain level of standardization and comparability of the results. In addition, the development and validation of a fluorescent microsphere immunoassay (Luminex technology) has been described that allows multiplex determination of sCD30 along with other molecules in the same sample and opens new analytical perspectives [117].

6.9.3 MOLECULES INVOLVED IN CYTOTOXICITY

Molecules involved in cytotoxicity, such as perforin, granzyme B, and FasL, have been extensively investigated in relation to the occurrence of rejection. The analytical procedures are based mostly on the determination of mRNA by microarray—or sensitive PCR—techniques. Both peripheral blood and urine may be used for this purpose. Combined upregulation of multiple genes was reported to detect acute rejection with a high sensitivity [118,119]. Aquino-Dias et al. presented data in support of the ability of the perforin, granzyme B, and FasL gene expression to distinguish acute rejection not only from the absence of pathology but also from acute tubular nephropathy and toxicity by CNIs [120]. Serial measurements of granzyme B and perforin seem to have the potential to detect acute rejection approximately 1 week prior to its clinical recognition [121–123], which would support earlier intervention and probably improve the long-term clinical outcome. However, diagnostic specificity seems to be limited due to the coincidence of increased gene expression in patients with infections such as human polyomavirus BK or cytomegalovirus [6]. Combination with biomarkers of donor-specific alloreactivity may be helpful to overcome this drawback. In addition, as already discussed for other potential biomarkers, not all studies have reported consistent findings [124]. Preanalytical and assay standardization are critical steps to be approached in order to improve the informative value and open the way for incorporation into clinical practice.

6.9.4 BIOMARKERS OF TOLERANCE

For the identification of recipients who would benefit from immunosuppression minimization, indicators of tolerance may be helpful. T lymphocytes with immunosuppressive activity have been known for more than three decades. These "regulatory" T cells (Tregs) can prevent allograft rejection. Tregs may help in identifying not only "high-risk" patients who may need intensified immunosuppression but also "operational tolerant" patients in whom immunosuppression could be safely withdrawn. There is heterogeneity of Tregs, which has to be considered [125]. Analyzing Treg frequencies after transplantation was done to examine the tolerance-inducing potential of different immunosuppressive regimens. For example, there is evidence that mTOR inhibitors favor an increase in peripheral Tregs [125]. Calcineurin inhibition was shown to lower the repopulation and accumulation of peripheral Tregs, with the frequency of $CD4^+CD25^+Foxp3^+$ Tregs being negatively correlated with tacrolimus pre-dose concentrations [126]. Bouvy et al. demonstrated differential effects of rATG and basiliximab on the repopulation of Tregs [127]. Note that monitoring of Tregs by flow cytometry is not trivial, as is the assessment of Treg function, which can be performed by techniques such as the cytotoxic lymphocyte test, ELISPOT, mixed lymphocyte reaction, or the trans vivo delayed-type hypersensitivity test [125]. For determination of the natural Treg in human peripheral blood, a method based on Treg-specific DNA demethylation within the *FOXP3* locus seems to be useful. The need for a highly specialized laboratory currently precludes routine measurements. Most reports include a limited number of patients and investigate Tregs by different parameters, which makes the comparison of results difficult.

An emerging area of investigation is the role of B cells for which an involvement in maintenance of tolerance but not in induction has been suggested [128]. One further promising tool to characterize possible tolerant patients is gene expression [129]. Kidney graft recipients exhibit unique peripheral blood transcriptional patterns. A signature, designated as the "tolerance footprint," was able to separate tolerant recipients from patients under chronic rejection [130]. In addition, studies have reported on the identification of a B-cell signature associated with renal transplant tolerance [131]. The difference in expression patterns was related to the immune response and could constitute the basis for a future diagnostic test of tolerance in order to adapt the immunosuppressive therapy. The gene expression patterns vary in recipients of different solid organs. For heart transplantation, the FDA has approved a gene expression test that helps to identify the absence of heart transplant rejection, and this test is now commercially available (AlloMap, XDx Expression Diagnostics, Brisbane, CA, USA).

In general, the role of the potential biomarkers for prediction of tolerance is not sufficiently elucidated and is subject to active research. Comprehensive summaries on current knowledge about biomarkers of immune activation and tolerance are provided in Chapters 8 and 10.

6.10 CONCLUSIONS

Guidance of immunosuppressive therapy in transplantation is currently moving from a level of mostly empiric to advanced individualized therapy. Supported by modern high-throughput OMICS technologies, new knowledge is rapidly developing, and a vast number of new biomarkers have entered analytical and clinical research as new candidates. From the standpoint of therapy optimization, biomarkers that can detect under- and over-immunosuppression early as well as drug toxicity are needed. However, based on this overview, there is still a lack of a reliable marker. Not one of the potential candidate biomarkers can meet all or even the majority of the requirements described in the introduction of this chapter. Careful analytical validation, multicenter cross-validation, assay standardization, and commercialization are critical steps on the way to introduction in clinical practice. Some biomarkers, such as the NFAT regulated gene expression "cyclosporine monitoring," IFN-γ ELISPOT, and sCD30 assays, offer an advanced level of standardization due to the availability of commercial kits. Sanchez et al. reported on the development of an external proficiency program for the IFN-γ ELISPOT to evaluate laboratory performance [90].

The procedures to investigate some parameters, such as donor-specific antibodies, cell-free DNA, mRNA expression, CD28 and CD26 expression on activated T cells, as well as sCD30, do not need cell isolation or in vitro stimulation, thus providing a result in a quicker and easier manner. For some biomarkers, such as sCD30 and cell-free DNA, attempts had been made to automate the analytic measurement step.

During recent years, it has become clear that no single biomarker will be able to distinguish patients with stable clinical outcome, who are candidates for therapy minimization or even for withdrawal from such with inappropriately managed therapy and at risk for rejection, infections, malignancy, and drug toxicity. It is obvious that the definition of individually adequate immunosuppression is a very complex issue that depends on different disease entities, donor and recipient factors, comedication, environmental aspects, etc. An immunosuppressive scheme that is optimal for the transplanted organ is not necessarily optimal for the individual as a whole. A promising approach to overcome this complex situation is the use of a combination of biomarkers complementing TDM to guide individualized immunosuppression. Which are the best markers is not clearly established, but it seems obvious that such a net should include (1) markers for immune activation specifically triggered by the allograft, such as donor-specific antibodies or T-cell response after stimulation with donor-specific antigens; (2) biomarkers for estimation of the global state of immunosuppression; (3) organ integrity markers specific for the allograft; (4) markers of organ damage by drug toxicity; and (5) biomarkers of tolerance. In addition, it can be assumed that introduction of pharmacogenetic and pharmacodynamic biomarkers will support in particular the choice of a personalized initial therapy as well as the identification of individual unresponsiveness to single drugs. Moreover, given that patients respond individually to treatments or changes in treatments, it can be suggested that sequential monitoring rather than single-point monitoring will be needed to guide the therapy. For example, monitoring would be necessary not only prior to a minimization procedure but also after its initiation for early detection of the risk of rejection and to allow intervention before clinical symptoms appear.

In summary, although there has been major progress in the development of new biomarkers for the management of immunosuppressive therapy, and although the needs and goals are clearly recognized, there is still work to be done in order to deliver reliable tools and strategies to the practicing clinician.

REFERENCES

[1]   Olbricht CJ. Why do we need biomarkers in solid organ transplantation. Clin Chim Acta 2012;413:1310–1.

[2]   Budde K, Matz M, Dürr M, Glander P. Biomarkers of over-immunosuppression. Clin Pharmacol Ther 2011;90:316–22.

[3]   Wieland E, Olbricht CJ, Süsal C, Gurragchaa P, et al. Biomarkers as a tool for management of immunosuppression in transplant patients. Ther Drug Monit 2010;32:560–72.

[4]   Wieland E, Shipkova M, Oellerich M. Biomarkers in transplantation medicine: guide to the next level in immunosuppressive therapy. Clin Chim Acta 2012;413:1309.

[5]   Sood S, Testro AG. Immune monitoring post liver transplant. World J Transplant 2014;4:30–9.

[6]   Heidt S, San Segundo D, Shankar S, Mittal S, et al. Peripheral blood sampling for the detection of allograft rejection: biomarker identification and validation. Transplantation 2011;92:1–9.

[7]   Ashton-Chess J, Giral M, Soulillou JP, Brouard S. Can immune monitoring help to minimize immunosuppression in kidney transplantation? Transpl Int 2009;22:110–9.

[8]   Cravedi P, Heeger PS. Immunologic monitoring in transplantation revisited. Curr Opin Organ Transplant 2012;17:26–32.

[9]   Wiesner RH, Fung JJ. Present state of immunosuppressive therapy in liver transplant recipients. Liver Transpl 2011;17(Suppl. 3):S1–S9.

[10] Page EK, Dar WA, Knechtle SJ. Biologics in organ transplantation. Transpl Int 2012;25:707–19.

[11] Clatworthy MR. Targeting B cells and antibody in transplantation. Am J Transplant 2011;11:1359–67.

[12] Roussey-Kesler G, Giral M, Moreau A, Legendre C, et al. Clinical operational tolerance after kidney transplantation. Am J Transplant 2006;6:736–46.

[13] Capron A, Lerut J, Latinne D, Rahier J, et al. Correlation of tacrolimus levels in peripheral blood mononuclear cells with histological staging of rejection after liver transplantation: preliminary results of a prospective study. Transpl Int 2012;25:41–7.

[14] Capron A, Mourad M, De Meyer M, De Pauw L, et al. CYP3A5 and ABCB1 polymorphisms influence tacrolimus concentrations in peripheral blood mononuclear cells after renal transplantation. Pharmacogenomics 2010;11:703–14.

[15] Yano I. Pharmacodynamic monitoring of calcineurin phosphatase activity in transplant patients treated with calcineurin inhibitors. Drug Metab Pharmacokinet 2008;23:150–7.

[16] Millán O, Brunet M, Campistol JM, Faura A, et al. Pharmacodynamic approach to immunosuppressive therapies using calcineurin inhibitors and mycophenolate mofetil. Clin Chem 2003;49:1891–9.

[17] Blanchet B, Hulin A, Duvoux C, Astier A. Determination of serine/threonine protein phosphatase type 2B PP2B in lymphocytes by HPLC. Anal Biochem 2003;312:1–6.

[18] Fukudo M, Yano I, Masuda S, Fukatsu S, et al. Pharmacodynamic analysis of tacrolimus and cyclosporine in living-donor liver transplant patients. Clin Pharmacol Ther 2005;78:168–81.

[19] Koefoed-Nielsen PB, Karamperis N, Højskov C, Poulsen JH, et al. The calcineurin activity profiles of cyclosporin and tacrolimus are different in stable renal transplant patients. Transpl Int 2006;19:821–7.

[20] Sanquer S, Amrein C, Grenet D, Guillemain R, et al. Expression of calcineurin activity after lung transplantation: a 2-year follow-up. PLoS One 2013;8:e59634.

[21] Fukudo M, Yano I, Katsura T, Ito N, et al. A transient increase of calcineurin phosphatase activity in living-donor kidney transplant recipients with acute rejection. Drug Metab Pharmacokinet 2010;25:411–7.

[22] Blanchet B, Hurtova M, Roudot-Thoraval F, Costentin CE, et al. Deficiency in calcineurin activity in liver transplantation candidates with alcoholic cirrhosis or hepatocellular carcinoma. Liver Int 2009;29:1152–7.

[23] Carr L, Gagez AL, Essig M, Sauvage FL, et al. Calcineurin activity assay measurement by liquid chromatography-tandem mass spectrometry in the multiple reaction monitoring mode. Clin Chem 2014;60:353–60.

[24] Giese T, Zeier M, Schemmer P, Waldemar U, et al. Monitoring of NFAT-regulated gene expression in the peripheral blood of allograft recipients: a novel perspective toward individually optimized drug doses of cyclosporine A. Transplantation 2004;77:339–44.

[25] Sommerer C, Konstandin M, Dengler T, Schmidt J, et al. Pharmacodynamic monitoring of cyclosporine a in renal allograft recipients shows a quantitative relationship between immunosuppression and the occurrence of recurrent infections and malignancies. Transplantation 2006;82:1280–5.

[26] Sommerer C, Giese T, Schmidt J, Meuer S, et al. Ciclosporin A tapering monitored by NFAT-regulated gene expression: a new concept of individual immunosuppression. Transplantation 2008;85:15–21.

[27] Sommerer C, Zeier M, Meurer S, Giese T. Pharmacodynamic monitoring of CsA therapy in the early posttransplant period. Kidney Int (Suppl) 2011;1000 [Abstract #M0518].

[28] Glander P, Hambach P, Liefeldt L, Budde K. Inosine 5′-monophosphate dehydrogenase activity as a biomarker in the field of transplantation. Clin Chim Acta 2012;413:1391–7.

[29] Glander P, Braun KP, Hambach P, Bauer S, et al. Non-radioactive determination of inosine 5′-monophosphate dehydrogenase (IMPDH) in peripheral mononuclear cells. Clin Biochem 2001;34:543–9.

[30] Glander P, Sombogaard F, Budde K, van Gelder T, et al. Improved assay for the nonradioactive determination of inosine 5′-monophosphate dehydrogenase activity in peripheral blood mononuclear cells. Ther Drug Monit 2009;31:351–9.

[31] Budde K, Braun KP, Glander P, Therville N, et al. Pharmacodynamic monitoring of mycophenolate mofetil in stable renal allograft recipients. Transplant Proc 2002;34:1748–50.

[32] Glander P, Hambach P, Braun KP, Fritsche L, et al. Effect of mycophenolate mofetil on IMP dehydrogenase after the first dose and after long-term treatment in renal transplant recipients. Int J Clin Pharmacol Ther 2003;41:470–6.

[33] Glander P, Hambach P, Braun KP, Fritsche L, et al. Pre-transplant inosine monophosphate dehydrogenase activity is associated with clinical outcome after renal transplantation. Am J Transplant 2004;4:2045–51.

[34] Budde K, Glander P, Krämer BK, Fischer W, et al. Conversion from mycophenolate mofetil to enteric-coated mycophenolate sodium in maintenance renal transplant recipients receiving tacrolimus: clinical, pharmacokinetic, and pharmacodynamic outcomes. Transplantation 2007;83:417–24.

[35] Vethe NT, Bergan S. Determination of inosine monophosphate dehydrogenase activity in human CD4+ cells isolated from whole blood during mycophenolic acid therapy. Ther Drug Monit 2006;28:608–13.

[36] de Jonge H, Naesens M, Kuypers DR. New insights into the pharmacokinetics and pharmacodynamics of the calcineurin inhibitors and mycophenolic acid: possible consequences for therapeutic drug monitoring in solid organ transplantation. Ther Drug Monit 2009;31:416–35.

[37] Sombogaard F, van Schaik RH, Mathot RA, Budde K, et al. Interpatient variability in IMPDH activity in MMF-treated renal transplant patients is correlated with IMPDH type II 3757T > C polymorphism. Pharmacogenet Genomics 2009;19:626–34.

[38] Chiarelli LR, Molinaro M, Libetta C, Tinelli C, et al. Inosine monophosphate dehydrogenase variability in renal transplant patients on long-term mycophenolate mofetil therapy. Br J Clin Pharmacol 2010;69:38–50.

[39] Raggi MC, Siebert SB, Steimer W, Schuster T, et al. Customized mycophenolate dosing based on measuring inosine-monophosphate dehydrogenase activity significantly improves patients' outcomes after renal transplantation. Transplantation 2010;90:1536–41.

[40] Molinaro M, Chiarelli LR, Biancone L, Castagneto M, et al. Monitoring of inosine monophosphate dehydrogenase activity and expression during the early period of mycophenolate mofetil therapy in *de novo* renal transplant patients. Drug Metab Pharmacokinet 2013;28:109–17.

[41] Dostalek M, Gohh RY, Akhlaghi F. Inosine monophosphate dehydrogenase expression and activity are significantly lower in kidney transplant recipients with diabetes mellitus. Ther Drug Monit 2013;35:374–83.

[42] Fukuda T, Goebel J, Thøgersen H, Maseck D, et al. Inosine monophosphate dehydrogenase (IMPDH) activity as a pharmacodynamic biomarker of mycophenolic acid effects in pediatric kidney transplant recipients. J Clin Pharmacol 2011;51:309–20.

[43] Stracke S, Shipkova M, Mayer J, Keller F, et al. Pharmacokinetics and pharmacodynamics of mycophenolate sodium (EC-MPS) co-administered with cyclosporine in the early-phase post-kidney transplantation. Clin Transplant 2012;26:57–66.

[44] Vethe NT, Ali AM, Reine PA, Andersen AM, et al. Simultaneous quantification of IMPDH activity and purine bases in lymphocytes using LC-MS/MS: assessment of biomarker responses to mycophenolic acid. Ther Drug Monit 2014;36:108–18.

[45] Laverdière I, Caron P, Couture F, Guillemette C, et al. Liquid chromatography-coupled tandem mass spectrometry based assay to evaluate inosine-5′-monophosphate dehydrogenase activity in peripheral blood mononuclear cells from stem cell transplant recipients. Anal Chem 2012;84:216–23.

[46] Hartmann B. p70S6 kinase phosphorylation for pharmacodynamic monitoring. Clin Chim Acta 2012;413:1387–90.

[47] Hartmann B, Schmid G, Graeb C, Bruns CJ, et al. Biochemical monitoring of mTOR inhibitor-based immunosuppression following kidney transplantation: a novel approach for tailored immunosuppressive therapy. Kidney Int 2005;68:2593–8.

[48] Leogrande D, Teutonico A, Ranieri E, Saldarelli M, et al. Monitoring biological action of rapamycin in renal transplantation. Am J Kidney Dis 2007;50:314–25.

[49] Hartmann B, He X, Keller F, Fischereder M, et al. Development of a sensitive phospho-p70 S6 kinase ELISA to quantify mTOR proliferation signal inhibition. Ther Drug Monit 2013;35:233–9.

[50] Dekter HE, Romijn FP, Temmink WP, van Pelt J, et al. A spectrophotometric assay for routine measurement of mammalian target of rapamycin activity in cell lysates. Anal Biochem 2010;403:79–87.

[51] Dieterlen MT, Bittner HB, Klein S, von Salisch S, et al. Assay validation of phosphorylated S6 ribosomal protein for a pharmacodynamic monitoring of mTOR-inhibitors in peripheral human blood. Cytometry B Clin Cytom 2012;82:151–7.

[52] MacPhee IA. Pharmacogenetic biomarkers: cytochrome P450 3A5. Clin Chim Acta 2012;413:1312–7.

[53] Shuker N, Bouamar R, Weimar W, van Schaik RH, et al. ATP-binding cassette transporters as pharmacogenetic biomarkers for kidney transplantation. Clin Chim Acta 2012;413:1326–37.

[54] Dupuis R, Yuen A, Innocenti F. The influence of UGT polymorphisms as biomarkers in solid organ transplantation. Clin Chim Acta 2012;413:318–25.

[55] Hesselink DA, Bouamar R, Elens L, van Schaik RH, et al. The role of pharmacogenetics in the disposition of and response to tacrolimus in solid organ transplantation. Clin Pharmacokinet 2014;53:123–39.

[56] Passey C, Birnbaum AK, Brundage RC, Oetting WS, et al. Dosing equation for tacrolimus using genetic variants and clinical factors. Br J Clin Pharmacol 2011;72:948–57.

[57] Woillard JB, Kamar N, Rousseau A, Rostaing L, et al. Association of sirolimus adverse effects with m-TOR, p70S6K or Raptor polymorphisms in kidney transplant recipients. Pharmacogenet Genomics 2012;22:725–32.

[58] Wu TY, Peng Y, Pelleymounter LL, Moon I, et al. Pharmacogenetics of the mycophenolic acid targets inosine monophosphate dehydrogenases IMPDH1 and IMPDH2: gene sequence variation and functional genomics. Br J Pharmacol 2010;161:1584–98.

[59] Gensburger O, Van Schaik RH, Picard N, Le Meur Y, et al. Polymorphisms in type I and II inosine monophosphate dehydrogenase genes and association with clinical outcome in patients on mycophenolate mofetil. Pharmacogenet Genomics 2010;20:537–43.

[60] Ling XB, Sigdel TK, Lau K, Ying L, et al. Integrative urinary peptidomics in renal transplantation identifies biomarkers for acute rejection. J Am Soc Nephrol 2010;21: 646–53.

[61] Kurian SM, Heilman R, Mondala TS, Nakorchevski A, et al. Biomarkers for early and late stage chronic allograft nephropathy by proteogenomic profiling of peripheral blood. PLoS One 2009;4:e6212.

[62] García Moreira V, Prieto García B, Baltar Martín JM, Ortega Suárez F, et al. Cell-free DNA as a noninvasive acute rejection marker in renal transplantation. Clin Chem 2009;55:1958–66.

[63] Sigdel TK, Vitalone MJ, Tran TQ, Dai H, et al. A rapid noninvasive assay for the detection of renal transplant injury. Transplantation 2013;96:97–101.

[64] Beck J, Bierau S, Balzer S, Reiner A, et al. Digital droplet PCR for rapid quantification of donor DNA in the circulation of transplant recipients as a potential universal biomarker of graft injury. Clin Chem 2013;59:1732–41.

[65] Oellerich M, Schütz E, Kanzow P, Schmitz J, et al. Use of graft-derived cell-free DNA as an organ integrity biomarker to reexamine effective tacrolimus trough concentrations after liver transplantation. Ther Drug Monit 2014;36:136–40.

[66] Caro-Oleas JL, González-Escribano MF, González-Roncero FM, Acevedo-Calado MJ, et al. Clinical relevance of HLA donor-specific antibodies detected by single antigen assay in kidney transplantation. Nephrol Dial Transplant 2012;27:1231–8.

[67] Terasaki PI, Ozawa M, Castro R. Four-year follow-up of a prospective trial of HLA and MICA antibodies on kidney graft survival. Am J Transplant 2007;7:408–15.

[68] Fotheringham J, Angel C, Goodwin J, Harmer AW, et al. Natural history of proteinuria in renal transplant recipients developing *de novo* human leukocyte antigen antibodies. Transplantation 2011;91:991–6.

[69] Dieplinger G, Ditt V, Arns W, Huppertz A, et al. Impact of *de novo* donor-specific HLA antibodies detected by Luminex solid-phase assay after transplantation in a group of 88 consecutive living-donor renal transplantations. Transpl Int 2014;27:60–8.

[70] Wiebe C, Nickerson P. Posttransplant monitoring of *de novo* human leukocyte antigen donor-specific antibodies in kidney transplantation. Curr Opin Organ Transplant 2013;18:470–7.

[71] Sun Q, Cheng Z, Cheng D, Chen J, et al. *De novo* development of circulating anti-endothelial cell antibodies rather than pre-existing antibodies is associated with post-transplant allograft rejection. Kidney Int 2011;79:655–62.

[72] Breimer ME, Rydberg L, Jackson AM, Lucas DP, et al. Multicenter evaluation of a novel endothelial cell crossmatch test in kidney transplantation. Transplantation 2009;87:549–56.

[73] Zou Y, Stastny P, Süsal C, Döhler B, et al. Antibodies against MICA antigens and kidney-transplant rejection. N Engl J Med 2007;357:1293–300.

[74] Solgi G, Furst D, Mytilineos J, Pourmand G, et al. Clinical relevance of pre and post-transplant immune markers in kidney allograft recipients: anti-HLA and MICA antibodies and serum levels of sCD30 and sMICA. Transpl Immunol 2012;26:81–7.

[75] Shipkova M, Wieland E. Surface markers of lymphocyte activation and markers of cell proliferation. Clin Chim Acta 2012;413:1338–49.

[76] Brunet M. Cytokines as predictive biomarkers of alloreactivity. Clin Chim Acta 2012;413:1354–8.

[77] Barten MJ, Shipkova M, Bartsch P, Dhein S, et al. Mycophenolic acid interaction with cyclosporine and tacrolimus *in vitro* and *in vivo*: evaluation of additive effects on rat blood lymphocyte function. Ther Drug Monit 2005;27:123–31.

[78] van den Berg AP, Twilhaar WN, Mesander G, van Son WJ, et al. Quantitation of immunosuppression by flow cytometric measurement of the capacity of T cells for interleukin-2 production. Transplantation 1998;65:1066–71.

[79] Chen Y, McKenna GJ, Yoshida EM, Buczkowski AK, et al. Assessment of immunologic status of liver transplant recipients by peripheral blood mononuclear cells in response to stimulation by donor alloantigen. Ann Surg 1999;230:242–50.

[80] Millán O, Benitez C, Guillén D, Lopez A, et al. Biomarkers of immunoregulatory status in stable liver transplant recipients undergoing weaning of immunosuppressive therapy. Clin Immunol 2010;137:337–46.

[81] Millán O, Rafael-Valdivia L, Torrademé E, Lopez A, et al. Intracellular IFN-γ and IL-2 expression monitoring as surrogate markers of the risk of acute rejection and personal drug response in *de novo* liver transplant recipients. Cytokine 2013;61:556–64.

[82] Ashokkumar C, Bentlejewski C, Sun Q, Higgs BW, et al. Allospecific CD154+ B cells associate with intestine allograft rejection in children. Transplantation 2010;90:1226–31.

[83] Ashokkumar C, Talukdar A, Sun Q, Higgs BW, et al. Allospecific CD154+ T cells associate with rejection risk after pediatric liver transplantation. Am J Transplant 2009;9:179–91.

[84] Boleslawski E, BenOthman S, Grabar S, Correia L, et al. CD25, CD28 and CD38 expression in peripheral blood lymphocytes as a tool to predict acute rejection after liver transplantation. Clin Transplant 2008;22:494–501.

[85] Boleslawski E, Othman SB, Aoudjehane L, Chouzenoux S, et al. CD28 expression by peripheral blood lymphocytes as a potential predictor of the development of *de novo* malignancies in long-term survivors after liver transplantation. Liver Transpl 2011;17:299–305.

[86] Wieland E, Shipkova M, Martius Y, Hasche G, et al. Association between pharmacodynamic biomarkers and clinical events in the early phase after kidney transplantation: a single-center pilot study. Ther Drug Monit 2011;33:341–9.

[87] Augustine JJ, Hricik DE. T-cell immune monitoring by the ELISPOT assay for interferon gamma. Clin Chim Acta 2012;413:1359–63.

[88] Augustine JJ, Poggio ED, Heeger PS, Hricik DE. Preferential benefit of antibody induction therapy in kidney recipients with high pretransplant frequencies of donor-reactive interferon-gamma enzyme-linked immunosorbent spots. Transplantation 2008;86:529–34.

[89] Bestard O, Cruzado JM, Lucia M, Crespo E, et al. Prospective assessment of antidonor cellular alloreactivity is a tool for guidance of immunosuppression in kidney transplantation. Kidney Int 2013;84:1226–36.

[90] Sanchez AM, Rountree W, Berrong M, Ambrosia G, et al. The External Quality Assurance Oversight Laboratory (EQAPOL) proficiency program for IFN-gamma enzyme-linked immunospot (IFN-γ ELISpot) assay. J Immunol Methods 2014;409:31–43.

[91] Bestard O, Crespo E, Stein M, Lucia M, et al. Cross-validation of IFN-γ Elispot assay for measuring alloreactive memory/effector T cell responses in renal transplant recipients. Am J Transplant 2013;13:1880–90.

[92] Heidt S, Shankar S, Muthusamy AS, San Segundo D, et al. Pretransplant serum CXCL9 and CXCL10 levels fail to predict acute rejection in kidney transplant recipients receiving induction therapy. Transplantation 2011;91:e59–61.

[93] Rotondi M, Netti GS, Lazzeri E, Stallone G, et al. High pretransplant serum levels of CXCL9 are associated with increased risk of acute rejection and graft failure in kidney graft recipients. Transpl Int 2010;23:465–75.

[94] Fischereder M, Schroppel B. The role of chemokines in acute renal allograft rejection and chronic allograft injury. Front Biosci (Landmark Ed) 2009;14:1807–14.

[95] Kowalski RJ, Post DR, Mannon RB, Sebastian A, et al. Assessing relative risks of infection and rejection: a meta-analysis using an immune function assay. Transplantation 2006;82:663–8.

[96] Israeli M, Yussim A, Mor E, Sredni B, et al. Preceding the rejection: in search for a comprehensive post-transplant immune monitoring platform. Transpl Immunol 2007;18:7–12.

[97] Israeli M, Ben-Gal T, Yaari V, Valdman A, et al. Individualized immune monitoring of cardiac transplant recipients by noninvasive longitudinal cellular immunity tests. Transplantation 2010;89:968–76.

[98] Cabrera R, Ararat M, Soldevila-Pico C, Dixon L, et al. Using an immune functional assay to differentiate acute cellular rejection from recurrent hepatitis C in liver transplant patients. Liver Transpl 2009;15:216–22.

[99] Schulz-Juergensen S, Burdelski MM, Oellerich M, Brandhorst G. Intracellular ATP production in CD4+ T cells as a predictor for infection and allograft rejection in trough-level guided pediatric liver transplant recipients under calcineurin-inhibitor therapy. Ther Drug Monit 2012;34:4–10.

[100] Israeli M, Klein T, Brandhorst G, Oellerich M. Confronting the challenge: individualized immune monitoring after organ transplantation using the cellular immune function assay. Clin Chim Acta 2012;413:1374–8.

[101] Sánchez-Velasco P, Rodrigo E, Valero R, Ruiz JC, et al. Intracellular ATP concentrations of CD4 cells in kidney transplant patients with and without infection. Clin Transplant 2008;22:55–60.

[102] Kobashigawa JA, Kiyosaki KK, Patel JK, Kittleson MM, et al. Benefit of immune monitoring in heart transplant patients using ATP production in activated lymphocytes. J Heart Lung Transplant 2010;29:504–8.

[103] Ravaioli M, Morelli M, Del Gaudio M, Zanello M, et al. Immunosuppression monitoring by Cylex ImmuKnow test after liver transplantation: preliminary results of randomized prospective trial. Transpl Int 2011;24:227 [Abstract].

[104] Süsal C, Opelz G. Posttransplant sCD30 as a biomarker to predict kidney graft outcome. Clin Chim Acta 2012;413:1350–3.

[105] Velásquez SY, García LF, Opelz G, Alvarez CM, et al. Release of soluble CD30 after allogeneic stimulation is mediated by memory T cells and regulated by IFN-γ and IL-2. Transplantation 2013;96:154–61.

[106] Süsal C, Pelzl S, Döhler B, Opelz G. Identification of highly responsive kidney transplant recipients using pretransplant soluble CD30. J Am Soc Nephrol 2002;13:1650–6.

[107] Pelzl S, Opelz G, Daniel V, Wiesel M, et al. Evaluation of posttransplantation soluble CD30 for diagnosis of acute renal allograft rejection. Transplantation 2003;75:421–3.

[108] Süsal C, Döhler B, Sadeghi M, Salmela KT, et al. Posttransplant sCD30 as a predictor of kidney graft outcome. Transplantation 2011;91:1364–9.

[109] Weimer R, Süsal C, Yildiz S, Staak A, et al. Post-transplant sCD30 and neopterin as predictors of chronic allograft nephropathy: impact of different immunosuppressive regimens. Am J Transplant 2006;6:1865–74.

[110] Billing H, Sander A, Süsal C, Ovens J, et al. Soluble CD30 and ELISA-detected human leukocyte antigen antibodies for the prediction of acute rejection in pediatric renal transplant recipients. Transpl Int 2013;26:331–8.

[111] Halim MA, Al-Otaibi T, Al-Muzairai I, Mansour M, et al. Serial soluble CD30 measurements as a predictor of kidney graft outcome. Transplant Proc 2010;42:801–3.

[112] Kovač J, Arnol M, Vidan Jeras B, Bren AF, et al. Pretransplant soluble CD30 serum concentration does not affect kidney graft outcomes 3 years after transplantation. Transplant Proc 2010;42:4043–6.

[113] Chen Y, Tai Q, Hong S, Kong Y, et al. Pretransplantation soluble CD30 level as a predictor of acute rejection in kidney transplantation: a meta-analysis. Transplantation 2012;94:911–8.

[114] Barraclough KA, Staatz CE, Johnson DW, Gillis D, et al. A differential impact of mycophenolic acid, prednisolone, and tacrolimus exposure on sCD30 levels in adult kidney transplant recipients. Ther Drug Monit 2013;35:240–5.

[115] Spiridon C, Nikaein A, Lerman M, Hunt J, et al. CD30, a marker to detect the high-risk kidney transplant recipients. Clin Transplant 2008;22:765–9.

[116] Altermann W, Schlaf G, Rothhoff A, Seliger B. High variation of individual soluble serum CD30 levels of pre-transplantation patients: sCD30 a feasible marker for prediction of kidney allograft rejection? Nephrol Dial Transplant 2007;22:2795–9.

[117] Pavlov I, Martins TB, Delgado JC. Development and validation of a fluorescent microsphere immunoassay for soluble CD30 testing. Clin Vaccine Immunol 2009;16:1327–31.

[118] Vasconcellos LM, Schachter AD, Zheng XX, Vasconcellos LH, et al. Cytotoxic lymphocyte gene expression in peripheral blood leukocytes correlates with rejecting renal allografts. Transplantation 1998;66:562–6.

[119] Netto MV, Fonseca BA, Dantas M, Saber LT, et al. Granzyme B, FAS-ligand and perforin expression during acute cellular rejection episodes after kidney transplantation: comparison between blood and renal aspirates. Transplant Proc 2002;34:476–8.

[120] Aquino-Dias EC, Joelsons G, da Silva DM, Berdichewski AR, et al. Non-invasive diagnosis of acute rejection in kidney transplants with delayed graft function. Kidney Int 2008;73:877–84.

[121] Suthanthiran M, Ding R, Sharma V, Abecassis M, et al. Urinary cell messenger RNA expression signatures anticipate acute cellular rejection: a report from CTOT-04. Am J Transplant 2011;11(Suppl. 2):29.

[122] Simon T, Opelz G, Wiesel M, Ott RC, et al. Serial peripheral blood perforin and granzyme B gene expression measurements for prediction of acute rejection in kidney graft recipients. Am J Transplant 2003;3:1121–7.

[123] Veale JL, Liang LW, Zhang Q, Gjertson DW, et al. Noninvasive diagnosis of cellular and antibody-mediated rejection by perforin and granzyme B in renal allografts. Hum Immunol 2006;67:777–86.

[124] Graziotto R, Del Prete D, Rigotti P, Anglani F, et al. Perforin, Granzyme B, and fas ligand for molecular diagnosis of acute renal-allograft rejection: analyses on serial biopsies suggest methodological issues. Transplantation 2006;81(8):1125–32.

[125] Schlickeiser S, Sawitzki B. Peripheral biomarkers for individualizing immunosuppression in transplantation-regulatory T cells. Clin Chim Acta 2012;413:1406–13.

[126] San Segundo D, Fernández-Fresnedo G, Ruiz JC, Rodrigo E, et al. Two-year follow-up of a prospective study of circulating regulatory T cells in renal transplant patients. Clin Transplant 2010;24:386–93.

[127] Bouvy AP, Klepper M, Kho MM, Boer K, et al. The impact of induction therapy on the homeostasis and function of regulatory T cells in kidney transplant patients. Nephrol Dial Transplant 2014;29:1587–97.

[128] Dugast E, Chesneau M, Soulillou JP, Brouard S. Biomarkers and possible mechanisms of operational tolerance in kidney transplant patients. Immunol Rev 2014;258:208–17.

[129] Braza F, Soulillou JP, Brouard S. Gene expression signature in transplantation tolerance. Clin Chim Acta 2012;413:1414–8.

[130] Brouard S, Mansfield E, Braud C, Li L, et al. Identification of a peripheral blood transcriptional biomarker panel associated with operational renal allograft tolerance. Proc Natl Acad Sci U S A 2007;104:15448–53.

[131] Newell KA, Asare A, Kirk AD, Immune Tolerance Network ST507 Study Group Identification of a B cell signature associated with renal transplant tolerance in humans. J Clin Invest 2010;120:1836–47.

Graft-derived cell-free DNA as a marker of graft integrity after transplantation

7

Michael Oellerich[1], Julia Beck[2], Philipp Kanzow[1,3], Jessica Schmitz[1], Otto Kollmar[4], Philip D. Walson[1], and Ekkehard Schütz[2]

[1]*Department of Clinical Pharmacology, University Medicine Göttingen, Göttingen, Germany;*
[2]*Chronix Biomedical GmbH, Göttingen, Germany;* [3]*Department of Preventive Dentistry,
Periodontology and Cardiology, University Medicine Göttingen, Göttingen, Germany;*
[4]*Department of General Visceral and Paediatric Surgery, University Medicine Göttingen,
Göttingen, Germany*

7.1 INTRODUCTION

Approximately 30,000 patients per year in the United States receive a transplanted organ. There are another 100,000 on US waiting lists due to the shortage of donor organs and approximately 200,000 living graft recipients. In the European Union, approximately 64,000 patients were on the waiting list in 2012, of which approximately 6% died while waiting for an organ [1,2]. The discrepancy between donor availability and patients waiting for organs mandates continuing attempts to both increase donor numbers and maximize transplantation outcomes.

Short-term graft survival has improved greatly in the past few decades largely as a result of a number of improvements in organ procurement, preservation, and transport, surgical techniques, and especially the use of potent new immunosuppressive drugs and drug combinations. The selection and initial dosing of immunosuppressant drugs (ISDs) is guided by protocols that have been tested in randomized controlled trials [3]. Dosing is then adjusted in individual patients based mostly on therapeutic drug monitoring (TDM) results [4], various measures of clinical response, and routine laboratory tests.

Although the use of new ISDs with TDM-assisted dose adjustments has greatly improved transplant outcomes, short-term graft survival has improved much more than long-term outcomes [5]. The two main factors that still limit long-term outcomes in solid organ transplantation are irreversible chronic allograft dysfunction and the adverse effects of chronic or excessive ISD treatment, such as renal toxicity, cardiovascular disease, opportunistic infections, and malignancies.

Transplant patients often suffer from graft rejection. For example, the frequency of acute rejection of liver transplants within 3 years is approximately 22%, whereas for

M. Oellerich & A. Dasgupta (Eds): Personalized Immunosuppression in Transplantation.
DOI: http://dx.doi.org/10.1016/B978-0-12-800885-0.00007-2

heart and lung transplants, 3-year rejection rates are close to 50% [1]. Long-term (i.e., 10 years) kidney transplant survival, especially with grafts from deceased donors, is still only approximately 50% [6].

7.2 CAUSES OF CHRONIC ALLOGRAFT DYSFUNCTION

Chronic allograft dysfunction can result from a number of both immunologic and non-immunologic causes [7].

Immunologic causes include acute rejection episodes that are most likely to be associated with poor human leukocyte antigen (HLA) matching, prior sensitization, and delayed graft function. Subacute and chronic alloimmune responses are more likely to be associated with antibody-mediated rejection (AMR), which can also be a result of insufficient immunosuppression. Inadequate immunosuppression may result from unpredictable individual differences in ISD pharmacokinetics or individually different ISD concentrations needed to suppress the immune system or poor patient adherence to dosing recommendations.

Non-immunologic causes of chronic organ dysfunction include the use of grafts from older donors or poor quality grafts. Poor quality grafts can be associated with cadaveric donors, preservation or ischemic injury, and peritransplant injuries causing delayed graft function. Graft injury leading to chronic dysfunction can occur from a number of causes, including hypertension, hyperlipidemia, or the chronic toxic effects of ISDs such as cyclosporine or tacrolimus [8]. Disease recurrence (e.g., hepatitis C) and polyomavirus (BK)-associated nephropathy may also contribute to chronic allograft dysfunction.

Although acute rejection episodes are most often controlled with steroids and other ISDs, they still occur and can cause acute graft loss or lead to sensitization causing chronic graft damage. As reviewed in a consensus report by Kobashigawa et al. representing the views of 71 participants from 42 heart transplant centers [9], the rapid diagnosis of primary graft dysfunction (PGD) is especially important after heart transplantation (HTx), but there are no universally accepted methods available as yet for either the diagnosis or management of PGD after HTx.

7.3 NEED FOR BIOMARKERS

Because existing methods used to guide therapy are not sufficient to provide individual patients with adequate and not excessive immune suppression, a number of attempts have been made to develop biomarkers that would complement TDM and preserve allograft function through personalized immunosuppression [10,11]. To achieve this, practical biomarkers are needed, with reasonable turnaround times and costs, that can accurately and repeatedly assess solid organ function and detect early graft injury because traditional tests (e.g. serum chemistry, liver function tests (LFTs), and cardiac enzymes) of solid organ function are inadequate for this purpose.

Reliable biomarkers should be useful for the pre-transplantation prediction of the risks for rejection; for the assessment of the minimal ISD exposure necessary to suppress the immune response; to assess (near) tolerance; and for the early detection of ongoing, undiagnosed graft injury that can lead to either acute rejection or chronic allograft dysfunction.

7.4 VALUE OF CONVENTIONAL TDM

The use of TDM to guide ISD dosing is based on the fact that drug concentrations or drug exposures (as measured, e.g., by area under time–concentration curve) can better reflect pharmacodynamic (PD) effects than do administered ISD doses [12]. However, the usefulness of TDM has been well established in randomized controlled trials only for some drugs (e.g., calcineurin and mTOR inhibitors) and for selected patients treated with some other ISDs (e.g., azathioprine). TDM is not fully established for mycophenolic acid (MPA). It seems to be useful to monitor MPA, particularly in patients with reduced calcineurin inhibitor (CNI) therapy, with CNI switch or withdrawal, mycophenolate mofetil (MMF) monotherapy, and patients with high immunological risk [13,14]. For ISDs like belatacept, TDM is not established.

7.4.1 LIMITATIONS OF TDM

Generally, TDM has limitations because it is more useful to prevent toxicity than to predict efficacy. The main problem of conventional TDM is that concentrations do not precisely predict the effects of ISDs on immune cells in individual patients. There are wide inter- and intraindividual differences in the immediate- and long-term suppression of immune function as well as in the individual intralymphocyte ISD concentrations seen at any given ISD plasma or blood concentration [15,16]. In part, these differences may be explained by the synergistic and antagonistic effects of concomitant drugs as well as by pharmacogenetic differences in metabolism or cellular transport. There are many additional clinical issues involved complicating the accurate prediction of the PD efficacy of ISD concentrations in individual patients, including the number of days post-transplantation, the type of organ transplanted, the degree of mismatch, and the amount of ischemia reperfusion injury or other factors that affect graft quality [17].

Analytical issues also cause difficulties in the prediction of the effects of ISD concentrations as discussed in detail in Chapter 2. When adjusting ISD doses in individual patients, it is important for the treating clinicians to know whether the assays being used differ from those that were used to establish the ISD therapeutic (or target) ranges being applied. Furthermore, method-specific interferences and cross-reactivity issues can influence the interpretation of the results. This is illustrated (Figure 7.1) by a study showing that everolimus dosage adjustments recommended based on fluorescent polarization immunoassay results differed significantly from those based on liquid chromatography tandem mass spectrometry assay (LC–MS/MS) results for the same samples [18].

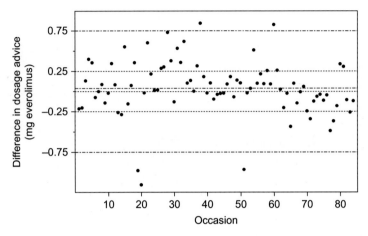

FIGURE 7.1

Differences in recommended change in the dose (in mg of everolimus) that would be recommended based on results of two different analytical methods using method adapted therapeutic ranges.

With permission from Moes et al. [18].

Poor compliance with ISD dosing is one major cause of graft failure, not only in adolescents but also in other age groups, but TDM is of limited use in detecting intermittent compliance [19]. TDM results cannot identify those patients who take their medications only during the days prior to clinic visits.

7.5 BIOMARKERS FOR IMMUNE MONITORING AS SUPPLEMENT TO TDM

A number of additional or alternative methods are being investigated in an attempt to assess the ability of any given ISD concentration/dose or ISD combinations to suppress rejection in individual transplant patients. Such methods include immune monitoring biomarkers (see Chapters 6, 8, 10, and 11) that are being investigated for their potential to improve solid organ transplant outcomes. Promising methods use biomarkers for immunological risk assessment (i.e., prediction of predisposition to acute rejection), tolerance prediction, and to better identify individuals with adequate but not excessive immune suppression [10,11]. These biomarkers, many of which are available only on an investigational basis, include assessment of other ISD PD effects on drug target enzymes (e.g., calcineurin inhibition), in vitro measures of the activation or proliferation of various T-cell populations, soluble molecules (e.g., sCD30 or donor-specific antibodies), functional T-cell assays (e.g., Cylex), or cytokines (e.g., interleukin-2 expression in CD8$^+$ T cells, NFAT-regulated gene expression), which are discussed in other chapters.

7.5.1 MINIMIZATION OF ISD EXPOSURE AND ASSESSMENT OF GRAFT FUNCTION

Minimization of ISD drug exposure is desired to decrease the risk of excessive immune suppression with subsequent infections and malignancies; however, exposure must also be adequate to suppress acute rejection episodes that can lead to immune sensitization with subsequent long-term, chronic transplant rejection and graft failure [20,21]. Identification of the minimum ISD concentration necessary to suppress rejection requires a way to reliably measure the earliest signs of rejection-related organ damage [5]. Currently used methods are not adequate to do this. For example, conventional LFTs such as aspartate aminotransferase (AST), alanine aminotransferase, alkaline phosphatase, γ-glutamyl transferase (GGT), bilirubin, and lactic dehydrogenase are not diagnostic for acute cellular liver rejection [22,23]. Serum creatinine (SCr) and creatinine clearance are of very limited use in identifying renal damage [24], in part because SCr is a relatively nonspecific measure of renal function that can be elevated with dehydration or altered by a number of factors, including body habitus, diet, medications, and malnutrition [25]. Renal biopsy results suggested that the false-positive (not rejection-related) SCr elevation rates were 0.65 in a series of 107 patients reported by Suthanthiran et al. [26]. However, approximately 50% of kidney function may be lost before an increase in SCr is seen [27]. Other, less commonly used measures of renal function, including inulin clearance, cystatin C, beta trace protein, and radiolabeled compounds, also have limitations [28]. In HTx the status of troponins remains controversial and neither cardiac enzyme measurements nor echocardiography results are adequate to predict early cardiac graft dysfunction [9]. In addition, although considered the gold standard, biopsies can all damage the grafts, can take days to process, are expensive, and are burdening for the patient. A major weakness of biopsy assessment lies in the large subjective component of the evaluation procedure. In a study on the comparability of endomyocardial biopsies (EMB) [29], there was only a panel concordance of 28.4% for ISHLT (International Society for Heart and Lung Transplantation System of Grading of Rejection) grade greater than or equal to 2R. These results confirm that EMB is far from being a fully standardized objective procedure.

As discussed later and in other chapters, the pre-transplantation prediction of the predisposition to post-transplant acute rejection might be useful to design personalized immunosuppressive regimens [30]. What is mostly desirable are monitoring methods that can identify candidates for ISD minimization and those who would need more robust immunosuppression. Methods are needed that can be used to improve longer-term graft survival, including biomarkers that can predict the risk for graft loss, identify the presence of even subclinical rejection, and rapidly, reliably, and directly interrogate graft integrity. To be clinically useful, the latter biomarkers must be available on the same day at a reasonable cost and should allow for both the continuous adjustment of personalized treatment regimens and the identification of minimal necessary drug exposures in patients with long-term stable graft function.

7.6 MOLECULAR METHODS: BIOPSY AND CELLULAR APPROACHES

Biopsy tissue is used to directly assess graft damage in solid organ transplant grafts. The histology of the graft tissue obtained can be assessed using consensus diagnostic criteria, such as is done with the Banff criteria for kidney transplant rejection [31]. In the case of documented or suspected anti-donor AMR, these criteria also include microcirculation lesions, and complement factor C4d in capillaries. However, the usefulness of the histological evaluation of biopsies, even when such consensus criteria are used, is subject to both subjective interpretation and sampling errors that can occur because the signs of rejection may not be uniform in all parts of the graft [29–33].

A number of new, molecular-based methods that use biopsy tissue are also being investigated to diagnose or predict the risk of rejection, including expression microarray tests of antibody-mediated kidney graft rejection (ABMR), which can emerge several years after transplantation [34]. In kidney transplantation, ABMR leads to the development of transplant glomerulopathy, and it is a major cause of kidney transplant failure [35].

Halloran et al. described a molecular pathology test based on the observation that donor HLA-specific antibody is a major risk factor for late graft loss [36,37]. The test identifies ABMR by assigning a score based on the amount of transcripts present in kidney biopsies that are mostly expressed in endothelial or natural killer cells or that are interferon-γ inducible. This molecular expression-based score was shown to be more strongly associated with graft failure than were conventional (Banff consensus-based) assessments.

Currently, only panel-reactive antibody and HLA genotype/serotype are used pre-transplant to avoid transplant mismatch [38]. There is no biomarker in routine clinical use that can reliably predict, at the time of transplantation, what the likelihood is of post-transplant acute cellular rejection. However, Hollander et al. described a biomarker panel that allowed for the prediction of acute cardiac graft rejection using donor heart tissue and pre-transplant recipient blood gene expression [30]. Their donor heart tissue panel included 25 transcripts of several well-known immunologic pathways, including vascular endothelial growth factor, epidermal growth factor receptor (EGFR) signaling, and mitogen-activated protein kinase, as well as 18 transcripts mostly involved in integrin-mediated cell surface interactions measured in pre-transplant recipient's blood. EGFR expression might stimulate the accumulation of macrophages and lymphocytes within cardiac tissue, which can accelerate a more aggressive immune response in the recipient. The results suggest that individuals showing a greater number of circulating activated lymphocytes are predisposed to developing heart graft rejection. They suggested that, provided the validity of this approach is verified, patients with a higher likelihood of developing acute rejection might be given higher initial ISD doses to prevent rejection. However, although perhaps not as relevant for liver transplant (LTx) as for kidney or heart grafts, it is logical to assume that donor characteristics (e.g., quality of the match and organ quality) that are not evaluated by this method would also affect graft survival.

In another molecular approach, Suthanthiran et al. used both biopsy specimens (410 biopsies from 220 recipients) and mRNA isolated from urinary sediment cells in 4300 samples from 485 kidney allograft recipients to develop a potential noninvasive test for acute kidney allograft cellular rejection [26]. These authors reported that a three-gene expression signature (CD3ε mRNA, IP-10 mRNA, and 18S rRNA) measured in urinary cells could be used to (1) distinguish acute cellular and acute AMR and (2) both diagnose acute cellular kidney allograft rejection and predict its progression. These authors also showed that urinary tract infections did not affect the signature and that the average trajectory of changes of the signature in repeated samples showed a sharp rise weeks before biopsies demonstrated signs of cellular rejection. However, the usefulness of the test in individual kidney transplant patients or to evaluate individual events has yet to be demonstrated, whereas a number of concerns have been raised about the validity and clinical utility of this approach [39–42]. A major disadvantage of this approach is the fact that this test cannot be used to diagnose AMR [39]. Furthermore, the described signature is also elevated in patients with polyomavirus type BK (BKV) infection [40].

7.6.1 CELL-FREE MOLECULAR METHODS

Acellular molecular diagnostic methods have also been examined, which include the use of urine or plasma microRNAs (miRNA), donor-derived urinary chromosome Y cell-free DNA (cfDNA), as well as massive parallel sequencing and droplet digital PCR (ddPCR) to measure donor-derived cfDNA in plasma.

The miRNAs are short, noncoding RNA sequences that have been investigated as potential biomarkers in a number of diseases. These nucleic acids are present in both plasma and urine. Their expression differs among and between organs and organ regions. They have been investigated for their potential use in transplantation despite a number of unanswered questions about both the role of miRNAs in organ transplantation and their basic biology, including their regulation, association with host genes, and their specific targets. Their potential use to assess donor organ quality and predict short- and long-term graft survival as well as acute rejection, chronic allograft dysfunction, and transplant tolerance has been reviewed by Mas et al. [5]. However, although they may have potential, as yet no miRNA tests have been proven to be clinically useful in the management of individual transplant patients.

7.6.1.1 Graft-derived cell-free chromosome Y-specific DNA

The initial methods to noninvasively detect graft rejection used gender mismatched donor/recipient pairs to identify increased donor-derived, graft DNA in the blood or urine of transplant recipients. Lo et al. were the first to demonstrate the presence of donor-derived DNA sequences in the plasma of liver and kidney transplant recipients [43]. In samples from 8 female liver and 28 female kidney recipients, the presence of DNA in plasma originating from a male donor was reported.

Sigdel et al. used a Y-chromosome (HSY)-specific dPCR to measure urinary, donor-derived cfDNA as a surrogate marker of kidney transplant injury in 63 female patients (41 stable and 22 with allograft injury) who had received grafts from male donors [44]. Patients with acute rejection had significantly higher values than patients with stable graft function or with chronic allograft injury. No difference between patients with acute rejection and those with human BKV infection was found, suggesting that urinary graft DNA was a non-rejection-specific, universal marker of kidney graft injury. An obvious, serious limitation of measuring HSY cfDNA is that it can only be applied to male/female donor/recipient pairs. In addition, as opposed to acute rejection, urine might not be the best sample source to search for chronic renal allograft injury because changes in renal excretion will influence urinary cfDNA concentrations. Finally, there are also problems associated with HSY chimerism [45], and these methods are only applicable to renal grafts.

7.6.1.2 Donor-specific cfDNA methods as liquid biopsies

Measurement of graft-derived, plasma cell-free DNA (GcfDNA) that does not require donor/recipient gender mismatch is a general, noninvasive test being used for the early detection of acute rejection. It involves the parallel determination of cfDNA from both donor and recipient in plasma, which can be used for any type of solid organ grafts.

Recently, massive whole-genome, shotgun, or targeted sequencing has been done to identify reads with donor- and recipient-specific single-nucleotide polymorphism (SNP) calls, which are used to calculate the percentage of donor (graft) DNA. Then the percentage of graft DNA is monitored over time and compared to values obtained in graft recipients who have long-term stable graft function as well as either no evidence of rejection or even operational tolerance. Any increase in the percentage of graft DNA can be identified and indicate graft damage from rejection or other causes.

In a study of HTx patients, Snyder et al. used shotgun sequencing to demonstrate the proof of the concept that graft-derived DNA could be used to detect early graft rejection [46]. GcfDNA percentages were statistically significantly lower in plasma samples ($n = 23$) from stable HTx patients (mean, 0.5%; range, $\leq 2.0\%$) than either in samples ($n = 15$) from patients just prior to a rejection episode (mean, 1.6%; range, $\leq 4.6\%$) or in samples ($n = 6$) from patients during rejection episodes (mean, 2.9%; range, 0.4–4.5%). They presented graphically the percentage of donor DNA over time for one HTx patient prior to and after a grade 3A rejection episode, showing that donor DNA increased substantially 3 months before rejection was proven by biopsy. Such an early indication would allow for individual adaptation of immunosuppressive therapy to prevent full-blown rejection. However, the routine use of these massive sequencing methods is limited by the time required (days), the cost of the methods, and the need to have access to donor DNA. The last limitation is a major problem in many countries, including those in the European Union, because of patient confidentiality laws. Furthermore, donor DNA is often not available for patients who received their transplants several years ago.

7.6.1.3 GcfDNA assay based on ddPCR

A new method has been developed using ddPCR that overcomes the limitations of other cell-free, graft DNA methods, particularly the long turnaround time (days), expensive, deep sequencing methods [47]. This method measures GcfDNA as a "liquid biopsy" to directly interrogate graft integrity. It is being used to identify rejection episodes and to directly measure the effects of ISDs in donor/recipient pairs without access to donor DNA. This method provides a rapid (same day), practical, cost-effective, universal way to directly interrogate donor organs using only reasonable blood sample volumes (~5–10 mL) without need to have access to DNA from the donor. This novel method has the potential to become a routine assay for the measurement of graft integrity.

The assay introduced by Beck et al., instead of inferring GcfDNA from SNP calls obtained by shotgun sequencing of the genome, used a small preselected library of approximately 41 SNPs that have a reported minor allele frequency (MAF) of greater than 40% [47]. The MAF is the frequency at which a less common allele occurs in a population. The most useful SNP assays are those homozygous in both donor and recipient but heterologous between the graft and recipient (AA/BB or BB/AA). SNPs homozygous in the patient and heterozygous in the graft (i.e., AA/AB or BB/AB) can be used also, but they have less sensitivity. Based on general population genomics, approximately 12.5% of assays selected for high MAF will be homozygous with heterologous alleles in graft and recipient, whereas another 25% will have a heterozygous difference.

From the first blood sample of an individual patient, the white blood cells (WBCs) that contain only the genomic DNA of the recipient are collected in addition to the plasma, which contains both cfDNA of the recipient and the graft. Special tubes, preventing degranulation of WBCs, are available for situations in which the sample cannot be processed within 4 h. The DNA extracted from WBCs is first used to identify homozygous SNPs from the library of greater than 40 selected SNPs. The first plasma sample of an individual patient is used to detect those SNPs for which the graft carries the heterologous allele in either homozygous or heterozygous state. In this initial assays selection, the best informative assay combination for the individual patient is obtained, which is then used for all subsequent plasma samples. By focusing the screening on a preselected set of SNPs and the later testing only on the informative subset, the method is more cost and time efficient compared to high-throughput sequencing or microarray hybridization.

The quantification of GcfDNA is performed with ddPCR [48] to calculate the percentage of donor DNA in the sample, where at least three independent SNP assays are used [47]. Due to the low amount of cfDNA extractable from the plasma samples, a preamplification step is performed in order to generate enough DNA to use 50–100 ng in each independent ddPCR assay. In ddPCR, each processed sample is partitioned into 20,000 droplets, into which template molecules are separated, and amplification occurs in each individual droplet. PCR is then performed on a thermal cycler using TaqMan hydrolysis probes. After PCR amplification, each droplet provides a specific fluorescent (positive) or a nonfluorescent (negative) signal for either allele in different fluorescence channels, indicating whether the graft or recipient target cfCNA was present or not. The positive and negative droplets are then counted, and Poisson statistics are used to calculate the average number of target molecules present in the droplets, which leads to the percentage of GcfDNA present in the circulation.

This assay had a mean recovery of added DNA of 94% (standard deviation, 13%) with an imprecision of 4–14% when controls were used that contained 2% minor allele [47]. The provisional cutoff value for GcfDNA after LTx was set at less than 10% based on results from a group of 10 stable adult LTx recipients, all of whom had values of less than 6.8%. Although not discussed further in this chapter, results in our ongoing studies were less than 0.5% in stable post kidney transplant patients and were less than 0.6% in stable post HTx patients.

Data (GcfDNA percentages, LFTs, ISD concentrations, and clinical events) from samples obtained at multiple time points after LTx are presented here for a number of adult LTx patients who were studied initially (see Figures 7.2–7.4 and 7.8).

ISD concentrations were measured using a published LC–MS/MS assay [49]. The LFTs were measured in the accredited hospital clinical laboratory using standard, automated techniques (Abbott Architect), and all patients were treated according to a standard post-LTx protocol.

7.6.1.4 Use of GcfDNA to identify rejection episodes

One complicated patient was reported (Figure 7.2), who had been re-transplanted, received protocol-driven immunosuppressive therapy during and after surgery, and received standard of care ISD dosing adjusted using results of routine TDM monitoring to reach target tacrolimus concentrations [50]. The patient also received CellCept

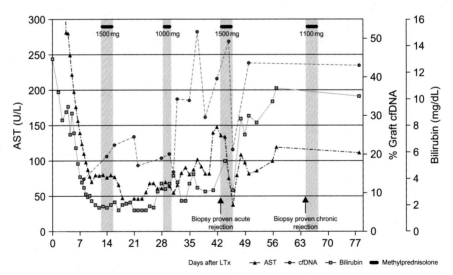

FIGURE 7.2

LTx patient with several rejection episodes. GcfDNA, AST, and bilirubin values are shown over time (days) post LTx. Methylprednisolone doses and tacrolimus target concentrations (shaded area) are also indicated. Results show that during rejection episodes, there was an increase in GcfDNA days before increases were seen in AST or bilirubin. *These figures are reproduced in color in the color plate section.*

With permission from Beck et al. [50].

(MMF, 1 g twice per day) and multiple methylprednisolone boluses for multiple rejection episodes. This patient had biopsy-proven acute rejection episodes that subsequently resulted in chronic rejection. As shown in Figure 7.2, there was a steep increase in GcfDNA up to 50%, which started several days before AST and bilirubin increased.

These results suggest that, as also shown by Snyder et al. in HTx patients [46], GcfDNA can rapidly identify rejection episodes. In this case, GcfDNA was more useful than were the traditional LFTs.

7.6.1.5 Use of GcfDNA to monitor responses to ISD dosing changes

Both LFTs and GcfDNA results are also shown for a patient (Figure 7.3) who was transplanted because of alcoholic hepatic cirrhosis. An initial infection led to use of decreased tacrolimus doses and concentrations resulting in an increase in GcfDNA percentage as well as AST. Subsequently, multiple infections demanding decreased tacrolimus doses finally led to the complete replacement of tacrolimus with only MPA and steroids. After these changes, GcfDNA increased to very high levels, and the patient developed biopsy-proven rejection. After tacrolimus was restarted, there was a rapid drop in GcfDNA, whereas the rate of AST decrease was much slower. GcfDNA in this case clearly reflected (retrospectively) the presence of insufficient immune suppression.

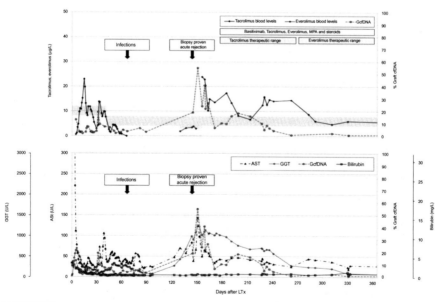

FIGURE 7.3

GcfDNA, LFTs, and ISD concentrations are shown for a patient who had an infection that resulted in decreases in ISD dosing, which led to an acute rejection episode that responded to increased ISD exposure. *These figures are reproduced in color in the color plate section.*

Adapted from Kanzow [51].

7.6.1.6 Use of GcfDNA to monitor marginal donor graft integrity

The lack of adequate numbers of organ donors has led to the increasing use of grafts from marginal donors. This complicates the interpretation of traditional LFT results because LFTs are not adequate to diagnose liver graft integrity [52]. The ability of GcfDNA to directly assess graft integrity may be especially useful in the management of such patients who receive grafts from marginal donors.

We recently reported retrospective GcfDNA results from such a patient who was transplanted because of alcoholic hepatic cirrhosis and received a graft from a donor who had died from HELLP (hemodialysis, elevated liver enzymes, low platelet count) syndrome [53]. Initial protocol treatment also consisted of basiliximab, tacrolimus, CellCept, and methylprednisolone.

In this patient, there was a rapid initial decrease in GcfDNA. The rate of decrease was similar to that observed in LTx patients who received grafts from nonmarginal donors (see Figure 7.2), which suggested that the pre-transplant graft damage was rapidly reversed and was consistent with this patient's eventual successful engraftment. During the period prior to stabilization, there were increases in GcfDNA that correctly rapidly reflected both immune-mediated (i.e., rejection) and non-immune-related (i.e., a traumatic hematoma) graft damage. As a result of a fall, the patient developed a post-traumatic liver hematoma with presumed liver ischemia that was associated with an approximately 90% increase in the percentage of graft DNA that was secondary to ischemic rather than immune-mediated organ damage. However, as would be predicted, increases in ISD concentrations were followed by decreases in GcfDNA when immune-related rejection was present but not when the increased GcfDNA was due to a non-rejection-associated cause (i.e., a hematoma). Despite a complicated course, the patient eventually was discharged from the hospital and was doing well more than 9 months after transplantation.

The ability of GcfDNA to rapidly, reliably, and directly monitor graft damage, regardless of cause, could be useful to improve outcomes in LTx patients, perhaps especially in the growing number of patients who receive grafts from marginal donors where pre-engraftment damage can already be extensive.

7.6.1.7 Specificity of GcfDNA for graft integrity

Results shown in Figure 7.4 are from a patient without rejection who developed post-LTx cholangiopathy. This patient was transplanted for cirrhosis as a result of hepatitis C virus (HCV) and received the same ISD protocol dosing with TDM as the other patients discussed previously. HCV copies at the time of transplantation were 1.9×10^5 U/mL and were 3×10^6 U/mL on day 151. The patient's HCV infection was stable on day 147; the day when cholestasis due to post-LTx cholangiopathy was eventually diagnosed to have occurred.

Increased LFTs were noted, first both GGT and AST increased, followed by increases in bilirubin concentrations. These LFT elevations all persisted despite major increases in tacrolimus doses and subsequent concentrations. GcfDNA, however, remained low, as would be expected in cholestasis with no signs of significant hepatocellular damage (as opposed to rejection). These findings suggest that

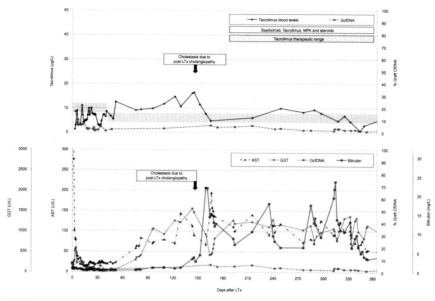

FIGURE 7.4

GcfDNA, LFTs, and ISD concentrations in a HCV+ patient who had an episode of cholestasis post-LTx. The therapeutic (target) ranges used to adjust ISD dosing are shown as shaded areas. *These figures are reproduced in color in the color plate section.*

Adapted from Kanzow [51].

GcfDNA had a higher specificity than traditional LFTs for the assessment of actual graft integrity.

The use of GcfDNA to assess the effects on graft integrity of therapeutic tacrolimus concentrations in LTx recipients with a number of clinical conditions, only some of which are associated with graft injury, was retrospectively assessed. Results obtained in 18 patients on days 8–30 after LTx with various single and multiple causes of elevated LFTs with or without graft dysfunction were examined. GcfDNA values in LTx patients with hepatitis C infection (HCV+), cholestasis without rejection, low (<8 µg/L) tacrolimus concentrations, and rejection episodes were compared to values (cutoff 10%) obtained in a historical control group ($n = 10$) of stable adult LTx patients without any clinical or laboratory indications of graft dysfunction or rejection (Figure 7.5) [47].

As shown in Figure 7.5, stable HCV− LTx patients had normal (i.e., <10%) GcfDNA values when their trough tacrolimus concentrations were greater than or equal to 8 µg/L. However, a number of stable HCV− patients (5/11) with low tacrolimus concentrations (<8 µg/L) had elevations of GcfDNA, indicating organ injury. HCV+ patients also had elevated GcfDNA values, suggesting virus-associated organ damage. This damage was even more evident in HCV+ patients who also had subtherapeutic (<8 µg/L) tacrolimus concentrations. Patients with acute rejection,

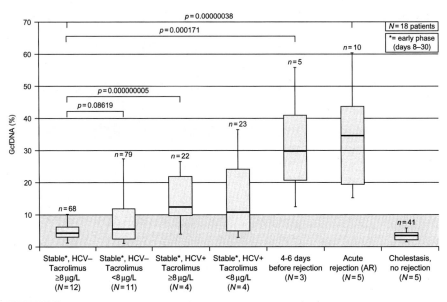

FIGURE 7.5

GcfDNA percentages obtained early after transplantation in LTx patients ($N = 18$) who had a variety of clinical conditions and either therapeutic or subtherapeutic trough tacrolimus concentrations measured. Results are compared to illustrate the potential usefulness of GcfDNA to assess the PD effects of tacrolimus in a number of different clinical situations [51,54]. The five patients with cholestasis had no signs of significant hepatocellular damage. Boxes represent median with interquartile, whiskers the 5th–95th percentile, and n the number of contributing GcfDNA values.

regardless of HCV status, had the highest GcfDNA values (~50%), and the increases in GcfDNA were noted 6–10 days before acute graft rejection was diagnosed. Patients with no signs of significant hepatocellular damage suffering from intrahepatic cholestasis ($n = 2$), drug-induced cholestasis ($n = 1$), or post-LTx cholangiopathy ($n = 2$) had GcfDNA values less than 10% (Figure 7.5). Changes observed with AST, GGT, and bilirubin showed more overlap between the described groups, rendering these tests less specific [51].

The increase in GcfDNA prior to the clinical diagnosis of rejection episodes in these LTx patients is similar to that reported by Snyder et al. in HTx patients using the more complex massive sequencing methods [46].

7.6.1.8 Use of GcfDNA to define therapeutic (or target) concentrations

Because the minimal effective concentration is what defines the bottom of therapeutic (or target) ranges, and because GcfDNA is a direct measure of organ damage, we used GcfDNA to examine the minimally effective tacrolimus concentration for LTx patients as shown in Figure 7.6 [55].

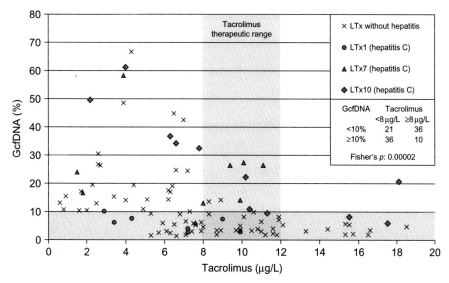

FIGURE 7.6

GcfDNA percentages are plotted against trough tacrolimus blood concentrations.

With permission from Oellerich et al. [55].

In Figure 7.6, GcfDNA values are compared to trough tacrolimus blood concentrations obtained on days 5–30 post-LTx. Interpretation of the GcfDNA percentages in the first 5 days post-transplant were assumed to be complicated by the presence of graft damage from collection, transport, and reperfusion. In addition, the cutoff values used were based on samples from stable LTx patients many months postsurgery rather than during this period. Although there were some potentially important differences between HCV$^+$ and HCV$^-$ patients, GcfDNA was elevated in the majority of patients, with tacrolimus concentrations below the bottom of the target range recommended by a European Consensus Conference [56] and used by our transplant surgeons during this period (i.e., 8–12 μg/L). The data presented in Figure 7.6 were analyzed using receiver operating characteristic analysis to re-examine the bottom of the tacrolimus therapeutic range in the first 8–30 days after LTx, with a GcfDNA percentage less than 10% assumed to reflect the desired PD effect of tacrolimus [55]. This analysis suggested that the bottom of the tacrolimus therapeutic range during days 5–30 in adult LTx patients was 6.8 μg/L.

This result is almost identical to that of another, independent report (Figure 7.7) on early tacrolimus exposure after LTx [23]. These authors, in this totally independent study, reported that graft survival was better with mean trough tacrolimus concentrations of 7–10 ng/mL than with less than 7 ng/mL ($p = 0.008$) or with 10–15 ng/mL ($p = 0.016$). Furthermore, tacrolimus trough concentrations of greater than 7 ng/mL on the day of protocol biopsies were associated with fewer patients classified as having moderate/severe rejection (23.8%) compared to patients with troughs of less than

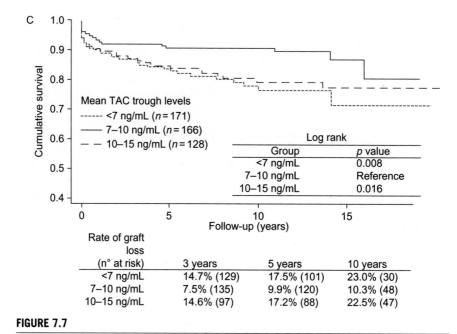

Rate of graft loss (n° at risk)	3 years	5 years	10 years
<7 ng/mL	14.7% (129)	17.5% (101)	23.0% (30)
7–10 ng/mL	7.5% (135)	9.9% (120)	10.3% (48)
10–15 ng/mL	14.6% (97)	17.2% (88)	22.5% (47)

FIGURE 7.7

The 3-, 5-, and 10-year cumulative survival curves for LTx patients who had trough tacrolimus concentrations either less than 7, 7–10 or 10–15 ng/mL are compared.

With permission from Rodriguez-Perálvarez et al. [23].

7 ng/mL (41.2%, $p = 0.004$). Only tacrolimus concentrations less than 7 ng/mL were associated with liver graft rejection-related mortality [23].

Taken together, these results suggest that GcfDNA results could be used to predict graft outcome and that any elevations in GcfDNA associated with low ISD concentrations after LTx may have negative implications for long-term graft survival because it is known that uncontrolled organ damage can be associated with immune sensitization and chronic allograft dysfunction.

7.6.1.9 Use of GcfDNA to monitor effects of ISD combinations and dosing change

A number of infectious as well as immune and surgical conditions require changes in ISD doses or combinations during both the initial days to weeks after LTx and months later. Examples include the use of reduced doses of CNIs (with or without changes in concomitant MPA doses) or the switch from tacrolimus to everolimus in patients with renal compromise. Assessment of the adequacy of immune suppression is especially problematic during such periods because therapeutic or target ranges may not be applicable in such settings.

We therefore examined the relationship between the ISD concentrations and GcfDNA percentages obtained in LTx recipients during clinically indicated

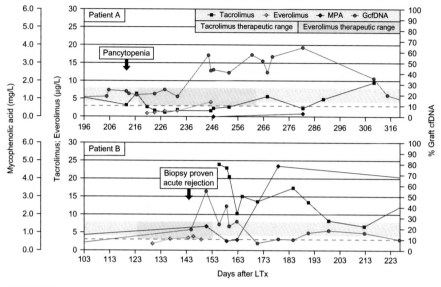

FIGURE 7.8

GcfDNA, LFTs, and ISD in patients whose IS therapies were switched. *These figures are reproduced in color in the color plate section.*

Adapted from Kanzow [51].

tacrolimus/everolimus switches in patients both with and without concomitant MPA treatment. Results were examined graphically and used to compare the effects of ISD concentrations and clinical events on GcfDNA (Figure 7.8). Tacrolimus, everolimus, and MPA concentrations were all measured using routine LC–MS/MS methods [49,57], and GcfDNA percentages were measured using ddPCR [47]. GcfDNA changes during tacrolimus/everolimus switches with or without concomitant MPA were correlated with rejection episodes but were both highly variable and not well predicted by tacrolimus or everolimus concentrations (Figure 7.8).

The clinical course is graphically presented for two selected LTx patients who underwent clinically indicated tacrolimus/everolimus switches with or without concomitant MPA therapy (Figure 7.8). ISD concentrations obtained were retrospectively compared to GcfDNA results. ISD (tacrolimus, everolimus, and MPA) concentrations and published therapeutic ranges, as well as rejection episodes and other clinical events, are displayed graphically to demonstrate the ability of GcfDNA to measure individual responses to complicated changes in ISD doses and combination regimens.

Data from one LTx patient enrolled in the study (patient A) were collected during and after an attempted switch from tacrolimus to everolimus. Initially when both tacrolimus and everolimus concentrations were below their respective target ranges (see Figure 7.8), the GcfDNA increased to greater than 10%, which is consistent with what would be expected in subclinical rejection. Based on the patient's clinical condition and LFTs (and not the GcfDNA results), the clinicians managing this patient stopped the switch and gave high-dose tacrolimus. This resulted in supratherapeutic tacrolimus concentrations and decreasing GcfDNA.

GcfDNA increased in a further patient (patient B) during a rejection episode that occurred when everolimus concentrations were below the therapeutic range (in combination with MPA). GcfDNA normalized only after the patient was switched back from everolimus to tacrolimus doses that resulted in supratherapeutic tacrolimus concentrations (also in combination with MPA). During ISD switches, when both tacrolimus and everolimus were being given (with or without MPA and methylprednisolone), the tacrolimus, everolimus, and MPA concentrations that were required to prevent or control elevations of GcfDNA in these and other similar patients varied widely and were not well predicted by published "therapeutic ranges."

Although the GcfDNA results were not made available or used to make therapeutic decisions in these patients, these results suggest that GcfDNA could be used to monitor the need for, and effects of, changes in ISD regimens during switches or whenever combinations of ISDs are used.

The ability to safely minimize or stop ISD therapy requires a way to reliably and rapidly diagnose changes in graft integrity after any change in dose or drug regimen. Although not yet proven in controlled, prospective multicenter trials, GcfDNA results might be especially useful during attempts at ISD minimization.

7.6.2 GcfDNA LIMITATIONS

There are some practical limitations to the dd GcfDNA methods used for these LTx studies, including the need for access to droplet digital equipment and qualified personnel required to produce reliable results and interpret them. The cost of an individual test is moderate and much less than that of massive sequencing. In addition, there are many other possible uses of droplet digital DNA techniques, including the diagnosis and management of cancer and detection of minimal residual disease [58], as well as in use in monitoring immune function [59]. The cutoff ranges must be established for each analytical method, organ type, time post-transplant, and perhaps even for different ethnic groups studied.

Note that the data presented for LTx patients presented in Figures 7.2–76 and 7.8 were for the relative percentage of graft to recipient cfDNA (graft cfDNA/graft + donor cfDNA). This ratio can be affected by the amounts of both donor and recipient cfDNA present in plasma samples. Methods to accurately quantify actual cfDNA amounts are being perfected [60]. Because this ratio is determined by the circulating amount of both graft and recipient DNA, the percentage would decrease whenever there was damage to more recipient than graft cells. Graft recipients can develop a number of clinical conditions, such as severe infections, that might increase the amount of circulating, cell-free, recipient DNA more than the amount of graft DNA and thereby lower the ratio. For these and other reasons, until further studies are done, it is still not known whether GcfDNA quantification will prove to be more or less clinically useful than the GcfDNA percentage alone [61].

7.7 CONCLUSIONS

The use of GcfDNA has tremendous potential to improve solid organ transplant outcomes. Organ transplants are also genome transplants—a fact that opens up the possibility of monitoring for allograft injury through cfdDNA measurements in recipients [62]. Results suggest that this GcfDNA method can be used as a "liquid biopsy" to directly interrogate graft integrity and to early detect acute rejection episodes in the days to months after transplantation. It also can be used to measure the therapeutic effects of ISDs in individual patients after transplantation; including during periods of ISD combination therapy and during minimization attempts. Changes in GcfDNA over time appeared to be useful to assess the effects of both clinical conditions and therapeutic interventions in transplanted organs and therefore may provide a way to individualize ISD dosing regimens and improve outcomes.

The direct measurement of organ integrity can lead to earlier detection of cellular or AMR that could help provide more effective, individualized therapy. This could be used to more effectively prevent full-blown rejection and ongoing graft damage that if undiagnosed or diagnosed too late can result in chronic allograft dysfunction and graft failure. This would be especially useful during ISD minimization attempts.

GcfDNA has major advantages over other tests used in solid organ transplantation, such as biopsies, LFTs, SCr, or cardiac echocardiographs (ECHOs). Biopsies are invasive, have major risks, are expensive, and are subject to both sampling errors and subjective interpretations. LFTs are not specific and are inadequate to predict the effects of immune suppression after LTx. SCr may not increase until after major rejection-associated tissue damage has occurred, and ECHOs cannot reliably detect early cardiac rejection.

GcfDNA has the potential to be a cost-effective, short turnaround-time test to directly assess the health of donor organs. It could be used alone to improve long-term graft survival or as a complement to a number of other pre- and post-transplant monitoring approaches that are currently being used. It might be especially useful to monitor graft function in response to therapeutic decisions made on the basis of other biomarkers. It would also help in situations such as compliance problems where TDM is inadequate. It could reduce the use of biopsies and replace less specific conventional organ function tests. It has special promise as a way to monitor minimization attempts in patients who appear to be immune tolerant or nearly tolerant. Finally, it might be useful to guide initial ISD regimen selection in patients who need more aggressive therapy because they have an increased risk for acute rejection or in patients who need less aggressive dosing because of increased risk or the presence of infections (Table 7.1).

Such truly personalized immune suppression requires a way to establish both minimal and maximal concentrations of single and combination ISD regimens. This will require the identification of optimal biomarker combinations. It has to be established which baseline values are most useful to select initial drug regimens or to tailor tolerance-permissive immune suppressive regimens. Methods such as GcfDNA can directly, rapidly, and cost-effectively measure organ integrity in response to changes in clinical status and pharmacologic treatments. When combined with better methods to predict

Table 7.1 Use of GcfDNA in Transplantation

Identification of recipients
- at risk of acute rejection or for late graft loss
- with ongoing undetected graft injury leading to chronic allograft dysfunction
- where TDM is inadequate (e.g., compliance problems, especially in adolescents)
- for clarification of nonspecific elevation of conventional organ function tests
- to guide changes in immunosuppression
- to achieve personalized immunosuppression (e.g., by minimization or more potent immunosuppression)

subjects at risk for either acute or late rejection and to measure individual changes in immune responses, the use of GcfDNA provides an effective tool for truly personalized immunosuppression. This in turn should allow a shift in emphasis in transplantation away from reaction and more toward prevention, which in turn should then make immunosuppressive drugs safer and reduce the cost of transplant health care.

All potentially useful methods must of course be carefully validated in prospective, well-controlled, multicenter clinical trials before any specific biomarker, combination, or approach can be used routinely in the clinical setting. Perhaps equally important, any proposed approaches must be shown to be practical and cost-effective to be useful. There is little benefit to identify a sophisticated panel that nobody can or will be able to pay for. Taken together, because of its benefits as liquid biopsy, GcfDNA will enable a close surveillance of transplant recipients and therefore promises to be a major part of future, more effective management in solid organ transplantation.

ACKNOWLEDGMENTS

Two of the authors are full-time employees (JB and ES) of Chronix Biomedical GmbH, the company that owns the rights to the proprietary GcfDNA ddPCR method described, and two of the authors (MO, advisory board member; and PDW) are paid consultants to Chronix Biomedical GmbH. Some of this work was the subject of the doctoral thesis of another author (PK). The assistance of many unnamed employees of both the Institute for Clinical Chemistry, University Medical Center Göttingen, and Chronix Biomedical GmbH is gratefully acknowledged, as is the support of both BMBF and Niedersachsen Professorship (MO, JS) grants. Finally, the participation of the patients who made the studies possible, as well as their families, their organ donors, and all the professionals who provided their medical care, is greatly appreciated.

REFERENCES

[1] Organ Procurement and Transplantation Network (OPTN) and Scientific Registry of Transplant Recipients (SRTR). OPTN/SRTR. 2010; Annual Data Report. Rockville, MD: Department of Health and Human Services, Health Resources and Services Administration, Healthcare Systems Bureau, Division of Transplantation; 2011.

[2] Eurotransplant International Foundation. Annual Report 2012, <http://www.eurotransplant.org/cms/mediaobject.php?file=AR2012.pdf> [accessed 08.05.14].

[3] Taylor AL, Watson CJ, Bradley JA. Immunosuppressive agents in solid organ transplantation: mechanisms of action and therapeutic efficacy. Crit Rev Oncol Hematol 2005;56:23–46.

[4] Kahan BD, Keown P, Levy GA, Johnston A. Therapeutic drug monitoring of immunosuppressant drugs in clinical practice. Clin Ther 2002;24:330–50.

[5] Mas VR, Dumur CI, Scian MJ, Gehrau RC, et al. MicroRNAs as biomarkers in solid organ transplantation. Am J Transplant 2013;13:11–19.

[6] Schröppel B, Heeger PS. Gazing into a crystal ball to predict kidney transplant outcome. J Clin Invest 2010;120:1803–6.

[7] Pascual M, Theruvath T, Kawai T, Tolkoff-Rubin N, et al. Strategies to improve long-term outcomes after renal transplantation. N Engl J Med 2002;346:580–90.

[8] Land WG. Chronic allograft dysfunction: a model disorder of innate immunity. Biomed J 2013;36:209–28.

[9] Kobashigawa J, Zuckermann A, Macdonald P, Consensus Conference Participants Report from a consensus conference on primary graft dysfunction after cardiac transplantation. J Heart Lung Transplant 2014;33:327–40.

[10] Wieland E, Olbricht CJ, Süsal C, Guurragchaa P, et al. Biomarkers as a tool for management of immunosuppression in transplant patients. Ther Drug Monit 2010;32:560–72.

[11] Sagoo P, Perucha E, Sawitzki B, Tomiuk S, et al. Development of a cross-platform biomarker signature to detect renal transplant tolerance in humans. J Clin Invest 2010;120:1848–61.

[12] Koch-Weser J. Serum drug concentrations as therapeutic guides. N Engl J Med 1972;287:277–81.

[13] van Gelder T, Le Meur Y, Shaw LM, Oellerich M, et al. Therapeutic drug monitoring of mycophenolate mofetil in transplantation. Ther Drug Monit 2006;28:145–54.

[14] Kuypers DR, Le Meur Y, Cantarovich M, The Transplantation Society (TTS) Consensus Group on TDM of MPA Consensus report on therapeutic drug monitoring of mycophenolic acid in solid organ transplantation. J Am Soc Nephrol 2010;5:341–58.

[15] Crettol S, Venetz JP, Fontana M, Aubert JD, et al. Influence of ABCB1 genetic polymorphisms on cyclosporine intracellular concentration in transplant recipients. Pharmacogenet Genomics 2008;18:307–15.

[16] Falck P, Asberg A, Guldseth H, Bremer S, et al. Declining intracellular T-lymphocyte concentration of cyclosporine a precedes acute rejection in kidney transplant patients. Transplantation 2008;85:179–84.

[17] Robles Piedras AL, De la O, Arciniega M, Reynoso Vázquez J. Clinical pharmacology and therapeutic drug monitoring of immuno-suppressive agents Rath T, editor. Current issues and future direction in kidney transplantation. InTech; 2014.

[18] Moes DJ, Press RR, de Fijter JW, Guchelaar HJ, et al. Liquid chromatography-tandem mass spectrometry outperforms fluorescence polarization immunoassay in monitoring everolimus therapy in renal transplantation. Ther Drug Monit 2010;32:413–9.

[19] Rianthavorn P, Ettenger RB, Malekzadeh M, Marik JL, et al. Noncompliance with immunosuppressive medications in pediatric and adolescent patients receiving solid-organ transplants. Transplantation 2004;77:778–82.

[20] van Sandwijk MS, Bemelman FJ, Ten Berge IJ. Immunosuppressive drugs after solid organ transplantation. Neth J Med 2013;71:281–9.

[21] Beimler J, Morath C, Zeier M. Modern immunosuppression after solid organ transplantation (German). Internist 2014;55:212–22.

[22] Rodriguez-Perálvarez M, Germani G, Tsochatzis G, Rolando N, et al. Predicting severity and clinical course of acute rejection after liver transplantation using blood eosinophil count. Transplant Int 2012;25:555–63.

[23] Rodriguez-Perálvarez M, Germani G, Papastergiou V, Tsochatzis E, et al. Early tacrolimus exposure after liver transplantation: relationship with moderate/severe acute rejection and long-term outcome. J Hepatol 2013;58:262–70.

[24] Prigent A. Monitoring renal function and limitations of renal function tests. Semin Nucl Med 2008;38:32–46.

[25] Stevens LA, Levey AS. Measured GFR as a confirmatory test for estimated GFR. J Am Soc Nephrol 2009;20:2305–13.

[26] Suthanthiran M, Schwartz JE, Ding R, Abecassis M, et al. Urinary-cell mRNA profile and acute cellular rejection in kidney allografts. N Engl J Med 2013;369:20–31.

[27] American Society of Nephrology American society of nephrology renal research report. J Am Soc Nephrol 2005;16:1886–903.

[28] Filler G, Yasin A, Medeiros M. Methods of assessing renal function. Pediatr Nephrol 2014;29:183–92.

[29] Crespo-Leiro MG, Zuckermann A, Bara C. Concordance among pathologists in the second Cardiac Allograft Rejection Gene Expression Observational Study (CARGO II). Transplantation 2012;94:1172–7.

[30] Hollander Z, Chen V, Sidhu K, Lin D, et al. Predicting acute cardiac rejection from donor heart and pre-transplant recipient blood gene expression. J Heart Lung Transplant 2013;32:259–65.

[31] Solez K, Racusen LC. The Banff classification revisited. Kidney Int 2013;83:201–6.

[32] Regev A, Berho M, Jeffers LJ, Milicowski C, et al. Sampling error and intraobserver variation in liver biopsy in patients with chronic HCV infection. Am J Gastroenterol 2002;97:2614–8.

[33] Lefkowitch JH. Liver biopsy assessment in chronic hepatitis. Arch Med Res 2007;38:634–43.

[34] Taner T, Stegall MD, Heimbach JK. Antibody-mediated rejection in liver transplantation: current controversies and future directions. Liver Transpl 2014;20:514–27.

[35] Puttarajappa C, Shapiro R, Tan HP. Antibody-mediated rejection in kidney transplantation: a review. J Transplant 2012:193724.

[36] Halloran PF, Pereira AB, Chang J. Microarray diagnosis of antibody-mediated rejection in kidney transplant biopsies: an international prospective study (INTERCOM). Am J Transplant 2013;13:2865–74.

[37] Sellares J, Reeve J, Loupy A, Mengel M, et al. Molecular diagnosis of antibody-mediated rejection in human kidney transplants. Am J Transplant 2013;13:971–83.

[38] Lachmann N, Todorova K, Harald Schulze H, Schonemann C. Luminex® and its applications for solid organ transplantation, hematopoietic stem cell transplantation, and transfusion. Transfus Med Hemother 2013;40:182–9.

[39] Schaub S, Hirt-Minkowski P. Urinary-cell mRNA and acute kidney-transplant rejection. N Engl J Med 2013;369:1858.

[40] Dharnidharka VR, Storch GA, Brennan DC. Urinary-cell mRNA and acute kidney-transplant rejection. N Engl J Med 2013;369:1858–9.

[41] Manrai AK, Kohane IS, Szolovits P. Urinary-cell mRNA and acute kidney-transplant rejection. N Engl J Med 2013;369:1859.

[42] Galichon P, Hertig A, Rondeau E. Urinary-cell mRNA and acute kidney-transplant rejection. N Engl J Med 2013;369:1859–60.

[43] Lo YMD, Tein MSC, Pang CCP, Yeung CK, et al. Presence of donor-specific DNA in plasma of kidney and liver-transplant recipients. Lancet 1998;351:1329–30.

[44] Sigdel TK, Vitalone MJ, Tran TQ, Dai H, et al. A rapid noninvasive assay for the detection of renal transplant injury. Transplantation 2013;96:97–101.

[45] Hubacek JA, Vymetalova Y, Bohuslavova R, Kocik M, et al. Detection of donor DNA after heart transplantation: how far could it be affected by blood transfusion and donor chimerism? Transplant Proc 2007;39:1593–5.

[46] Snyder TM, Khush KK, Valantine HA, Quake SR, et al. Universal noninvasive detection of solid organ transplant rejection. PNAS 2011;108:6229–34.

[47] Beck J, Bierau S, Balzer S, Andag R, et al. Digital droplet PCR for rapid quantification of donor DNA in the circulation of transplant recipients as a potential universal biomarker of graft injury. Clin Chem 2013;59:1732–41.

[48] Hindson BJ, Ness KD, Masquelier DA, Belgrader P, et al. High-throughput droplet digital PCR system for absolute quantitation of DNA copy number. Anal Chem 2011;86:8604–10.

[49] Streit F, Armstrong VW, Oellerich M. Rapid liquid chromatography–tandem mass spectrometry routine method for simultaneous determination of Sirolimus, Everolimus, Tacrolimus, and Cyclosporin A in whole blood. Clin Chem 2002;48:955–8.

[50] Beck J, Bierau S, Balzer S, Andag R, et al. Rapid and cost effective measurement of circulating cell free graft DNA for the early detection of liver transplant rejection. Clin Chem 2013;59(Suppl.):A-93.

[51] Kanzow P. Zirkulierende Nukleinsäuren im zellfreien Plasma von LTx-Patienten als Frühmarker einer Schädigung des Spenderorgans. Doctoral thesis, UMG Göttingen; 2014.

[52] Rodriguez-Perálvarez M, Germani G, Darius T, Lerut J, et al. Tacrolimus trough levels, rejection and renal impairment in liver transplantation: a systematic review and meta-analysis. Am J Transplant 2012;12:2797–814.

[53] Kanzow P, Kollmar O, Schütz E, Oellerich M, et al. Graft-derived cell-free DNA as an early organ integrity biomarker after transplantation of a marginal HELLP syndrome donor liver. Transplantation 2014;98:e43–5.

[54] Oellerich M, Kanzow P, Beck J, Schmitz J, et al. Graft-derived cell-free DNA (GcfDNA) as a sensitive measure of individual graft integrity after liver transplantation. Am J Transplant 2014;14(Suppl.):874.

[55] Oellerich M, Schütz E, Kanzow P, Schmitz J, et al. Use of graft-derived cell-free DNA as an organ integrity biomarker to reexamine effective tacrolimus trough concentrations after liver transplantation. Ther Drug Monit 2014;36:136–40.

[56] Wallemacq P, Armstrong VW, Brunet M, Haufroid V, et al. Opportunities to optimize tacrolimus therapy in solid organ transplantation: report of the European consensus conference. Ther Drug Monit 2009;31:139–52.

[57] Streit F, Shipkova M, Armstrong VW, Oellerich M. Validation of a rapid and sensitive liquid chromatography tandem mass spectrometry method for free and total mycophenolic acid. Clin Chem 2004;50:152–9.

[58] Beck J, Hennecke S, Bornemann-Kolatzki K, Urnovitz HB, et al. Genome aberrations in canine mammary carcinomas and their detection in cell-free plasma DNA. PLoS One 2013;8:e75485.

[59] Schmitz J, Götze S, Andag R, Brockmöller J, et al., Droplet digital PCR (ddPCR) for quantitative analysis of Treg-specific demethylation region (TSDR) in peripheral blood compared to flow cytometry (FACS). Clin Chem 2014;60(Suppl.):S106.

[60] Beck J, Schmitz J, Kanzow P, Kollmar O, et al. Absolute quantification of graft derived cell-free DNA (GcfDNA) early after liver transplantation (LTx) using droplet digital PCR. Clin Chem 2014;60(Suppl.):S194–5.

[61] Lo YMD. Transplantation monitoring by plasma DNA sequencing. Clin Chem 2011;57:941–2.

[62] De Vlaminck I, Valantine HA, Snyder TM, Strehl C, et al. Circulating cell-free DNA enables noninvasive diagnosis of heart transplant rejection. Sci Transl Med 2014;6:241ra77.

Biomarkers of tolerance in kidney transplantation

8

Daniel Baron, Magali Giral, and Sophie Brouard

INSERM, Nantes, France, CHU de Nantes, ITUN, Nantes, France, and Université de Nantes,
Faculté de Médecine, Nantes, France

8.1 INTRODUCTION

Transplantation is the treatment of choice for end-stage renal diseases. It is one of the revolutionary fields in modern medicine that has saved thousands of lives. According to current estimates, 18,000 recipients live with a transplanted kidney in Europe, and up to 2700 patients are transplanted each year in France. As quality of life is improved and length of life is also significantly prolonged after kidney transplantation, its application has been progressively and successfully extended to new indications, particularly in aged patients [1]. Furthermore, there is compelling evidence of continuous improvement in kidney transplant recipient and transplant survival during the past two decades [2] that is attributed to not only a general improvement in surgical techniques and clinical management, diagnostic tools, and control of infectious and neoplasia [3] but also better control of the alloimmune response to immunosuppression [4,5].

Although the incidence of acute rejection has drastically decreased to less than 10% in most transplant centers [6], immunosuppressant drugs have only a marginal effect on chronic rejection because long-term graft loss rates remain unmodified [4,7–9]. The cost for immunosuppressant drugs is approximately 1110 Euros monthly for a patient [10]. Lifelong immunosuppression therapy is far from harmless; it is associated with nephrotoxicity [11,12] and numerous other side effects, including infectious complications [13–18], malignancies [3,19], and metabolic disorders [20] that contribute substantially to morbidity and mortality among transplant recipients [21]. Of major concern, cardiovascular diseases [22], opportunistic infections [13], and malignancies [23] are underscored as particularly deleterious, accounting for 70% of deaths in patients with well-functioning kidney allograft. Thus, ironically, long-term survival of kidney transplant recipients, which initially benefited from modern immunosuppressive treatments, may now be principally limited by the effects of long-term exposure to these drugs [4,9,15,16].

M. Oellerich & A. Dasgupta (Eds): Personalized Immunosuppression in Transplantation.
DOI: http://dx.doi.org/10.1016/B978-0-12-800885-0.00008-4
© 2016 Elsevier Inc. All rights reserved.

For these reasons, achieving a state of long-term graft acceptance in the absence of immunosuppressant drugs—a situation known as "tolerance" [24]—is thus increasingly regarded as an ideal solution. Since the first experimental demonstration more than 60 years ago that nonresponsiveness to foreign antigens is possible [25], tolerance has been widely achieved in numerous rodent models [26], including models of renal transplantation [27]. However, the possibility to reach this "Holy Grail" of renal transplantation in humans [28], by manipulating host immunological mechanisms, is more difficult [29–32]. To date, successful induction of clinical tolerance in renal transplantation has been rarely achieved, and most promising intents relied on concurrent stem cell transplantation and achievement of mixed bone marrow chimerism [33,34]. Successful treatment has been reported only for a very small number of patients enrolled in the early phase of clinical protocols [35–42], and the applicability of these protocols to a broader population is still limited.

Therefore, "spontaneous operational tolerance" exists in humans [43] and refers to rare noncompliant recipients and others deliberately removed from immunosuppressants who do not develop rejection even long after the event [44]. These cases provide the proof that tolerance can be achieved [45] and represent a unique opportunity to dissect the mechanism implicated in the development or maintenance of this status and identify relevant biomarkers [46]. Elucidation of the related mechanisms is a prerequisite to induce this state, and the identification of biomarkers of tolerance, the individualization of immunosuppressant, and real-time monitoring of posttransplant immune responses may help to achieve this goal [47].

8.2 DEFINITION OF THE CLINICAL STATUS OF OPERATIONAL TOLERANCE

The original definition of Medawar in the 1950s referred to nonresponsiveness to antigens [48]. In animal studies, tolerance may be defined as good long-standing graft function in the presence of a competent immune system, with no signs of graft immune injury. The latter definition is obviously not useful in human transplantation; therefore, "operational tolerance" is the term most widely used. Given that no biopsy can be performed, kidney transplant recipients who have been successfully weaned from immunosuppressants and have maintained stable graft function for 1 year or more are referred to as functionally or operationally tolerant [49–51]. These cases are usually observed by chance when transplanted recipients no longer take their immunosuppressant drugs but do not experience organ rejection. Spontaneously tolerant patients stop their immunosuppressive treatment for two major reasons: noncompliance and the occurrence of deleterious side effects of the immunosuppressive drugs (drug toxicity or malignancy) [49–51]. The precise prevalence of tolerance among kidney recipients is currently unknown. These cases are rare (<1% of kidney transplanted recipients) [52]; it is estimated that there are currently 100 cases throughout the world [43]. This number is certainly higher because a substantial portion of the compliant kidney recipients could be in fact tolerant [44]. Such patients can maintain excellent graft function for decades [49,53,54]. The majority of them received immunosuppressant treatment in the past involving azathioprine and corticosteroids, and they do not differ from other transplant recipients as to whether they received a kidney from a deceased or living donor. Also, the number of human leukocyte antigen (HLA) incompatibilities is similar to that for other transplant recipients [49,52,55–59]. If the individual parameters and history of these patients are extremely variable [49–51], several interesting features could emerge from their careful follow up. First, operational tolerance can develop even in the presence of either HLA mismatches at baseline or anti-HLA antibodies during follow up, as well as in patients who have experienced acute rejection. Second, tolerant cases had not been nonspecifically immunosuppressed because they did not present any significantly increased risk for either opportunistic/severe infections or cancers, but they showed responses to vaccination comparable to the general population. Third, the operational tolerance process has been shown to be metastable over time, as demonstrated by a non-negligible proportion of patients who lose their graft for immunological reasons or simply due to physiological age defects. Finally, operational tolerance corresponds to an immunocompetent situation [60] associated with immune regulation, as shown by a decrease of the donor-reactive delayed-type hypersensitivity response specific to the donor [58,61].

8.3 TECHNICAL CONSIDERATIONS ON THE BIODETECTION OF TOLERANCE

The research on these tolerant patients is intense [46], and many studies have tried to dissect the phenotype of tolerance in kidney transplantation in order to understand its mechanisms and also to be able to identify patients under conventional immunosuppression who may have developed tolerance to their transplant. Indeed, establishing biomarkers [62,63] of operational tolerance may provide tools to select patients who are eligible for enrolment in trials of immunosuppression (IS) drug weaning or withdrawal, as well as surrogate endpoints for tolerance induction trials.

8.3.1 BIOMARKERS AND LIMITS OF CONVENTIONAL TESTS

Biomarkers, as defined by the Biomarkers Definition Working Group, are characteristics that can be measured objectively and evaluated as an indicator of a normal biological process, a pathogenic process, or a pharmacological response to a therapeutic intervention [64]. Ideally, a biomarker is accurate and reproducible, with high sensitivity and specificity as well as high positive and negative predictive values. A biomarker should also be widely available, rapid, easy to use, and inexpensive if it is to find a place in routine clinical practice [64]. Biomarker discovery is an active domain of research in kidney transplantation [65] to establish molecular diagnostics [66] personalized medicine [67,68], especially by improving post-transplant monitoring [69,70] and prediction of long-term outcome [71].

For defining a state of operational tolerance, biomarkers should be assessable noninvasively by using, for example, peripheral blood or urine [72], the latter being minimally invasive. Currently, the allograft biopsy remains the "gold standard" for assessing the status of the graft [73], but this invasive procedure is not suitable for monitoring the graft on a regular, sometimes daily, basis. Evaluation of graft function is thus based on creatinine and proteinuria levels. They give essential information on kidney function and allow the medical staff to adapt the patient's treatment. Therefore, these parameters lack specificity because they can vary under normal physiological conditions as well as with disease [74]. For instance, the rate of production of creatinine is dependent on muscle mass, which is subject to the major modifying effects of age, gender, and ethnicity. Although widely used in clinical practice of kidney injury, they correlate poorly with actual kidney function and offer little useful prognostic information regarding the likelihood of organ failure or recovery. Moreover, they provide no information about the immune status of the organ recipient. Thus, there is still an urgent need to develop new biomarkers of tolerance [75]. Therefore, most of the studies on operationally tolerant kidney patients are very heterogeneous due to the techniques, controls used, or the various clinical profiles of the patients [49–51,58,61,76–91]. Moreover, the cohorts studied are small, which prevents a robust statistical approach. These considerations markedly contribute to the difficulty for generalization and standardization of the results [68]. Finally, the lack of biopsies is a problem in these patients because some indications of graft deterioration may not be detected [51]. In the search for new biomarkers, there are three major dilemmas that have to be considered: the technology to be used, the origin of the samples, and the control population.

8.3.2 CHOICE OF TECHNOLOGY

A major barrier to clinical tolerance is the absence of a method to detect it prospectively. In animal models, donor and third-party skin grafting has been used as a robust test, but this is not a practical clinical approach for many reasons. In humans, many immunologic assays have been used as surrogate tests to monitor the immune response after transplantation [62,63]. Tests of antigen-specific T-cell responses (mixed lymphocyte reaction and limiting dilution) have not been shown to predict the development of tolerance or to be helpful guides for immunosuppressant withdrawal. More recent tests of precursor frequency (enzyme-linked immunosorbent spot, tetramer analysis, and others [92,93]), although promising during therapy with immunosuppressants, have not yet been applied in tolerant patients. Benefiting from advances in genomic science [66,94], very sensitive molecular techniques have become available to quantify relevant gene expression patterns and protein signatures in biologic samples [95,96]. They have been of added value [97] to characterize spontaneously tolerant transplant recipients [98] and establish a tolerance gene signature [99,100].

8.3.3 CHOICE OF SPECIMEN

Regarding the origin of the samples, peripheral blood, graft biopsy [77], and urine have all been used for analysis [89]. In kidney transplantation, the graft biopsy is recognized as the gold standard for rejection diagnosis [73]. However, in most cases, operationally tolerant patients refuse biopsy, and it is ethically questionable to perform a biopsy of a fully functional graft. Cellular infiltrates have been reported to be very low in tolerant kidney graft [77] and would therefore probably not yield a great deal of information [101]. Analyzing the peripheral blood [72,102] has the advantage of being less invasive and less expensive than biopsy, which makes it the main method used to analyze gene profiles [72]. Blood is a promising source of diagnostic markers and therapeutic molecules [103,104], but it probably does not always reflect what is happening in the graft [105]. In kidney transplantation, analyzing urine may have several advantages [72,102]: Its collection is noninvasive and inexpensive, and urine is in direct contact with the grafted organ, which could give relevant information on kidney function [106,107]. Unfortunately, high variability in concentration and volume makes the quantification of biomarkers often difficult and occasionally unreliable.

8.3.4 CHOICE OF CONTROL

The other significant dilemma is choosing the right control population, which is not easy for tolerant patients [65,108]. On the one hand, these patients have been grafted and have good graft function, so we might suppose that stable patients under immunosuppressant treatment would be the best control, but the absence of immunosuppressive drugs in the tolerant patients could influence the results. On the other hand, the absence of treatment makes tolerant patients similar to healthy individuals, but we cannot ignore the absence of transplantation in the latter group. Comparison of tolerant patients with patients undergoing chronic transplant rejection has also been performed, but these patients are clinically very different. Moreover, it cannot be excluded that some tolerant patients could present functionally undetectable subclinical graft lesions, and the absence of systematic kidney biopsies for these tolerant patients prevents any conclusions from being drawn. Faced with the lack of the perfect control population, the use of multiple controls may be the best alternative.

In approximately the past 10 years, a number of studies have been conducted to identify new, robust, tolerance biomarkers, and two major consortia have been involved in the discovery of such biomarkers: the Immune Tolerance Network (ITN) in the United States (http://www.immunetolerance.org) and the Indices of Tolerance (IOT) in Europe (http://www.risetfp6.org/). The existence of such consortia is essential because operationally tolerant patients are rare (as previously stated, <100 known in the world), and so it is the only way to develop multicenter studies and to have access to larger cohorts of patients.

8.4 A B-CELL SIGNATURE PREDOMINATES IN BLOOD FROM TOLERANT RECIPIENTS

Concentrated efforts, especially using phenotypic and transcriptomic analyses [78,86,89,91,109], led to the identification of B-cell feature distinguishing tolerant patients from other recipients.

8.4.1 TOLERANT PATIENTS OVEREXPRESS B-CELL BIOMARKERS

Our group and others have analyzed the transcriptome of peripheral blood mononuclear cells. These five analyses revealed an increased expression of B-cell-related genes in tolerant patients compared to stable patients [78,86,89,91,109]. In a princeps study [109], tolerance was characterized by a footprint of genes signing immune quiescence and implicating the overexpression of B-cell markers such as CD79a, CD79b, CD19, or CD20 [109]. Such enrichment of B-cell markers was also reported in other studies: 23 genes (77%) [110], 6 genes (60%) [91], and 24 genes (69%) [86]. These genes were especially involved in the proliferation, activation, and maturation of B cells [90], in accordance with the higher number of B cells in these patients [85]. Also, many genes expressed by naive and transitional/immature B cells were overrepresented in tolerant patients, confirming the enrichment of these subsets in this group [89]. Some of these genes could be commonly identified between the different studies [86], such as the CD20 protein, which was reported to be strongly expressed in blood from tolerant recipients in three of the five transcriptomic studies [86,89,91] and also detected in their urine [89]. Because the number of samples in each of the studies was relatively low, the significance of these results was assessed through a meta-analysis [111]. The high number of samples analyzed (96 samples from 50 tolerant recipients from three independent multicentric cohort: French, United Kingdom, and United States) led to the identification, for the first time, of a specific gene signature. This signature could unequivocally distinguish tolerant from other recipients (>90% accuracy) through cross-validation and was remarkably enriched in B-cell-related genes. Of interest, these markers linked to B cells were among the best discriminative ones between tolerant and stable recipients. A minimal selection of the top 20 genes, mostly enriched in B-cell markers, yielded similar performances of discrimination and could be validated in an independent set of 18 samples, including new tolerant cases. These data provide proof of principle that tolerance can be identified among transplanted recipients by the use of a 20-gene predictor, mostly centered on B cells [111]. Hence, these biomarkers could be used to detect tolerance and stratify kidney recipients in clinics. First, they may help for a better follow up of the tolerant recipients. Several lines of evidences indicate that tolerance is likely not a stable situation for "entire life" [109]. In such situation, these biomarkers could predict future graft loss, and immunotherapy could be reinstated before the first clinical symptoms appear. Second, these biomarkers may help to monitor recipients under IS regimens. Among stable cases, those detected as having a low risk of rejection would be highly eligible for progressive IS weaning.

8.4.2 TOLERANT PATIENTS EXPAND SPECIFIC B-CELL SUBSETS

Accordingly, cellular analysis by flow cytometry reported an increase in absolute number of B cells in tolerant patients compared to immunosuppressed recipients [85]. This finding has been further replicated and validated by three studies [89–91]. This increase was associated with an enrichment in naive and transitional B-cell subsets in the peripheral blood mononuclear cells of tolerant patients [89,91] and a lack of plasma cells attributed to a default in B-cell differentiation and a higher sensibility to apoptosis in the late stages of differentiation [112]. Phenotypic analysis identifies a global inhibitory profile with a diminution of CD32a/CD32b ratio, increased expression of BANK1 (which negatively modulates CD40-mediated AKT activation), and augmentation of CD1d CD5 expressing B cells [90], which are considered to be regulatory phenotypes [113]. These studies thus support the fact that operationally tolerant recipients display a strong B-cell signature. This feature is unique to kidney tolerant recipients because it is not observed in liver tolerant patients [86]. Currently, the exact reasons for the expansion of the different B-cell subsets in the blood of tolerant recipients are unknown. Therefore, it is interesting to note that recipients with end-stage renal disease have a significant reduction in the peripheral total B-cell count [114–116]. Also, after transplantation, patients are treated with a strong IS therapy, which guarantees a stable function of the graft but strongly alters the immune system. However, some patients who stopped their treatments managed to tolerate their kidney allograft and are subject to a strong immune reconstitution with an increase of naive or immature B cells in their blood compared to stable recipients. This phenomenon is observed in kidney transplantation tolerance mediated by mixed chimerism with a repopulation of transitional B cells in tolerant recipients [31]. Accordingly, a recent study suggested that B cells could play a role in the maintenance of tolerance but not in its induction and that their development may be due to the progressive weaning off IS, which may allow regulatory populations to emerge [58]. These data suggest that the repopulation by immature and naive B cells could be a feature facilitating tolerance in kidney transplantation [117], and they reinforce the essential role of the B-cell compartment [118].

8.5 AN UNSUSPECTED ROLE FOR B CELL IN OPERATIONAL TOLERANCE

The implication of the B-cell compartment in the development and/or maintenance was further evidenced by the tolerogenic property of these cells. In a rat model of long-term cardiac allograft [119], tolerant rodents were shown to display an increased number of B cells in their blood, a blockade in the IgM-to-IgG switch recombination process, and they overexpressed BANK-1 and CD32b. Most important, B cells from tolerant rats were able to transfer tolerance [119]. Thus, as observed in humans [90], tolerant rats have an accumulation of B cells exhibiting an inhibited and regulatory profile [37], strengthening their role in the maintenance of transplantation tolerance. These observations strongly support the fact that B cells may exert regulatory functions in tolerance. Indeed, B cells with immune-regulating function (Bregs) largely contribute to immune regulation [120,121], and although currently limited, such regulatory B cells could also play a crucial role in the development and maintenance of tolerance to allograft [110,118,122–125]. The term "regulatory B cells" was first introduced following the identification of Bregs as an interleukin-10 (IL-10)-producing B-cell subset [126]. Therefore, a unique marker defining a Breg phenotype has not yet been described, and consistent differences have been reported between murine and human Bregs [113,126,127]. The pathways by which regulatory Bregs exert immunosuppressive functions essentially include the secretion of two cytokines, IL-10 and transforming growth factor-β (TGF-β) [113,126–129], or the production of the serine protease granzyme B (GrB) [130].

In the setting of operational tolerance, the identification of Breg subsets producing TGF-β [91], IL-10 [89,123], or GrB [131] brings mechanistic considerations linking B cells to suppressed immunity in tolerance to allograft. An increase of TGF-β-producing B cells was observed in tolerant recipients [91]. This suggests that B cells of tolerant patients had a skewed cytokine response, with a higher propensity for TGF-β production than B cells from other study groups [91]. These results are corroborated by a regulatory profile with marked increase of TGF-β expression [88] and the implication of the TGF-β pathway in operationally tolerant recipients [82]. This production of TGF-β in B cells could be regulated by an increase of miR142-3p through a negative feedback loop [84]. Although IL-10 was detected for all study groups (tolerant and stable recipients), no difference in production was observed [91]. Indeed, polyclonal activation of total B cells revealed no difference in cytokine secretion in all groups of transplanted patients [90,91]. By contrast, stimulation of transitional B cells showed an enrichment in IL-10-secreting B cells in tolerant and healthy donors compared to stable patients [89,112]. These results could be explained by the fact that transitional B cells constituted only 0–5% of total B cells [132]. Consequently, this response could be undetectable in total B cells. Although these transitional B cells could represent a regulatory B-cell population based on their increased IL-10 production [118], no difference in B-cell subsets (total, naive, and transitional cells) or inhibitory cytokines (IL-10 and TGF-β) was detected when compared to healthy controls [89]. This is corroborated by the observation that a functional B-cell regulatory compartment is preserved in blood from operationally tolerant and healthy volunteers, with normal capacity to phosphorylate signal transducer and activator of transcription 3 (STAT3) after activation [133]. Compared to stable recipients and healthy volunteers, because chronic rejection patients display B cells with impaired suppressive function (inability to efficiently inhibit autologous cell proliferation) [134] and a quantitative decrease of Bregs with a skew in their cytokine polarization (decreased IL-10/tumor necrosis factor-α ratio) [135], it is likely that B-cell-inducing tolerance could be explained by a preserved B-cell compartment. Recently, the regulatory function of Breg was evidenced by GrB rather than IL-10 production [131]. In this study, tolerant recipients harbored a higher number of B cells expressing GrB and displaying a CD19$^+$CD5$^+$CD27$^+$CD138$^+$ phenotype. These Bregs were able to actively inhibit effector T cells through a contact- and GrB-dependent pathway [131].

These data on B cells, with an increase of B-cell populations with regulatory properties and a decrease in plasma cells producing deleterious antibodies in tolerant patients, are very encouraging. They have been reproduced in varying studies in different cohorts of tolerant patients and strongly suggest that a critical balance of the B-cell compartment is essential in tolerance (Figure 8.1). Reconciling the function of

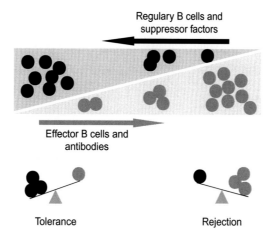

FIGURE 8.1

The balance between regulatory (Breg) and effector (Beff) functions of the B-cell compartment. This balance emphasizes the role of the number of Bregs in the development and maintenance of tolerance to kidney allograft. In the presence of too large numbers of Beffs (black circles), the regulatory mechanisms, consisting of Bregs (gray circles) and suppressive factors (cytokines and Gzb), are unable to attenuate the immune response, which therefore leads to graft rejection. However, in the presence of a sufficient number of Bregs, the mechanisms of regulation can suppress the immune response, which leads to graft tolerance.

these B cells with other regulatory cells such as Tregs [136] and with a concomitant role for T cells will not be difficult due to their well-documented interaction and the strong link between cellular and humoral immunity [137,138]. However, with the present data, it is difficult to determine whether the "B-cell signature of tolerance" preceded the development of tolerance and thus possibly contributed to its development or whether it arose after tolerance had developed and could reflect a tolerant state per se. These considerations should have important implications for the design of protocols of minimization of immunosuppressant therapy as well as tolerance-inducing regimens and assays for detecting tolerance.

8.6 POTENTIAL APPLICATIONS OF THE BIOMARKERS AND THE FUTURE FOR TOLERANCE RESEARCH

The data obtained on operational tolerant cases are of major importance for kidney transplantation. Indeed, on the one hand, the characterized biomarkers may help to identify, among cohorts of transplanted recipients or among cases having received a protocol of tolerance induction, the patients who have really developed a tolerance state. On the other hand, according to the preponderant role of the B-cell compartment in tolerance to kidney allograft, therapies that aims at favoring specific "pro-tolerogenic" B-cell subsets could help to develop new protocols and induce this state.

8.6.1 PERSONALIZED MINIMIZATION OF IMMUNOSUPPRESSANT THERAPY

Currently, minimization of immunosuppressant therapy in kidney recipients remains a risky procedure (irreversible graft damage), and appropriate selection of patients is a necessity for the safety of the strategy [139]. Although histological examination of graft biopsies is the gold standard for assessing recipient status [73], this procedure is invasive and cannot be easily repeated in stable recipients. Thus, the development of a "B-cell" biomarker signature as a diagnostic test of tolerance [111] opens up the possibility of rationally designed immunosuppressant-weaning protocols by improving individual monitoring [139] and clinical decision aids [140]. The principle is based on the assumption that among stable recipients under immunosuppressant therapy, some patients could have developed tolerance and thus may harbor the related biomarkers [109]. These patients presenting "low risk" of rejection [139] may be the ideal candidates for progressive minimization of immunosuppressant therapy.

Current data identify 7% of stable recipients under immunosuppressant therapy who accurately display the tolerance gene signature [111]. This finding is in agreement with previous reports showing that tolerance is rarely observed in large cohorts of kidney transplant recipients [52], and only a small percentage of the stable recipients (5–10%) are expected to be tolerant [82,91,109]. Remarkably, among these stable patients, some cases on weaning ("minimally immunosuppressed" under corticosteroid monotherapy) harbor this gene signature [91,109,111] and also an indirect T-cell response close to that of tolerant patients [58], demonstrating that *prope* tolerance [141] is achievable through minimization of immunosuppressant therapy. Despite the low number of potentially tolerant among stable recipients, this strategy remains advantageous with regard to drug costs and quality of life (IS side effects).

Nevertheless, although currently limited, some convincing arguments suggest that higher numbers of "eligible low-risk" patients could be detected as tolerance could develop over time. Indeed, if immature and naive B-cell subsets and related tolerance-associated transcripts are detectable within the first year post-transplantation [142], they in fact seem to increase over time to reach levels comparable to those observed in operational tolerant 10 years post-transplantation [143]. These data thus suggest that under immunosuppression, the critical threshold to achieve operational tolerance depends on a long period (a decade) after transplantation. This is of major interest because weaning protocols for stable kidney transplant should be aimed at patients with a long follow up. To date, most of the attempts to minimize immunosuppressant therapy, or even to induce tolerance, have been performed soon after transplantation—after 1 year or less [144–146]—and have been associated with a significant increase of rejection. Of course, such studies do not provide formal proof that operational tolerance can be achieved in these patients, and the fact that some stable patients are really tolerant is a hypothesis that only a weaning/minimization of immunosuppression could confirm. Only prospective studies on very large cohorts and at later time will satisfy the "proof of concept" of this hypothesis.

Finally, the development of this tolerance signature was not observed in all recipients and largely depended on the IS treatment used [143]. Because intrinsic differences between the different immunosuppressant drugs on the immune system exist [147], this finding suggests that different immunosuppressant schedules modulate the immune cell populations that participate in the graft acceptance. This observation deserves further investigation on the use of "tolerance-permissive" IS regimens.

8.6.2 PERMISSIVE B-CELL THERAPIES TO INDUCE TOLERANCE

According to the potential pivotal role of the B-cell compartment, B-cell-directed therapy is emerging as a key component in achieving transplantation tolerance and long-term graft survival [148]. Currently, a B-cell approach for tolerance induction is promising, but further investigation on how these cell populations regulate allo-immune response is necessary [149]. Moreover, this strategy may be limited due to the prohibitive costs, availability (with only a few centers capable of amplifying cell populations to sufficient numbers), and issues of standardization and biologics regulation [150]. As an alternative, the existence of some specific "tolerance-permissive" immunosuppressant regimens may help to expand specific B-cell subsets [117,151,152]. In this context, the application of the tolerance gene signature for the immune monitoring of patients should be a great advantage to identify potentially tolerant recipients and could also help to develop new permissive regimens.

In nonhuman primate (cynomolgus macaque) studies, long-term allograft acceptance has been achieved by augmenting traditional immunotherapy with B-cell depleting antibodies [151,153]. For instance, rituximab (a monoclonal antibody to CD20) plus cyclosporine prolonged cardiac graft survival by inhibition of DSA production and attenuation of chronic rejection [153]. Accordingly, an induction immunotherapy regimen, consisting of rabbit anti-thymocyte globulin (thymoglobulin) and rituximab, also promoted long-term islet allograft survival in macaques maintained on rapamycin monotherapy [151]. The B-cell reconstitution began 100 days after transplantation, and long-term survivors exhibited immature and transitional B cells in contrast with early rejectors [151].

Similar observations were also made in humans, when kidney transplant recipients undergoing rituximab-mediated B-cell depletion for desensitization experienced reconstitution with transitional B cells while the donor HLA-specific memory B-cell repopulation was significantly delayed [154]. Another potent lymphocyte-depleting agent used as induction therapy, the anti-CD52 monoclonal antibody alemtuzumab, led to a strong depletion of the B-cell compartment followed by rapid repopulation up to levels exceeding baseline [117]. Interestingly, lymphocyte reconstitution was characterized by a rapid and marked transient increase in transitional B cells and cells with phenotypic characteristics of regulatory B cells, as well as a long-term dominance in naive B cells [117]. Finally, in a model of tolerance induction based on a combined kidney and bone marrow transplantation, B-cell reconstitution with a high frequency of peripheral transitional B cells was observed in tolerant recipients (three out of the four patients) [152], indicating that the involvement of B-cell subsets in the mechanisms of tolerance is not limited to operational tolerance but also concerns patients with therapeutic-induced tolerance.

Currently, these studies support that selective use or pairing of B-cell-depleting agents can generate tolerance-promoting B-cell phenotypes and eliminate factors leading to chronic rejection. Because B-cell depletion is inadequate for preventing xeno-specific antibodies [155] and has mixed results in desensitization [156–158], further evaluation is needed to optimize its use in transplantation.

8.7 CONCLUSIONS

The results summarized in this chapter are encouraging. Research efforts by scientists of the European IOT and American ITN consortia in the establishment of multicentric cohorts of tolerant kidney recipients is a major step toward our understanding of tolerance, and its detection has been realized in the past decade. The identification and cross-validation of the expansion of B-cell subsets and related gene markers have been achieved, creating opportunities for their future clinical application. Moreover, the fact that some of these B-cell subsets present proven regulatory functions adds to the crucial role of this compartment in the development and maintenance of the tolerance status.

The described biomarkers and functional assay will help to develop new strategies, to identify tolerant patients, and can be used to shape the drug-weaning protocols of transplanted patients. Large-scale clinical studies are now warranted to validate the utility of this tolerance signature as a means to identify tolerant cases among long-term kidney recipients with stable graft function, to determine the timing of appearance of the observed tolerant footprint post-transplantation, and to test the stability of this profile over time. These analyses will be especially helpful to identify an optimal window for future protocols. Currently, minimization of immunosuppressant therapy and induction trials have unfortunately concentrated on the early post-transplantation period, which could explain the discouraging results from most attempts. Although not proven so far, recent data suggest that tolerance is a long process to develop. Future protocols could thus consider later favorable periods, when spontaneous tolerance is to be the most probably naturally achieved. In such a favorable window, minimizing of immunosuppressant or inducing tolerance is easier.

Altogether, these results may be helpful to establish individualized therapy for kidney transplant recipients and may enable improvement in long-term graft outcomes. Of course, B cell is not the unique feature operating in tolerance, and there are several emerging reports evidencing the role of other regulatory subsets. Immunologic tolerance is a multifaceted situation involving a large array of participants and regulations. It is certain that adopting an integrated view of multiple data sources (cellular, immunologic, phenotypic, genetic, epigenetic proteomic, metabolomic, etc.) by a system biology approach will help to model tolerance and to determine why a graft is accepted by one recipient but not by another. This approach will be facilitated by the accelerated improvement of immunological and molecular techniques and also of analysis. Regarding what has been achieved to date on the road to the "Holy Grail," personalized medicine for kidney transplant recipients might underpin clinical practice for the coming decade.

REFERENCES

[1] Wolfe RA, Ashby VB, Milford EL, Ojo AO, et al. Comparison of mortality in all patients on dialysis, patients on dialysis awaiting transplantation, and recipients of a first cadaveric transplant. N Engl J Med 1999;341:1725–30.

[2] Pascual M, Theruvath T, Kawai T, Tolkoff-Rubin N, et al. Strategies to improve long-term outcomes after renal transplantation. N Engl J Med 2002;346:580–90.

[3] Dantal J, Hourmant M, Cantarovich D, Giral M, et al. Effect of long-term immunosuppression in kidney-graft recipients on cancer incidence: randomised comparison of two cyclosporin regimens. Lancet 1998;351:623–8.

[4] Opelz G. Influence of treatment with cyclosporine, azathioprine and steroids on chronic allograft failure. The Collaborative Transplant Study. Kidney Int Suppl 1995;52:S89–92.

[5] Vincenti F, Kirk AD. What's next in the pipeline. Am J Transplant 2008;8:1972–81.

[6] Hardinger KL, Brennan DC. Novel immunosuppressive agents in kidney transplantation. World J Transplant 2013;3:68–77.

[7] Hariharan S, McBride MA, Cherikh WS, Tolleris CB, et al. Post-transplant renal function in the first year predicts long-term kidney transplant survival. Kidney Int 2002;62:311–8.

[8] Hariharan S, Stablein DE. Improvements in long-term renal transplant graft survival. Am J Transplant 2005;5:630–1.

[9] Nankivell BJ, Borrows RJ, Fung CL, O'Connell PJ, et al. The natural history of chronic allograft nephropathy. N Engl J Med 2003;349:2326–33.

[10] Earnshaw SR, Graham CN, Irish WD, Sato R, et al. Lifetime cost-effectiveness of calcineurin inhibitor withdrawal after *de novo* renal transplantation. J Am Soc Nephrol 2008;19:1807–16.

[11] Casey MJ, Meier-Kriesche HU. Calcineurin inhibitors in kidney transplantation: friend or foe? Curr Opin Nephrol Hypertens 2011;20:610–5.

[12] Ojo AO, Held PJ, Port FK, Wolfe RA, et al. Chronic renal failure after transplantation of a nonrenal organ. N Engl J Med 2003;349:931–40.

[13] Fishman JA, Rubin RH. Infection in organ-transplant recipients. N Engl J Med 1998;338:1741–51.

[14] Fishman JA. Infection in solid-organ transplant recipients. N Engl J Med 2007;357:2601–14.

[15] Morelon E, Stern M, Kreis H. Interstitial pneumonitis associated with sirolimus therapy in renal-transplant recipients. N Engl J Med 2000;343:225–6.

[16] Morelon E, Stern M, Israel-Biet D, Correas JM, et al. Characteristics of sirolimus-associated interstitial pneumonitis in renal transplant patients. Transplantation 2001;72:787–90.

[17] Rabot N, Buchler M, Foucher Y, Moreau A, et al. CNI withdrawal for post-transplant lymphoproliferative disorders in kidney transplant is an independent risk factor for graft failure and mortality. Transpl Int 2014;27:956–65.

[18] Soulillou JP, Giral M. Controlling the incidence of infection and malignancy by modifying immunosuppression. Transplantation 2001;72:S89–93.

[19] London NJ, Farmery SM, Will EJ, Davison AM, et al. Risk of neoplasia in renal transplant patients. Lancet 1995;346:403–6.

[20] Halloran PF. Immunosuppressive drugs for kidney transplantation. N Engl J Med 2004;351:2715–29.

[21] Halloran PF, Bromberg J, Kaplan B, Vincenti F. Tolerance versus immunosuppression: a perspective. Am J Transplant 2008;8:1365–6.

[22] Miller LW. Cardiovascular toxicities of immunosuppressive agents. Am J Transplant 2002;2:807–18.

[23] Rama I, Grinyo JM. Malignancy after renal transplantation: the role of immunosuppression. Nat Rev Nephrol 2010;6:511–9.

[24] Lechler RI, Garden OA, Turka LA. The complementary roles of deletion and regulation in transplantation tolerance. Nat Rev Immunol 2003;3:147–58.

[25] Billingham RE, Brent L, Medawar PB. Actively acquired tolerance of foreign cells. Nature 1953;172:603–6.

[26] Kingsley CI, Nadig SN, Wood KJ. Transplantation tolerance: lessons from experimental rodent models. Transpl Int 2007;20:828–41.

[27] Jovanovic V, Lair D, Soulillou JP, Brouard S. Transfer of tolerance to heart and kidney allografts in the rat model. Transpl Int 2008;21:199–206.

[28] Schroeder RA, Marroquin CE, Kuo PC. Tolerance and the "Holy Grail" of transplantation. J Surg Res 2003;111:109–19.

[29] Ashton-Chess J, Brouard S, Soulillou JP. Is clinical tolerance realistic in the next decade? Transpl Int 2006;19:539–48.

[30] Fehr T, Sykes M. Tolerance induction in clinical transplantation. Transpl Immunol 2004;13:117–30.

[31] Girlanda R, Kirk AD. Frontiers in nephrology: immune tolerance to allografts in humans. J Am Soc Nephrol 2007;18:2242–51.

[32] Page EK, Dar WA, Knechtle SJ. Tolerogenic therapies in transplantation. Front Immunol 2012;3:198.

[33] Auchincloss Jr. H. In search of the elusive Holy Grail: the mechanisms and prospects for achieving clinical transplantation tolerance. Am J Transplant 2001;1:6–12.

[34] Millan MT, Shizuru JA, Hoffmann P, jbakhsh-Jones S, et al. Mixed chimerism and immunosuppressive drug withdrawal after HLA-mismatched kidney and hematopoietic progenitor transplantation. Transplantation 2002;73:1386–91.

[35] Kawai T, Cosimi AB, Spitzer TR, Tolkoff-Rubin N, et al. HLA-mismatched renal transplantation without maintenance immunosuppression. N Engl J Med 2008;358:353–61.

[36] Kawai T, Cosimi AB, Sachs DH. Preclinical and clinical studies on the induction of renal allograft tolerance through transient mixed chimerism. Curr Opin Organ Transplant 2011;16:366–71.

[37] Leventhal J, Abecassis M, Miller J, Gallon L, et al. Chimerism and tolerance without GVHD or engraftment syndrome in HLA-mismatched combined kidney and hematopoietic stem cell transplantation. Sci Transl Med 2012;4:124ra28.

[38] Leventhal J, Abecassis M, Miller J, Gallon L, et al. Tolerance induction in HLA disparate living donor kidney transplantation by donor stem cell infusion: durable chimerism predicts outcome. Transplantation 2013;95:169–76.

[39] Leventhal JR, Mathew JM, Salomon DR, Kurian SM, et al. Genomic biomarkers correlate with HLA-identical renal transplant tolerance. J Am Soc Nephrol 2013;24:1376–85.

[40] Scandling JD, Busque S, jbakhsh-Jones S, Benike C, et al. Tolerance and chimerism after renal and hematopoietic-cell transplantation. N Engl J Med 2008;358:362–8.

[41] Scandling JD, Busque S, jbakhsh-Jones S, Benike C, et al. Tolerance and withdrawal of immunosuppressive drugs in patients given kidney and hematopoietic cell transplants. Am J Transplant 2012;12:1133–45.

[42] Sharabi Y, Sachs DH. Mixed chimerism and permanent specific transplantation tolerance induced by a nonlethal preparative regimen. J Exp Med 1989;169:493–502.

[43] Orlando G, Hematti P, Stratta RJ, Burke III GW, et al. Clinical operational tolerance after renal transplantation: current status and future challenges. Ann Surg 2010;252:915–28.

[44] Ashton-Chess J, Giral M, Brouard S, Soulillou JP. Spontaneous operational tolerance after immunosuppressive drug withdrawal in clinical renal allotransplantation. Transplantation 2007;84:1215–9.

[45] Newell KA. Clinical transplantation tolerance. Semin Immunopathol 2011;33:91–104.

[46] Dugast E, Chesneau M, Soulillou JP, Brouard S. Biomarkers and possible mechanisms of operational tolerance in kidney transplant patients. Immunol Rev 2014;258:208–17.

[47] Sawitzki B, Reinke P, Pascher A, Volk HD. State of the art on the research for biomarkers allowing individual, tailor-made minimization of immunosuppression. Curr Opin Organ Transplant 2010;15:691–6.

[48] Aiba Y, Yamazaki T, Okada T, Gotoh K, et al. BANK negatively regulates Akt activation and subsequent B cell responses. Immunity 2006;24:259–68.

[49] Brouard S, Pallier A, Renaudin K, Foucher Y, et al. The natural history of clinical operational tolerance after kidney transplantation through twenty-seven cases. Am J Transplant 2012;12:3296–307.

[50] Roussey-Kesler G, Giral M, Moreau A, Subra JF, et al. Clinical operational tolerance after kidney transplantation. Am J Transplant 2006;6:736–46.

[51] Soulillou JP, Giral M, Brouard S. Operational tolerance in kidney transplantation-improved terminology may enable more precise investigation. Transplantation 2013;96:e36–8.

[52] Zoller KM, Cho SI, Cohen JJ, Harrington JT. Cessation of immunosuppressive therapy after successful transplantation: a national survey. Kidney Int 1980;18:110–4.

[53] Starzl TE, Murase N, Demetris AJ, Trucco M, et al. Lessons of organ-induced tolerance learned from historical clinical experience. Transplantation 2004;77:926–9.

[54] Weil III R, Starzl TE, Porter KA, Kershaw M, et al. Renal isotransplantation without immunosuppression. Ann Surg 1980;192:108–10.

[55] Burlingham WJ, Grailer AP, Fechner Jr. JH, Kusaka S, et al. Microchimerism linked to cytotoxic T lymphocyte functional unresponsiveness (clonal anergy) in a tolerant renal transplant recipient. Transplantation 1995;59:1147–55.

[56] Christensen LL, Grunnet N, Rudiger N, Moller B, et al. Indications of immunological tolerance in kidney transplantation. Tissue Antigens 1998;51:637–44.

[57] Fischer T, Schobel H, Barenbrock M. Specific immune tolerance during pregnancy after renal transplantation. Eur J Obstet Gynecol Reprod Biol 1996;70:217–9.

[58] Haynes LD, Jankowska-Gan E, Sheka A, Keller MR, et al. Donor-specific indirect pathway analysis reveals a B-cell-independent signature which reflects outcomes in kidney transplant recipients. Am J Transplant 2012;12:640–8.

[59] Uehling DT, Hussey JL, Weinstein AB, Wank R, et al. Cessation of immunosuppression after renal transplantation. Surgery 1976;79:278–82.

[60] Ballet C, Roussey-Kesler G, Aubin JT, Brouard S, et al. Humoral and cellular responses to influenza vaccination in human recipients naturally tolerant to a kidney allograft. Am J Transplant 2006;6:2796–801.

[61] VanBuskirk AM, Burlingham WJ, Jankowska-Gan E, Chin T, et al. Human allograft acceptance is associated with immune regulation. J Clin Invest 2000;106:145–55.

[62] Najafian N, Albin MJ, Newell KA. How can we measure immunologic tolerance in humans? J Am Soc Nephrol 2006;17:2652–63.

[63] Newell KA, Larsen CP. Tolerance assays: measuring the unknown. Transplantation 2006;81:1503–9.

[64] Lachenbruch PA, Rosenberg AS, Bonvini E, Cavaille-Coll MW, et al. Biomarkers and surrogate endpoints in renal transplantation: present status and considerations for clinical trial design. Am J Transplant 2004;4:451–7.

[65] Heidt S, Wood KJ. Biomarkers of operational tolerance in solid organ transplantation. Expert Opin Med Diagn 2012;6:281–93.

[66] Naesens M, Sarwal MM. Molecular diagnostics in transplantation. Nat Rev Nephrol 2010;6:614–28.

[67] Roedder S, Vitalone M, Khatri P, Sarwal MM. Biomarkers in solid organ transplantation: establishing personalized transplantation medicine. Genome Med 2011;3:37.

[68] Sawitzki B, Pascher A, Babel N, Reinke P, et al. Can we use biomarkers and functional assays to implement personalized therapies in transplantation? Transplantation 2009;87:1595–601.

[69] Nickerson P. Post-transplant monitoring of renal allografts: are we there yet? Curr Opin Immunol 2009;21:563–8.

[70] Townamchai N, Safa K, Chandraker A. Immunologic monitoring in kidney transplant recipients. Kidney Res Clin Pract 2013;32:52–61.

[71] Brouard S, Ashton-Chess J, Soulillou JP. Surrogate markers for the prediction of long-term outcome in transplantation: Nantes Actualite Transplantation (NAT) 2007 meeting report. Hum Immunol 2008;69:2–8.

[72] Chowdhury P, Hernandez-Fuentes MP. Non-invasive biomarkers to guide management following renal transplantation: the need for a multiplatform approach. Curr Opin Organ Transplant 2013;18:1–5.

[73] Sis B, Mengel M, Haas M, Colvin RB, et al. Banff '09 meeting report: antibody mediated graft deterioration and implementation of Banff working groups. Am J Transplant 2010;10:464–71.

[74] Bellomo R, Kellum JA, Ronco C. Defining acute renal failure: physiological principles. Intensive Care Med 2004;30:33–7.

[75] Londono MC, Danger R, Giral M, Soulillou JP, et al. A need for biomarkers of operational tolerance in liver and kidney transplantation. Am J Transplant 2012;12:1370–7.

[76] Baeten D, Louis S, Braud C, Braudeau C, et al. Phenotypically and functionally distinct CD8+ lymphocyte populations in long-term drug-free tolerance and chronic rejection in human kidney graft recipients. J Am Soc Nephrol 2006;17:294–304.

[77] Becker LE, de Oliveira BF, Conrad H, Schaier M, et al. Cellular infiltrates and NFkappaB subunit c-Rel signaling in kidney allografts of patients with clinical operational tolerance. Transplantation 2012:729–37.

[78] Braud C, Baeten D, Giral M, Pallier A, et al. Immunosuppressive drug-free operational immune tolerance in human kidney transplant recipients: Part I. Blood gene expression statistical analysis. J Cell Biochem 2008;103:1681–92.

[79] Braudeau C, Racape M, Giral M, Louis S, et al. Variation in numbers of CD4 + CD25highFOXP3+ T cells with normal immuno-regulatory properties in long-term graft outcome. Transpl Int 2007;20:845–55.

[80] Braudeau C, Ashton-Chess J, Giral M, Dugast E, et al. Contrasted blood and intragraft toll-like receptor 4 mRNA profiles in operational tolerance versus chronic rejection in kidney transplant recipients. Transplantation 2008;86:130–6.

[81] Brouard S, Dupont A, Giral M, Louis S, et al. Operationally tolerant and minimally immunosuppressed kidney recipients display strongly altered blood T-cell clonal regulation. Am J Transplant 2005;5:330–40.

[82] Brouard S, Le BA, Dufay A, Gosselin M, et al. Identification of a gene expression profile associated with operational tolerance among a selected group of stable kidney transplant patients. Transpl Int 2011;24:536–47.

[83] Danger R, Thervet E, Grisoni ML, Puig PL, et al. PARVG gene polymorphism and operational renal allograft tolerance. Transplant Proc 2012;44:2845–8.

[84] Danger R, Pallier A, Giral M, Martinez-Llordella M, et al. Upregulation of miR-142-3p in peripheral blood mononuclear cells of operationally tolerant patients with a renal transplant. J Am Soc Nephrol 2012;23:597–606.

[85] Louis S, Braudeau C, Giral M, Dupont A, et al. Contrasting CD25hiCD4 + T cells/ FOXP3 patterns in chronic rejection and operational drug-free tolerance. Transplantation 2006;81:398–407.

[86] Lozano JJ, Pallier A, Martinez-Llordella M, Danger R, et al. Comparison of transcriptional and blood cell-phenotypic markers between operationally tolerant liver and kidney recipients. Am J Transplant 2011;11:1916–26.

[87] Moraes-Vieira PM, Silva HM, Takenaka MC, Monteiro SM, et al. Differential monocyte STAT6 activation and CD4(+)CD25(+)Foxp3(+) T cells in kidney operational tolerance transplanted individuals. Hum Immunol 2010;71:442–50.

[88] Moraes-Vieira PM, Takenaka MC, Silva HM, Monteiro SM, et al. GATA3 and a dominant regulatory gene expression profile discriminate operational tolerance in human transplantation. Clin Immunol 2012;142:117–26.

[89] Newell KA, Asare A, Kirk AD, Gisler TD, et al. Identification of a B cell signature associated with renal transplant tolerance in humans. J Clin Invest 2010;120:1836–47.

[90] Pallier A, Hillion S, Danger R, Giral M, et al. Patients with drug-free long-term graft function display increased numbers of peripheral B cells with a memory and inhibitory phenotype. Kidney Int 2010;78:503–13.

[91] Sagoo P, Perucha E, Sawitzki B, Tomiuk S, et al. Development of a cross-platform biomarker signature to detect renal transplant tolerance in humans. J Clin Invest 2010;120:1848–61.

[92] Najafian N, Salama AD, Fedoseyeva EV, Benichou G, et al. Enzyme-linked immunosorbent spot assay analysis of peripheral blood lymphocyte reactivity to donor HLA-DR peptides: potential novel assay for prediction of outcomes for renal transplant recipients. J Am Soc Nephrol 2002;13:252–9.

[93] Poggio ED, Clemente M, Hricik DE, Heeger PS. Panel of reactive T cells as a measurement of primed cellular alloimmunity in kidney transplant candidates. J Am Soc Nephrol 2006;17:564–72.

[94] Perkins D, Verma M, Park KJ. Advances of genomic science and systems biology in renal transplantation: a review. Semin Immunopathol 2011;33:211–8.

[95] Hoffmann SC, Pearl JP, Blair PJ, Kirk AD. Immune profiling: molecular monitoring in renal transplantation. Front Biosci 2003;8:e444–62.

[96] Sigdel TK, Gao X, Sarwal MM. Protein and peptide biomarkers in organ transplantation. Biomark Med 2012;6:259–71.

[97] Braza F, Soulillou JP, Brouard S. Reconsidering the bio-detection of tolerance in renal transplantation. Chimerism 2013;4:15–17.

[98] Danger R, Racape M, Soulillou JP, Brouard S. What can we learn from the transcriptional characterization of spontaneously tolerant transplant recipients? Curr Opin Organ Transplant 2010;15:435–40.

[99] Braza F, Soulillou JP, Brouard S. Gene expression signature in transplantation tolerance. Clin Chim Acta 2012;413:1414–8.

[100] Hernandez-Fuentes MP, Lechler RI. A 'biomarker signature' for tolerance in transplantation. Nat Rev Nephrol 2010;6:606–13.

[101] Demetris AJ, Lunz III JG, Randhawa P, Wu T, et al. Monitoring of human liver and kidney allograft tolerance: a tissue/histopathology perspective. Transpl Int 2009;22:120–41.

[102] Hilton R, Hernandez-Fuentes M. Biomarkers of tolerance: hope or hype? Trends Transplant 2010;4:68–77.

[103] Ilie M, Hofman V, Long-Mira E, Selva E, et al. "Sentinel" circulating tumor cells allow early diagnosis of lung cancer in patients with chronic obstructive pulmonary disease. PLoS One 2014;9:e111597.

[104] Villeda SA, Plambeck KE, Middeldorp J, Castellano JM, et al. Young blood reverses age-related impairments in cognitive function and synaptic plasticity in mice. Nat Med 2014;20:659–63.

[105] Ashton-Chess J, Dugast E, Colvin RB, Giral M, et al. Regulatory, effector, and cytotoxic T cell profiles in long-term kidney transplant patients. J Am Soc Nephrol 2009;20:1113–22.

[106] Mas VR, Mas LA, Archer KJ, Yanek K, et al. Evaluation of gene panel mRNAs in urine samples of kidney transplant recipients as a non-invasive tool of graft function. Mol Med 2007;13:315–24.

[107] Muthukumar T, Dadhania D, Ding R, Snopkowski C, et al. Messenger RNA for FOXP3 in the urine of renal-allograft recipients. N Engl J Med 2005;353:2342–51.

[108] Perucha E, Rebollo-Mesa I, Sagoo P, Hernandez-Fuentes MP. Biomarkers of tolerance: searching for the hidden phenotype. Kidney Int Suppl 2011;1:40–6.

[109] Brouard S, Mansfield E, Braud C, Li L, et al. Identification of a peripheral blood transcriptional biomarker panel associated with operational renal allograft tolerance. Proc Natl Acad Sci U S A 2007;104:15448–53.

[110] Newell KA, Phippard D, Turka LA. Regulatory cells and cell signatures in clinical transplantation tolerance. Curr Opin Immunol 2011;23:655–9.

[111] Baron D, Ramstein G, Chesneau M, Echasseriau Y, et al. A common gene signature across multiple studies identifies biomarkers and functional regulation in tolerance to renal allograft. Kidney Int 2015 Jan 8 [E-pub ahead of print].

[112] Chesneau M, Pallier A, Braza F, Lacombe G, et al. Unique B cell differentiation profile in tolerant kidney transplant patients. Am J Transplant 2014;14:144–55.

[113] Bouaziz JD, Yanaba K, Tedder TF. Regulatory B cells as inhibitors of immune responses and inflammation. Immunol Rev 2008;224:201–14.

[114] Girndt M, Sester M, Sester U, Kaul H, et al. Molecular aspects of T- and B-cell function in uremia. Kidney Int Suppl 2001;78:S206–11.

[115] Pahl MV, Gollapudi S, Sepassi L, Gollapudi P, et al. Effect of end-stage renal disease on B-lymphocyte subpopulations, IL-7, BAFF and BAFF receptor expression. Nephrol Dial Transplant 2010;25:205–12.

[116] Smogorzewski M, Massry SG. Defects in B-cell function and metabolism in uremia: role of parathyroid hormone. Kidney Int Suppl 2001;78:S186–9.

[117] Heidt S, Hester J, Shankar S, Friend PJ, et al. B cell repopulation after alemtuzumab induction-transient increase in transitional B cells and long-term dominance of naive B cells. Am J Transplant 2012;12:1784–92.

[118] Redfield III RR, Rodriguez E, Parsons R, Vivek K, et al. Essential role for B cells in transplantation tolerance. Curr Opin Immunol 2011;23:685–91.

[119] Le Texier L, Thebault P, Lavault A, Usal C, et al. Long-term allograft tolerance is characterized by the accumulation of B cells exhibiting an inhibited profile. Am J Transplant 2011;11:429–38.

[120] Ashoor IF, Najafian N. Rejection and regulation: a tight balance. Curr Opin Organ Transplant 2012;17:1–7.

[121] Mauri C, Blair PA. Regulatory B cells in autoimmunity: developments and controversies. Nat Rev Rheumatol 2010;6:636–43.

[122] Adams AB, Newell KA. B cells in clinical transplantation tolerance. Semin Immunol 2012;24:92–5.

[123] Chesneau M, Michel L, Degauque N, Brouard S. Regulatory B cells and tolerance in transplantation: from animal models to human. Front Immunol 2013;4:497.

[124] Stolp J, Turka LA, Wood KJ. B cells with immune-regulating function in transplantation. Nat Rev Nephrol 2014;10:389–97.

[125] Zarkhin V, Chalasani G, Sarwal MM. The yin and yang of B cells in graft rejection and tolerance. Transplant Rev (Orlando) 2010;24:67–78.

[126] Mizoguchi A, Bhan AK. A case for regulatory B cells. J Immunol 2006;176:705–10.

[127] Lampropoulou V, Calderon-Gomez E, Roch T, Neves P, et al. Suppressive functions of activated B cells in autoimmune diseases reveal the dual roles of Toll-like receptors in immunity. Immunol Rev 2010;233:146–61.

[128] Yanaba K, Bouaziz JD, Haas KM, Poe JC, et al. A regulatory B cell subset with a unique CD1dhiCD5+ phenotype controls T cell-dependent inflammatory responses. Immunity 2008;28:639–50.

[129] Yanaba K, Bouaziz JD, Matsushita T, Tsubata T, et al. The development and function of regulatory B cells expressing IL-10 (B10 cells) requires antigen receptor diversity and TLR signals. J Immunol 2009;182:7459–72.

[130] Hagn M, Jahrsdorfer B. Why do human B cells secrete granzyme B? Insights into a novel B-cell differentiation pathway. Oncoimmunology 2012;1:1368–75.

[131] Chesneau M, Michel L, Chenouard A, Pallier A, et al. Tolerant kidney transplant patients display B cells with a CD5+ CD27+ CD138+ phenotype that express granzyme B and show regulatory properties. J Am Soc Nephrol 2014 [in press].

[132] Perez-Andres M, Paiva B, Nieto WG, Caraux A, et al. Human peripheral blood B-cell compartments: a crossroad in B-cell traffic. Cytometry B Clin Cytom 2010;78(Suppl. 1):S47–60.

[133] Silva HM, Takenaka MC, Moraes-Vieira PM, Monteiro SM, et al. Preserving the B-cell compartment favors operational tolerance in human renal transplantation. Mol Med 2012;18:733–43.

[134] Nouel A, Segalen I, Jamin C, Doucet L, et al. B cells display an abnormal distribution and an impaired suppressive function in patients with chronic antibody-mediated rejection. Kidney Int 2014;85:590–9.

[135] Cherukuri A, Rothstein DM, Clark B, Carter CR, et al. Immunologic human renal allograft injury associates with an altered IL-10/TNF-alpha expression ratio in regulatory B cells. J Am Soc Nephrol 2014;25:1575–85.

[136] Braza F, Dugast E, Panov I, Paul C, et al. Central role of CD45RA$^-$Foxp3^{hi} memory Tregs in clinical kidney transplantation tolerance. J Am Soc Nephrol 2015 [E-pub ahead of print].

[137] Parker A, Bowles K, Bradley JA, Emery V, et al. Management of post-transplant lymphoproliferative disorder in adult solid organ transplant recipients—BCSH and BTS Guidelines. Br J Haematol 2010;149:693–705.

[138] Wahl SM, Rosenstreich DL. Role of B lymphocytes in cell-mediated immunity. I. Requirement for T cells or T-cell products for antigen-induced B-cell activation. J Exp Med 1976;144:1175–87.

[139] Ashton-Chess J, Giral M, Soulillou JP, Brouard S. Can immune monitoring help to minimize immunosuppression in kidney transplantation? Transpl Int 2009;22:110–9.

[140] Brouard S, Giral M, Soulillou JP, Ashton-Chess J. Elaboration of gene expression-based clinical decision aids for kidney transplantation: where do we stand? Transplantation 2011;91:691–6.

[141] Calne R, Friend P, Moffatt S, Bradley A, et al. Prope tolerance, perioperative campath 1H, and low-dose cyclosporin monotherapy in renal allograft recipients. Lancet 1998;351:1701–2.

[142] Viklicky O, Krystufkova E, Brabcova I, Sekerkova A, et al. B-cell-related biomarkers of tolerance are up-regulated in rejection-free kidney transplant recipients. Transplantation 2013;95:148–54.

[143] Moreso F, Torres IB, Martinez-Gallo M, Benlloch S, et al. Gene expression signature of tolerance and lymphocyte subsets in stable renal transplants: results of a cross-sectional study. Transpl Immunol 2014;31:11–16.

[144] Abramowicz D, Del Carmen RM, Vitko S, del CD, et al. Cyclosporine withdrawal from a mycophenolate mofetil-containing immunosuppressive regimen: results of a five-year, prospective, randomized study. J Am Soc Nephrol 2005;16:2234–40.

[145] Ekberg H, Tedesco-Silva H, Demirbas A, Vitko S, et al. Reduced exposure to calcineurin inhibitors in renal transplantation. N Engl J Med 2007;357:2562–75.

[146] Pallardo LM, Oppenheimer F, Guirado L, Conesa J, et al. Calcineurin inhibitor reduction based on maintenance immunosuppression with mycophenolate mofetil in renal transplant patients: POP study. Transplant Proc 2007;39:2187–9.

[147] Salinas-Carmona MC, Perez LI, Galan K, Vazquez AV. Immunosuppressive drugs have different effect on B lymphocyte subsets and IgM antibody production in immunized BALB/c mice. Autoimmunity 2009;42:537–44.

[148] Vivek K, Mustafa MM, Rodriguez E, Redfield III RR, et al. Strategies for B-lymphocyte repertoire remodeling in transplantation tolerance. Immunol Res 2011;51:1–4.

[149] Newell KA, Chong AS. Making a B-line for transplantation tolerance. Am J Transplant 2011;11:420–1.

[150] Bluestone JA, Thomson AW, Shevach EM, Weiner HL. What does the future hold for cell-based tolerogenic therapy? Nat Rev Immunol 2007;7:650–4.

[151] Liu C, Noorchashm H, Sutter JA, Naji M, et al. B lymphocyte-directed immunotherapy promotes long-term islet allograft survival in nonhuman primates. Nat Med 2007;13:1295–8.

[152] Porcheray F, Wong W, Saidman SL, De VJ, et al. B-cell immunity in the context of T-cell tolerance after combined kidney and bone marrow transplantation in humans. Am J Transplant 2009;9:2126–35.

[153] Kelishadi SS, Azimzadeh AM, Zhang T, Stoddard T, et al. Preemptive CD20+ B cell depletion attenuates cardiac allograft vasculopathy in cyclosporine-treated monkeys. J Clin Invest 2010;120:1275–84.

[154] Kopchaliiska D, Zachary AA, Montgomery RA, Leffell MS. Reconstitution of peripheral allospecific CD19+ B-cell subsets after B-lymphocyte depletion therapy in renal transplant patients. Transplantation 2009;87:1394–401.

[155] Alwayn IP, Xu Y, Basker M, Wu C, et al. Effects of specific anti-B and/or anti-plasma cell immunotherapy on antibody production in baboons: depletion of CD20- and CD22-positive B cells does not result in significantly decreased production of anti-alphaGal antibody. Xenotransplantation 2001;8:157–71.

[156] Kozlowski T, Andreoni K. Limitations of rituximab/IVIg desensitization protocol in kidney transplantation: is this better than a tincture of time? Ann Transplant 2011;16:19–25.

[157] Munoz AS, Rioveros AA, Cabanayan-Casasola CB, Danguilan RA, et al. Rituximab in highly sensitized kidney transplant recipients. Transplant Proc 2008;40:2218–21.

[158] Ramos EJ, Pollinger HS, Stegall MD, Gloor JM, et al. The effect of desensitization protocols on human splenic B-cell populations *in vivo*. Am J Transplant 2007;7:402–7.

Intracellular concentrations of immunosuppressants

Heike Bittersohl and Werner Steimer

Institute of Clinical Chemistry and Pathobiochemistry,
Klinikum rechts der Isar der TU München, Munich, Germany

9.1 INTRODUCTION

Measurements of whole blood or plasma drug concentrations are commonly used for the monitoring of immunosuppressive therapy. Despite achieving therapeutic levels of immunosuppressive drugs, a considerable proportion of transplant patients still experience acute graft rejection [1,2]. The immunosuppressive site of action for calcineurin inhibitors (CNIs), proliferation signal inhibitors (PSIs), and mycophenolic acid (MPA) is inside the lymphocyte blood cells. CNIs inhibit the calcium/calmodulin-dependent phosphatase calcineurin (CN) by inhibiting its interaction with cyclosporine–cyclophilin and tacrolimus–FK506-binding protein 12 complexes. Sirolimus and its synthetically produced derivative everolimus (PSIs) inhibit the kinase mammalian target of rapamycin (mTOR). MPA acts as an antimetabolite immunosuppressant by inhibition of inosine monophosphate dehydrogenase (IMPDH). Due to the fact that the intracellular compartment of lymphocytes is the target site of drug action, whole blood or plasma concentrations can only serve as substitute markers. It is assumed that the content of immunosuppressants in lymphocytes is influenced by several drug transporters located on the lymphocyte cell membrane. For example, the activity of P-glycoprotein (P-gp), an ATP-dependent efflux pump that is encoded by the *ABCB1* gene in humans is influenced by genetic variants and can be inhibited or induced by comedication or other xenobiotics. Intra- and interindividual variabilities are the reason for unpredictable target-cell drug concentrations that are kept concealed by only measuring whole blood levels. A few years prior to immunosuppressants, intracellular drug measurement had been realized for antiretroviral agents after sensitive liquid chromatography–tandem mass spectrometry (LC–MS/MS) methods became available [3,4]. A good correlation between intracellular and free fraction [5] or plasma concentrations [6] has been observed, indicating that the intracellular monitoring might not be of great relevance for HIV-infected patients under therapy. However, reliable and sensitive methods for measurements of immunosuppressive drugs in lymphocytes have only been established recently, allowing the conduction of informative research studies. The aim of such studies is to evaluate whether

M. Oellerich & A. Dasgupta (Eds): Personalized Immunosuppression in Transplantation.
DOI: http://dx.doi.org/10.1016/B978-0-12-800885-0.00009-6

intracellular monitoring could better reflect effective drug concentrations and, as a consequence, might more clearly indicate under- and overdosing of immunosuppressants in transplant patients.

9.2 MEASURING INTRACELLULAR CONCENTRATIONS OF IMMUNOSUPPRESSANTS

Although measuring intracellular concentrations of various immunosuppressants appear to be superior to traditional determination of trough concentrations in whole blood (cyclosporine A, tacrolimus, sirolimus, and everolimus) or plasma (mycophenolic acid) determination of intracellular concentrations of immunosuppressants is technically more challenging than routine therapeutic drug monitoring (TDM) of immunosuppressants. This section discusses various issues related to the determination of intracellular concentrations of immunosuppressants.

9.2.1 ANALYTICAL TECHNIQUES

During the past two decades, a number of analytical methods for the analysis of very small amounts of immunosuppressive drugs have been developed, enabling intracellular drug monitoring. Masri et al. carried out the first investigation on intracellular cyclosporine A (CsA) concentrations in 1998 using density-gradient centrifugation on Ficoll–Hypaque for cell isolation. For the subsequent drug quantification, they utilized commercial monoclonal immunoassay on the TDx analyzer (Abbott Diagnostics), which in part, specific for the parent compound CsA [7]. Despite the rather small number of following studies, methods have been substantially improved to yield reliable data, allowing for investigations of drug pharmacokinetics at a lymphocyte cell level. However, LC–MS/MS-based methods have better analytical sensitivity and precision for determination of intracellular concentrations of various immunosuppressants.

9.2.1.1 Isolation of peripheral blood mononuclear cells and lymphocytes

Peripheral blood mononuclear cells (PBMCs) are blood cells with round nuclei, such as monocytes, lymphocytes, and macrophages. As the first step of most intracellular immunosuppressant quantification methods, mononuclear cells are isolated from peripheral blood. Commonly, this is achieved through density gradient centrifugation using a hydrophilic colloid. Polymers formed by the copolymerization of sucrose and epichlorohydrin or polyvinylpyrrolidone-coated colloidal silica are examples of hydrophilic colloids that can be purchased in different qualities. Saumet et al. [8] tested one conventional Ficoll–Paque gradient centrifugation and two commercial sampling devices: the Vacutainer cell tube (Becton Dickinson) and the Leucosep tube (Greiner Bio-One). By use of Leucosep tubes, an average of 82% of PBMCs in heparinized blood samples could be recovered; thus, this appeared to be the most efficient separation method.

In general, approximately 8 mL of anticoagulated peripheral venous blood is diluted with buffer solution and then carefully layered onto the separation medium and centrifuged (usually at 400 g for 30–40 min). Because of their low density, mononuclear cells and platelets are found on top of the separation medium. In contrast, red blood cells and granulocytes, which have a higher density, are found at the bottom of the tube. The PBMC layer is harvested by careful pipetting and washed twice with phosphate buffered saline solution (PBS) or cell medium to remove platelets and residual separation medium. Performing the PBMC isolation at 4°C [9] or adding P-gp inhibitors such as verapamil or quinidine [10–12] are techniques used for prevention of drug efflux from cells. After PBMC isolation, an aliquot is taken for cell counting to relate the intracellular drug concentration to the number of PBMCs in each sample.

By use of standard methods such as Ficoll–Paque density gradient centrifugation for PBMC, isolation recoveries yield on average $0.5-2 \times 10^6$ cells/mL blood taken. According to Ulmer and Flad [13], only 60–80% of the isolated cells are lymphocytes; the remaining cells are monocytes (20–40%) and polymorphonuclear cells (1–4%). Plebanksi [14] published a more detailed description of PBMC components, displaying a higher portion of lymphocytes (Table 9.1).

There are several methods for subsequent lymphocyte purification [15,16]. Protocols have been established to separate the target cells from monocytes by taking advantage of monocytes adhering to plastics. Another method for depletion of monocytes and macrophages is based on their high lysosomal enzyme content: L-leucine methyl ester (a lysosomotropic agent) is added and taken up by cytotoxic and phagotoxic cells. It accumulates in lysosomes, where it is converted into L-leucyl-L-leucine methyl ester, which is a toxic agent to the cells. Most lymphocytes remain unaffected by exposure to L-leucine methyl ester because of their lack of lysosomal enzymes. However, NK cells and cytotoxic T cells would also be depleted. Nevertheless, lymphocyte purification with the previously described methods has not been used in the context of intracellular measurement of immunosuppressants.

A convenient way to specifically isolate T lymphocytes has been applied by Falck et al. [10,17,18]: By use of Prepacyte, a layer containing more than 97% of

Table 9.1 Average Composition of PBMCs in a Healthy Adult Human

Cell Type	%	Frequencies (×10³ Cells, Isolated from 1 mL Blood)
T cells (CD3⁺)	60	300–1200
T helper cells (CD3⁺, CD4⁺)	70 of T cells	210–840
Cytotoxic T cells (CD3⁺, CD8⁺)	30 of T cells	90–360
Monocytes/macrophages (CD14⁺)	15	75–300
B cells (CD22⁺)	10	50–200
Natural killer (NK) cells (CD56⁺/CD16⁺)	15	75–300

Data from Peblanski [14].

lymphocytes with T lymphocytes comprising 88–96% of the resultant cell population can be harvested after preparation. The procedure involves negative separation via antibodies against specific antigens expressed on the surfaces of erythrocytes, B lymphocytes, mature myeloid cells such as granulocytes, monocytes, and platelets, causing agglutination of these cells but not the T lymphocytes.

Another technique for removal of unwanted cell types in PBMC is to label them with magnetic beads that are conjugated to specific antibodies against cell surface antigens. Thus, the labeled and unlabeled cells are applied to a column exposed to a magnetic field. Magnetically labeled cells are retained, whereas unlabeled cells pass through the column and can be collected for further sample preparation steps. This technique could be adapted for fast lymphocyte isolation, minimizing the exposure of lymphocytes to surrounding liquids and, thus, reducing the risk of drug leakage. Isolated lymphocytes can represent the target site of action much more precisely than the mixture of lymphocytes, monocytes, and macrophages and may therefore serve as a convenient matrix for measuring immunosuppressant drug exposure. A prerequisite, however, is the availability of analytical methods sensitive enough to cope with minimal drug quantities.

9.2.1.2 *Extraction and determination of intracellular immunosuppressive drugs*

After PBMC or lymphocyte isolation, an aliquot is taken for cell counting, eventually allowing the amount of drug present to be expressed as per 10^6 or 10^7 cells. Whereas Masri and Barbari used immunoassays [7] or high-performance liquid chromatography (HPLC) [19] for drug quantification, LC–MS/MS methods have been established for more recent investigations [9,20–22]. In most analytical assays, methanol containing the internal standard is added to the thawed PBMC/lymphocyte pellet, which is stored frozen after isolation from whole blood. Further cell lysis and analyte extraction is performed by long-term shaking. Falck et al. [10] implemented an additional subsequent purification step with solid phase extraction cartridges. Other authors add PBS to the cell pellet before storage at −20° or −80°C and perform a liquid–liquid extraction with an organic solvent after unfreezing the samples [9,19]. The use of deuterated internal standards, which have very similar physiochemical properties compared to the analyte compound, is highly recommended because such internal standards can correct for all losses and inefficiencies that might occur during the sample preparation process [23]. Especially during an extraction step, it is important to equally recover both the analyte and the internal standard for valid results. The extraction is finished with a centrifugation step, separating the solid remnants of cell lysis from the supernatant containing dissolved drug molecules. Afterwards, the supernatant is collected and dried under nitrogen or using a vacuum concentrator. For measurement via LC-MS/MS, the dry residue is reconstituted in a solvent suitable for liquid chromatography and injected into the liquid chromatography system. The present methods for isolation and purification of immunosuppressant drugs from PBMCs are rather laborious and time-consuming. However, they are a prerequisite for the detection of very low drug concentrations.

9.3 IMMUNOSUPPRESSANT DRUG CONCENTRATIONS IN PBMCs/LYMPHOCYTES

This section discusses the determination of concentrations of specific immunosuppressants (cyclosporine, tacrolimus, sirolimus, everolimus, and MPA) in PBMC/lymphocytes and the clinical implications of such results.

9.3.1 CYCLOSPORINE A

Introduction of CsA in the early 1980s greatly contributed to improving the long-term survival of patient and graft. Even today, it is still a cornerstone of the immunosuppressive therapy in solid organ transplant recipients. Due to a narrow therapeutic window and great inter- and intrapatient pharmacokinetic variation, TDM is required. In general, whole blood samples are used for CsA determination because the drug is highly bound to blood cells and plasma proteins. The distribution of CsA in blood is dependent on temperature, drug concentration, hematocrit, and lipoproteins. At body temperature, 60% of CsA can be found in plasma. Considering the association of CsA with lymphocytes, even at extremely high concentrations of up to 7000 ng/mL, this compartment remains nonsaturable [24,25]. Determination of CsA inside lymphocytes could give more relevant information on the drug's efficacy and further improve and individualize TDM.

Some early studies on intracellular CsA measurements were conducted by Barbari and Masri [7,26–30]. They observed great interindividual variation of CsA accumulation in lymphocytes and found no correlation between intracellular CsA levels, doses, and blood levels [7,26,27]. In later studies, it was shown that PBMC CsA levels were lower prior to rejection episodes compared to stable graft conditions in renal transplant patients, whereas whole blood concentrations revealed no difference between rejection and non-rejection groups [26,28,29]. An increase in hematocrit appeared to have an adverse effect on CsA lymphocyte binding [28]. These findings seem fully coherent and were partly consistent with results from studies performed by other investigators [17,31,32]. Nevertheless, these results must be interpreted carefully. The PBMC concentrations were approximately 1000-fold greater compared to those of studies using radioimmunoassay (RIA) or validated LC–MS/MS methods and, thus, lack verification from other working groups. Measurements were performed using an immunoassay with monoclonal antibodies originally intended for CsA determination in whole blood samples. Therefore, they may lack sensitivity for small drug amounts in a matrix other than whole blood.

In the course of several research studies on intracellular CsA concentrations, the influence of genetic polymorphisms with respect to drug-metabolizing enzymes and active drug efflux from lymphocytes by P-gp was additionally evaluated [17,18,31–33]. This influence on CsA pharmacokinetics is described in detail in Section 9.4.

Table 9.2 provides an overview of published studies on intracellular CsA measurements in transplant patients. In 2007, Lepage [21] conducted a study on a cohort of 20 stable renal transplant recipients. A monoclonal selective fluorescence

Table 9.2 Overview of Published Studies Regarding PBMC Trough CsA Concentrations

No. of Patients	Organ	Day of Measurement	Whole Blood CsA Concentration (C_0) (ng/mL)		PBMC CsA Concentration (at C_0) (ng/10^6 Cells)		References
			Mean ± SD	Range	Mean ± SD	Range	
20	Kidney	7.2 ± 4.9 months after transplantation	150–300 (target range)		3.8 ± 3.7	0.6–16.3	[21]
64	Various	Steady state	104	33–205	2.1	0.3–13.6	[31]
20/9[a]	Kidney	Steady state	349 ± 105	–	26.5 ± 17.3[b]	–	[17][c]
					(No rejection; $n = 5$)		
		Steady state	294 ± 62	–	8.6 ± 4.0[b]	–	
					(Rejection; $n = 4$)		
25	Kidney	Steady state	210 ± 81	–	25.5 ± 22	–	[18][c]
					(Elderly > 65; $n = 11$)		
			255 ± 92	–	12.9 ± 9.0	–	
					(Young; $n = 14$)		
10	Heart	17 ± 6 to 70 ± 8 days after transplantation	301	152–513	8.1	1.3–25	[33][c]
					(No rejection; $n = 7$)		
			316	153–564	10.1	1.5–39	
					(Mild rejection; $n = 3$)		

[a]C_0 published only for 9 patients who underwent a 12-h pharmacokinetic investigation.
[b]Intra-lymphocyte concentration is given in ng/mL.
[c]CsA PBMC concentrations determined in isolated T lymphocytes.

polarization immunoassay and an RIA were used to assess intracellular concentrations. The aim of the study was to monitor CsA in CD4$^+$ lymphocytes, the target compartment. Due to the complex cell separation technique and the limited assay sensitivity, it was possible to measure CsA in PBMCs but not in lymphocyte subsets. Concentrations varied from 0.6 to 16.3 ng per million PBMCs, and there was only a weak correlation with whole blood levels and no correlation with CsA doses. It remains unknown if a significant lack of correlation would have been found between PBMC and whole blood CsA concentrations if the PBMC isolation technique had resulted in a greater proportion of lymphocytes than reported in this study (lymphocyte/monocyte ratio = 1.28).

In the course of a study on *ABCB1* gene polymorphisms and P-gp activity [32], 24-h pharmacokinetic profiles of 19 healthy volunteers receiving a single oral dose of CsA microemulsion (Sandimmun Neoral) were recorded. Prior to the study, the author developed and fully validated a sensitive and selective analytical LC–MS/MS method specifically for the purpose of intracellular CsA determinations [22]. 27-Demethoxy-sirolimus is used as internal standard, and an online solid phase extraction is applied for further analyte purification. The method allows measurement of very small amounts of CsA down to 0.5 fg per PBMC in clinical samples. PBMC and whole blood pharmacokinetics followed parallel profiles for each participant, but no correlation was observed between CsA PBMC and whole blood concentrations taking all volunteers into account. Interindividual variability was significantly greater in PBMCs than in whole blood. Ansermot [32] proposed a single intracellular measurement as an interesting complement to routine whole blood TDM, but several factors influence CsA distribution in blood, such as nutrition, varying medication, or immune status, which requires more measurements during the patient follow-up period. Later studies with subsequent measurements of intracellular CsA demonstrated a significant intrapatient variability [17,33].

Using the same analytical method as that used by Ansermot et al. [32], CsA PBMC concentrations were measured in samples of 64 stable transplanted patients with various transplanted organs (kidney, liver, or lung) [31]. A moderate, but significant, correlation was observed between whole blood and intracellular CsA concentrations. This finding is contradictory to the hypothesis that whole blood levels do not predict intralymphocyte CsA concentrations. A nonhomogenous patient cohort was chosen with respect to type of transplant and comedication, and the treatment with P-gp inhibitors was found to have no influence on the PBMC CsA levels. Interestingly, 2 patients presented anti-HLA antibodies, which are associated with an increased risk for rejection. Both the intracellular and the whole blood CsA concentrations were lower compared to those in the rest of the patient population. An insufficient downregulation of the immune system might explain the development of anti-HLA antibodies.

Concurrent with the investigations by Ansermot and Crettol, Falck et al. developed an LC-MS/MS method to measure CsA and six CsA main metabolites, which was validated according to U.S. Food and Drug Administration guidelines [10]. The sample preparation comprises isolation of T lymphocytes using Prepacyte® and a solid phase extraction step. Lower limits of quantification were $0.25\,ng/10^6$ cells for intracellular and $2.5\,ng/mL$ for whole blood measurements. So far, it has been used for three follow-up studies [17,18,33]. Results, however, have been published for the parent compound only. A study including 20 kidney transplant patients [17] showed a significant decrease of intracellular CsA 1 week before acute rejection. The decrease was, on average, observed 3 days before the rejection, and it was clinically diagnosed by an increase of serum creatinine. In contrast, the corresponding CsA C_2 (concentration 2 h after dosing) whole blood concentrations showed no difference between rejection and non-rejection groups. The authors also measured intralymphocyte cyclosporine area under the concentration time curve (AUC_{0-12}) and found areas under the curve almost twice as high during stable phase compared to patients experiencing rejection ($p = 0.004$). Measured free plasma CsA fractions tended to be lower in the rejection group, but the observed trend showed no significance. This finding is in contrast to an earlier investigation, also performed with kidney transplant patients, that revealed a significant decrease of the free CsA fraction immediately prior to rejection episodes [34]. However, the study supports the hypothesis of a possible clinical benefit of intracellular CsA monitoring despite a low number of study participants.

In another study, also performed by Falck et al. [18], the authors investigated a possible difference in intracellular pharmacokinetics of CsA between elderly (>65 years) and younger renal transplant recipients. The portion of CsA available inside lymphocytes was greater in elderly patients, offering an explanation for the general lower rate of rejections among this age group. Recently, the LC-MS/MS method was applied to a pilot study involving 10 heart transplant recipients followed for several weeks after transplantation [33]. Surprisingly, the study failed to show any correlations between CsA concentrations in whole blood, intralymphocyte, and endomyocardial tissue samples. No decrease in intracellular CsA levels before rejection episodes was observed. However, there were only 2 patients in the small cohort who suffered only mild rejection episodes.

Despite the low number of studies and some controversial results, investigations of intracellular CsA levels remain interesting in terms of understanding the drug's pharmacokinetics and the respective clinical findings. Several drawbacks, such as small patient numbers, different immunosuppressive regimens, varying comedication, as well as few rejection episodes among study cohorts, make it difficult to obtain significant results. Currently, two powerful analytical methods have been published, one of which actually measures CsA concentrations in T lymphocytes. Therewith, the tool to perform informative studies is available. More and larger studies are needed to determine if intracellular CsA concentrations can describe the response to immunosuppressive therapy.

9.3.2 TACROLIMUS

Currently, tacrolimus is the most used immunosuppressive agent in solid organ transplantation. It presents a narrow therapeutic range and considerable interindividual variability with poor correlation between drug intake, blood concentrations, and clinical outcome [2,35]. Thus, TDM is necessary, and for practical reasons as well as lack of convincing data supporting more sophisticated pharmacokinetic strategies, trough whole blood concentrations (C_0) are generally used for adjusting the individual drug dosage [36].

Tacrolimus is principally bound to erythrocytes, with an approximate mean blood-to-plasma ratio of 15 [35]. The fraction of unbound protein able to diffuse into lymphocyte cells has been estimated to be $0.47 \pm 0.18\%$. Tacrolimus associated with lymphocytes ranged between 0.11 and 1.53%, being lower in patients who suffer rejection compared with stable organ transplant patients [37]. These values were found more than 10 years ago when highly sensitive LC–MS/MS methods for detection of minimal tacrolimus amounts were not yet available. Alternatively, patient blood was incubated with a radiolabeled tacrolimus derivative (^{3}H-dihydro-tacrolimus), which showed very similar distribution characteristics in blood compared with the real immunosuppressant tacrolimus [38]. The cells were isolated over a Ficoll gradient, and radioactivity was measured with a liquid scintillation counter. Despite this convenient solution to assess the amount of drug in the target compartment, several methodological barriers limit the significance of the gained results. For instance, the solvent in the ^{3}H-dihydro-tacrolimus solution added to the blood sample might alter the distribution pattern of the drug. In addition, the incubation of the blood sample in a non-physiological environment after spike addition could lead to biochemical changes of blood components.

In 2007, Barbari et al. [30] performed some of the first intracellular tacrolimus measurements using an immunoassay. Some extraordinarily high intralymphocyte tacrolimus concentrations were found, ranging from 1 to 16 pg per lymphocyte (data taken from diagram). To date, no other group has been able to repeat those results.

The following investigations on intracellular tacrolimus concentrations were performed by thorough PBMC isolation, cell counting, and drug determination via highly sensitive and validated LC-MS/MS methods [9,39–42]. A method established by Capron et al. [9] displayed a lower limit of quantification of 0.01 ng/mL, allowing measurement of the smallest concentrations down to 0.006 ng per 10^6 PBMCs. Capron et al. estimated the time needed to process 10 patient samples to be 5 or 6 h. This time frame is acceptable for study purposes and possible benefits, such as a better patient outcome, could even justify increased hands-on time in the routine laboratory.

The results of studies on intracellular tacrolimus measurements are summarized in Table 9.3. All authors found a lack of correlation between intracellular tacrolimus concentrations and the corresponding whole blood levels. These findings provide additional evidence for the assumption that whole blood concentrations rather serve as global drug exposure markers, whereas intracellular drug monitoring may more precisely determine whether a patient's immunosuppressant intake is sufficient.

Capron et al. [39] performed one study that included 96 kidney transplant patients who received MPA and steroids for immunosuppression along with tacrolimus. In 6 patients, rejection occurred during the first month after transplantation (5.76%). This tended to be associated with lower tacrolimus concentrations in PBMCs ($p = 0.094$). Tacrolimus PBMC concentrations correlated neither at day 7 post-transplantation

Table 9.3 Overview of Studies Published on Tacrolimus PBMC Concentrations

No. of Patients	Transplanted Organ	Day of Measurement[a]	Whole Blood Tacrolimus Concentration (C$_0$) (ng/mL)		Tacrolimus Concentration in PBMC (at C$_0$) (pg/10^6 Cells)		References
			Mean ± SD	Range	Mean ± SD	Range	
96	Kidney	1	13.4	11.9–15.0	–	–	[39]
		7	13.2	12.4–14.0	71.6 ± 19.4	–	
		Steady state	11.2	10.6–11.7	76.6 ± 19.9	–	
90	Liver	1	4.2 ± 1.6	1.0–4.5	28.7 ± 22.2	0–80.2	[40]
		3	6.8 ± 2.1	4.7–8.2	63.6 ± 49.8	10.9–287.4	
		5	8.8 ± 4.8	5.9–12.9	62.1 ± 40.6	10.0–214.7	
		7	8.9 ± 3.0	6.7–13.2	65.4 ± 41.8	10.1–185.6	
24	Heart	Steady state	8.1 ± 2.6	4.3–18.3	40.0 ± 29.0	5.0–150.0	[41]
10	Liver	1	6.9 ± 3.1	–	71.3 ± 78.5	–	[42]
		7	5.4 ± 3.1	–	39.5 ± 38.8	–	

[a]Days after organ transplantation or first administration of tacrolimus.

nor at steady state with whole blood concentrations. This suggests that drug determinations within the target cells might provide better insight into individual tacrolimus pharmacokinetics and may allow assessing the efficacy of intracellular compared to whole blood concentration measurements. Patients received concomitant therapies, including atorvastatin and proton pump inhibitors, which are inhibitors of P-gp, an efflux transporter present on the lymphocyte membrane. No influence on intracellular or whole blood levels could be observed. Interestingly, further biological parameters have been determined, and the hematocrit, the mean corpuscular volume, and the total amount of plasma protein revealed a negative correlation with intracellular tacrolimus concentrations. It can be assumed that the free tacrolimus fraction is greater in samples with low hematocrit and total protein content and might diffuse more readily into lymphocytes.

A later study, also performed by Capron et al. [40], included 90 patients who received liver transplant and tacrolimus-based immunosuppressive therapy. Clinical rejection established in 12 (10.8%) patients was characterized by a significantly lower mean tacrolimus PBMC concentration on days 5 and 7 after surgery ($p < 0.05$). In addition, intrahepatic tacrolimus concentrations were determined 1 week after surgery. The intrahepatic tacrolimus levels revealed a significant relationship with the histological staging of rejection and also with PBMC tacrolimus concentrations of day 5 but not with the respective tacrolimus whole blood levels.

In 2013, Lemaitre et al. [41] applied a validated LC-MS/MS method for tacrolimus determination in PBMCs of 24 cardiac transplant recipients. A greater interpatient variability for tacrolimus in PBMCs compared to the respective whole blood levels and, surprisingly, a positive correlation between PBMC tacrolimus concentrations and creatinemia were found. In contrast to findings from Capron et al. [39], no correlations with hematocrit or proteinemia were detected. Thus, there may be several factors regarding the type of organ transplanted that influence tacrolimus pharmacokinetics in blood.

Lemaitre et al. [42] explored the pharmacokinetics and pharmacodynamics of tacrolimus in 10 de novo liver transplant patients by measuring the CN activity as well as whole blood and intracellular tacrolimus concentrations. This combination of drug-level measurements and direct monitoring of drug effect seems to be a very valuable approach enabling the investigation of the relationship between drug concentration and reduction in CN activity. Interestingly, there was one study participant suffering acute cellular rejection (ACR) during the study period despite an adequate tacrolimus whole blood exposure. However, the patient's intracellular tacrolimus concentrations were four times lower compared to those of the mean study population. In addition, a raising CN activity from day 1 to day 7 after surgery was also observed in this patient. These findings suggest that measurement of tacrolimus directly at the target site could better predict the drug efficacy compared to whole blood measurements. Tacrolimus concentrations in PBMCs displayed a greater variability between patients, tended to be lower prior to ACR, and correlated with biological markers influencing the drug distribution in blood. However, despite these encouraging results, more studies on intracellular tacrolimus concentrations are required. The following two questions need to be addressed: Can a therapeutic range be defined, and could this kind of monitoring be relevant for both the early post-transplant period and periodic long-term examinations?

9.3.3 MYCOPHENOLIC ACID

MPA is often combined with CNIs in immunosuppressive drug regimens after organ transplantation. Unlike CsA or tacrolimus, it has no nephrotoxic side effects [43,44] and, hence, can be used to reduce the CNI dose. MPA is a selective, reversible inhibitor of IMPDH, an important enzyme in the de novo purine synthesis. B and T lymphocytes are highly dependent on IMPDH for cell proliferation, whereas other cell types can use salvage pathways. Therefore, MPA selectively inhibits lymphocyte proliferation and functions. MPA and its major metabolite MPA glucuronide, are substrates of the efflux protein multidrug resistance-associated protein 2 (MRP2) present in the lymphocyte membrane [45,46]. Varying activity (and polymorphisms) could result in different intralymphocyte drug concentrations, leading to different intensities of immunosuppression. Very little work has been done on measuring intracellular MPA. Bénech et al. [47] developed an LC–MS/MS method that featured a run time of 10 min and a lower limit of quantification of 0.24 ng per sample, but no results from patient samples have been published. A fast LC–MS/MS method with a run time of 6 min and a lower limit of quantification at 0.1 ng/mL has been established and applied in a clinical research study on kidney transplant patients [48]. First results in 40 patients showed MPA concentrations between 6.9 and 33.9 ng/10^6 cells. Interestingly, a poor correlation ($p = 0.165$) between pre-dose MPA plasma levels and the respective PBMC concentrations was found, indicating a possible benefit from intracellular measurements. The author reports that the described method is currently applied in a larger research study involving approximately 100 kidney transplant patients to investigate whether measurements of MPA in plasma (C_0 and AUC), intralymphocyte, or IMPDH activity as a marker of drug response serve as the best tool for predicting clinical outcomes in transplant patients.

9.3.4 PSIs: SIROLIMUS AND EVEROLIMUS

Sirolimus and its synthetically produced derivative everolimus are increasingly used for maintenance immunosuppression following solid organ transplantation, typically in combination with CsA and a corticosteroid. Compared to sirolimus, the newer drug everolimus has a shorter half-life, which results in twice-daily dosing compared to once-daily dosing of sirolimus, thus allowing more rapid achievement of a steady state [49].

Both agents have narrow therapeutic ranges and, as a result of highly variable intersubject pharmacokinetics, require TDM. TDM of whole blood samples is the current state of the art due to a great distribution in red blood cells. Sirolimus and everolimus trough concentrations prior to the dose are good surrogate markers of drug exposure and correlate with pharmacological response and clinical outcomes. The target trough whole blood levels are 3–8 ng/mL for everolimus and 4–12 or 12–20 ng/mL for sirolimus with or without concomitant CsA therapy, respectively [50–52]. To our knowledge, only one publication about intracellular sirolimus levels in PBMCs exists in the literature [19]. The study involved 42 kidney transplant patients from whom EDTA whole blood was collected at three different time points (C_0, pre-dose; C_1, 1 h post-dose; and C_2, 2 h post-dose) for whole blood and intracellular sirolimus determinations. PBMCs were isolated from an aliquot of whole blood by use of a Ficoll gradient and three subsequent washing steps. In addition, the lymphocyte count was determined with a flow cytometer. The isolation of sirolimus was performed with "MERI," a solution patented by the author. For drug determination, Masri used HPLC-ultraviolet or microparticle enzyme-linked immunoassay and observed higher values with the immunoassay compared to HPLC, which is possibly due to unspecific binding of antibodies to sirolimus metabolites. In contrast to blood levels and lymphocyte counts, the intracellular sirolimus concentrations for C_0, C_1, and C_2 and the number of lymphocytes showed a significant negative correlation. This finding could be related to a fast pharmacological drug response. However, the publication gives no information about a possible correlation or noncorrelation between intracellular and whole blood levels of sirolimus. Furthermore, the concentrations of PBMCs (ranging between 1 and 10 pg per cell; data taken from graph) appear to be several magnitudes too high. Earlier studies on CsA concentrations in PBMCs authored by Masri and Barbari et al. [7,26–30] also reported concentrations that were approximately 1000-fold higher compared to findings of other groups [17,31]. The reason might be the use of an immunoassay, which is intended for clinical routine use of whole blood samples containing much higher drug amounts.

First measurements of everolimus in PBMCs were performed by Roullet-Renoleau, who developed a sensitive LC–MS/MS method for this purpose [20]. The method was validated according to the requirements of the International Conference on Harmonization and applied to PBMC samples of 36 stable heart transplant patients. The measured concentrations of everolimus in PBMCs ranged between 0.04 and 0.47 ng/10^6 cells and correlated only moderately with the respective trough whole blood concentrations ($r^2 = 0.558, p = 0.0002$). Robertsen contributed another publication with regard to intracellular everolimus concentrations [53]. The pilot study included 12 renal transplant recipients from whom blood was drawn for a 12-h pharmacokinetic profile. Measurements were performed with an LC–MS/MS method used in the local clinical laboratory [54]. Deuterated everolimus was used as internal standard in order to compensate possible matrix effects. Concentrations of everolimus in PBMCs ranged between 9.1 and 29.9 pg/10^6 cells. The $\text{AUC}_{1–12}$ of whole blood and PMBCs showed a clear correlation (74 (51–130)$_{[\mu g*h/L]}$ vs. 225 (178–408)$_{[pg*h/million cells]}$; $r = 0.90, p < 0.01$). These results do not support the assumption of a more targeted drug monitoring within PBMCs compared to the rather global measurement in whole blood. However, the author observed a potential contamination of isolated PBMCs with erythrocytes as a conceivable source for inaccurate results. Unfortunately, the isolation technique for T lymphocytes used for previous investigations [17,18,33] was not applied.

In general, it may be questioned whether measurements of PSIs in PBMCs should be of great interest. In contrast to cyclosporine A and tacrolimus, both PSIs show a good relationship between trough level monitoring and clinical efficacy [52,55]. Therefore, the laborious and rather time-consuming measurement of drugs inside the lymphocytes seems to be interesting in terms of understanding the drug's pharmacokinetic characteristics in the target compartment, but it may be redundant for therapeutic monitoring. Nevertheless, the development of an analytical method for simultaneous determination of different immunosuppressive drugs in T lymphocytes would be highly beneficial. Widely used combination therapies could be assessed more efficiently by processing and analyzing only one specimen to determine several analytes in the same run. The different extent of drug accumulation inside the lymphocytes could be evaluated and possible physiological influences recognized.

9.4 DRUG TRANSPORT ACROSS LYMPHOCYTE CELL MEMBRANES: THE ROLE OF P-GLYCOPROTEIN

The bioavailability of a drug is influenced by its liberation, absorption, distribution, metabolism, and excretion. Active transport processes across various membranes play an important role in determining bioavailability at the site of action. Efflux transporters protect against intracellular accumulation of potentially toxic compounds. Most of these transporters belong to the ABC (ATP-binding cassette) family of membrane proteins. Although there are approximately 50 other members of this family of proteins, such as ABCC1, ABCC2 (MRP), and ABCG2 (breast cancer-related protein (BCRP)) [56], P-gp (ABCB1/MDR1) is by far the best examined transporter protein and is the major focus of this discussion. Considerable data exist, however, supporting the idea that other transporter proteins, such as MRP2, may be of relevance for other immunosuppressants such as MPA [45,46,57–62].

Many tissues host P-gp, including the small intestine, liver, kidneys, and the blood–brain barrier [63]. Common immunosuppressives such as CNIs (cyclosporine A and tacrolimus) and the mTOR inhibitors (sirolimus and everolimus) are, among many other drugs, substrates for P-gp. The pharmacodynamic targets of all these drugs are located within the lymphocyte. P-gp is of particular interest because it is located in the membrane of lymphocytes [64] and, thus, may influence intracellular concentrations at the site of action. This concentration could be more directly related to the immunosuppressive effect than whole blood concentrations [53].

9.4.1 MODIFIERS OF P-GP ACTIVITY

A number of factors have been identified as possible modifiers of P-gp activity. These factors are discussed in this section.

9.4.1.1 Coexpression with proteins of the cytochrome P450 3A family

Like cytochrome P450 3A4, P-gp is nonspecific for a large variety of drugs from many different indication areas. P-gp is coexpressed with enzymes of the cytochrome P450 3A family, which are responsible for the oxidative metabolism of many drugs and environmental compounds, thus contributing essentially to the detoxification of these substances along with P-gp. CYP3A4, CYP3A5 and P-gp are also expressed in lymphocytes.

Coregulation of P-gp and CYP3A4/CYP3A5 has been found in various tissues and organs [65]. For instance, 79% of the variability in *ABCB1* mRNA expression was explained by the corresponding *CYP3A5* expression levels in intestinal tissue in one study [66]. The nuclear pregnane X receptor (PXR) has been identified as the most probable reason for this strong coregulation of CYP3A and P-gp [65,67,68].

9.4.1.2 Induction and inhibition by concomitant drug therapy and endogenous substances

Both CYP3A4/5 and P-gp can be induced by substances acting as PXR ligands, such as rifampicin [67] or St. John's wort [69]. On the other hand, substrates with high affinity may also act as inhibitors. The calcium channel blocker verapamil, but also cyclosporine A, and many other drugs have been shown to exhibit a noticeable inhibitory activity [70].

It is interesting to note that the inhibition of P-gp has been used as a therapeutic concept, for instance, in HIV therapy [71,72]. It is clear that interacting comedication must be considered when interpreting the results of intracellular drug monitoring of immunosuppressives in lymphocytes.

9.4.1.3 Regulation by cytokines

It has also been reported that P-gp is regulated by cytokines in patients with ulcerative colitis. P-gp mRNA and protein expression depended on the extent of a clinical activity index. Cytokines IL-1b and IL-8 were upregulated [73]. The downregulation of *ABCB1* was attributed to the interaction of IL-8 and *ABCB1* in vitro [70]. Clinical events changing cytokine activity may therefore have to be considered as well when assessing the results of intracellular drug monitoring.

9.4.2 THE GENETICS OF P-GP (*ABCB1*)

P-gp is encoded by the human *ABCB1* gene. Since 1994 [74], several hundred single-nucleotide polymorphisms (SNPs) have been described within the *ABCB1* gene, including more than 100 SNPs in coding regions. Two SNPs in strong linkage disequilibrium have been studied most extensively: the synonymous *C3435T* and the non-synonymous *G2677T/A*. The functional significance of these polymorphisms on *ABCB1* mRNA levels, P-gp expression or activity in various tissues, as well as on the pharmacokinetics of different substrates is still unclear, and conflicting results have been reported [75]. In 2006, Cascorbi stated that there was only weak evidence for a significant impact on mRNA or protein expression in vivo [76].

The impact of *ABCB1* polymorphisms on immunosuppressive therapy has mostly been studied with regard to blood concentrations of immunosuppressants and clinical outcome. A meta-analysis that included a total of 1036 patients failed to identify a major effect of the *3435C > T* variant on cyclosporine pharmacokinetics. Despite minor ethnic differences and slightly lower AUCs in CC homozygotes, none of the changes translated into clinically relevant changes in outcome [77].

The results observed with tacrolimus are similar to those obtained with cyclosporine. *ABCB1* variants failed to show a significant influence on pharmacokinetic parameters. However, CYP3A5 status was repeatedly identified as influencing tacrolimus pharmacokinetics and clinical outcome [78,79]. Other studies, such as that by Cattaneo et al. [80], which showed an influence of *ABCB1* variations, were not controlled for CYP3A5. Considering the well-known coexpression with the CYP3A family (discussed previously), a combined analysis is strongly recommended when addressing the pharmacokinetics and clinical outcome of tacrolimus therapy [70].

However, there is ongoing discussion about the influence of *ABCB1* variations on clinical outcome. A recent study showed an influence of *CYP3A5* and *-3A4* but not *ABCB1* variations on tacrolimus dose requirements [81]. In contrast, another study reported an influence of the *ABCB1 3435C > T* polymorphism on *ABCB1* activity of T cells and the pharmacodynamic effect of tacrolimus [82]. Only few data are available regarding sirolimus. In general, no convincing data were found supporting an association of blood concentration or clinical outcome with *ABCB1* or haplotypes [78,79,83–85].

In summary, with respect to blood concentrations and clinical outcome, *ABCB1* genotypes have so far failed to provide pharmacokinetic predictions or clinically useful data in immunosuppressant therapy. However, blood concentrations of immunosuppressants do not reflect the concentrations at the site of action in the intracellular compartment of lymphocytes. Clinical outcome may be influenced by too many other factors to identify a genetic influence of variations in the *ABCB1* gene.

Therefore, recent studies using new, more sensitive technology such as LC–MS/MS have addressed the idea of intracellular concentration monitoring and associating these results with *ABCB1* genotypes. In 2007, Elens et al. [86] reported a significant correlation between intracellular levels of tacrolimus in liver cells and *ABCB1* genetic polymorphisms, whereas their impact on blood concentrations appeared negligible. The *1199G > A* and *2677G > T/A* SNPs resulted in a reduced activity of P-gp on tacrolimus.

In 2008, Crettol et al. [31] studied *ABCB1 61A > G, 1236C > T, 2677G > T, 1199G > A*, and *3435C > T* polymorphisms. They found cyclosporine intracellular lymphocyte concentrations in 64 renal, liver, and lung transplant patients that were 1.7-fold higher in *3435TT* carriers compared to *CC* carriers. *ABCB1 1199A* carriers presented a 1.8-fold decreased cyclosporine A intracellular concentration. In contrast, *ABCB1 61A > G, 1236C > T*, and *2677G > T* polymorphisms did not influence cyclosporine intracellular and blood concentrations. Interestingly, cyclosporine A intracellular concentration correlated only moderately with blood concentration ($r = 0.30$), and the effect of the *3435C > T* polymorphism on blood concentration was considerably lower than that on intracellular concentrations (1.2-fold vs. 1.7-fold). This finding is typical for other studies showing only minor effects on blood concentrations, possibly due to other major effects such as CYP3A4/5 activity in liver and intestine. Also in 2008, another study [32] found significant negative correlations between cyclosporine $t_{1/2}$ in PBMCs and P-gp activity in $CD4^+$ or $CD8^+$ cells in a subgroup of individuals with the *2677TT–3435TT* haplotype. Carriers of the *2677GG–3435CC* haplotype displayed a negative correlation between P-gp activity in $CD4^+$ cells and cyclosporine PBMC AUC_{0-24}. However, there was no correlation between P-gp activity in $CD4^+$ or $CD8^+$ cells and cyclosporine pharmacokinetic parameters in PBMCs when considering all subjects. The authors concluded that cyclosporine PBMC pharmacokinetics was influenced by P-gp activity, but cyclosporine whole blood concentrations did not predict PBMC drug levels, suggesting that despite values in the therapeutic range, some subjects could have inadequate intracellular drug levels.

In 2014, Dessilly et al. [87] performed an in vitro study in recombinant cell lines showing that the *ABCB1 1199G* wild-type allele resulted in a more efficient efflux of tacrolimus than the variant A allele. This supports previous clinical data [39,86]. It is important to note that this seems to be a substrate-specific behavior because cyclosporine and a number of other drugs, such as some anticancer medications, have been shown to react in the opposite manner with regard to the genetic variants tested. Recently, a study revealed a significant association between everolimus whole blood and PBMC concentrations, suggesting *ABCB1*-mediated efflux from PBMC to be of minor importance for the distribution of everolimus [53]. If this holds true, *ABCB1* genetic variation should have no significant effect on intracellular concentrations of everolimus.

9.5 CONSIDERATIONS REGARDING INTRACELLULAR DRUG MONITORING

Many factors influence *ABCB1* activity and can therefore influence intracellular concentrations of immunosuppressants in lymphocytes at the site of action. Methodological problems must still be addressed. Currently, intracellular drug concentrations are mostly analyzed in PBMCs. It is not clear, however, if *ABCB1* is equally expressed across different T-cell subsets. When interpreting the results of such studies, these influences will have to be taken into account. Regarding genetic variation, SNPs in *ABC* transporter genes are currently not suitable as biomarkers for solid organ transplantation [88]. However, they may be of particular interest in connection with the study of intracellular drug concentrations in PBMCs. Such monitoring at the site of action may provide improved outcome in the future.

Whether genotyping of transporter proteins, such as *ABCB1*, may be of clinical use can only be speculated at present because monitoring intracellular concentration at the site of action also incorporates many other factors, including any genetic influence. On the other hand, genotyping may provide early information on necessary dosing prior to the initiation of therapy and may therefore be used to speed up the process of finding an optimal individual dose. Both genotyping and intracellular monitoring, however, may become obsolete once pharmacodynamic monitoring with adequate biomarkers assessing the immune status becomes an option. For now, there is considerable room for improvement due to the lack of correlation between whole blood and intracellular concentrations as reported in many studies. Well-designed clinical studies are needed to achieve the aim of improved patient care by means of intracellular drug monitoring in immunosuppressive therapy.

9.5.1 DRUG BINDING PROTEINS IN THE LYMPHOCYTE CYTOPLASM

Cytoplasmic protein receptors in the lymphocyte cell, the so-called immunophilins, are able to bind IL-2-suppressing drugs such as tacrolimus, cyclosporine A, and sirolimus. The binding of tacrolimus to the immunophilin FK binding protein 12 (FKBP12) or CsA to cyclophilin and subsequent inhibition of nuclear factor of activated T-cells (NFAT) transcription by CN inhibition is very well understood. However, there are several other mechanisms in addition to these main pathways of drug action, and some of these mechanisms have been discovered in recent years [89–93]. Apart from the prominent binding proteins FKBP12 and cyclophilin, there are several other immunophilins in the lymphocyte cytoplasm, which can also form complexes with immunosuppressive drug molecules. Some complexes lead to a reduction in CN activity, whereas others have no effect. For example, the immunophilins FKBP12.6, FKBP51 [91], and ubiquitin [93] in complex with tacrolimus decrease the CN activity in human cells, whereas tacrolimus complexed with FKBP13 or FKBP25 does not contribute to the inhibition of CN phosphatase activity [92]. Measuring CN phosphatase activity has been proposed as a pharmacodynamic approach to optimize CNI drug dosing [94]. However, apart from CN inhibition and subsequent reduced NFAT transcription, NF-κB (another transcription factor) plays a key functional role in T-cell activation. Some authors could show that tacrolimus and cyclosporine A also prevent immune activation by blocking the NF-κB activation cascade in peripheral human T cells [90,95]. Therefore, investigation of CN activity only reveals some effects of the drug, whereas intracellular drug measurement considers the different drug effects in the lymphocyte cell.

The doses for a 50% inhibition of CN (IC_{50}) have been calculated for blood concentrations of tacrolimus and cyclosporine A as 18.9 ± 4.6 and 181 ± 74 ng/mL (mean $\pm$ SD), respectively. Thus, at therapeutic CNI levels, it can be assumed that the enzyme activity is only partially inhibited. Whereas high whole blood concentrations of CsA (≥ 1000 ng/mL) can almost completely inhibit CN activity, high tacrolimus concentrations lead to only partial enzyme inhibition [39]. Kung and Halloran [89] reported that the addition of exogenous FK506-binding protein enhances CN inhibition. Consequently, a lack of intracellular FKBP12 might be the reason for the incomplete CN inhibition by tacrolimus. It can be assumed that binding protein expression varies to a certain degree between and within individual patients. Thus, the number of drug molecules available for the intended enzyme inhibition might vary as well. This would help to explain varying drug level requirements in different patients.

However, intracellular drug concentration measurement includes all drug molecules inside the cell. Molecules leading to CN inhibition as well as those without immunosuppressive effect due to intracellular protein binding or cell membrane adsorption are quantified. Consequently, intralymphocyte drug monitoring should be considered as a surrogate marker of drug concentration at the target site, reflecting the pharmacokinetic situation more precisely than measuring plasma or whole blood.

9.5.2 LYMPHOCYTE INTRAPATIENT VARIATION OF WHITE BLOOD CELLS

Lymphocytes are the main component of PBMCs, the matrix used by most researchers for the measurement of intracellular immunosuppressant drug concentrations. Therefore, it is important to understand alterations in lymphocyte number and availability. In peripheral blood, 65–80% of the lymphocytes are T lymphocytes, 8–15% are B lymphocytes, and 10% are NK cells. Only 2% of the lymphocytes in the human organism are located in the blood, with the majority residing in the lymph nodes and the spleen. B and T lymphocytes can leave the circulating blood and shuttle between different compartments, a process that is called recirculation. Unlike B and T lymphocytes, NK cells are not able to recirculate from the blood via the lymph nodes and the thoracic duct back to the blood. Every day, all lymphocytes ($\sim0.5 \times 10^{12}$) circulate into the blood compartment and migrate back into the tissue. On average, they remain less than 1 h in the peripheral blood [96]. Despite the erythrocytes remaining in the vascular system and B and T lymphocytes shuttling between different compartments, immunosuppressant drug concentrations in whole blood and T lymphocytes/PBMCs follow parallel profiles with similar times to peak (t_{max}) and elimination half-lives ($t_{1/2}$) [17,18,32].

The total number of circulating lymphocytes also changes with a circadian rhythmicity, which is in antiphase with cortisol, an adrenal gland hormone. A peak (acrophase) at midnight and a trough at 8 a.m. can be observed. The circadian difference between peak and trough lymphocyte count can be calculated as peak concentration minus trough concentration divided by the daily mean concentration multiplied by 100. This has been found to be 67% in healthy middle-aged male subjects. Mean peak and trough lymphocyte counts were approximately 3000 and 2000 cells per microliter blood [97]. However, not all lymphocyte subsets show an increase during the night; numbers of NK cells, extrathymic T cells, $\gamma\delta$ T cells, and CD8$^+$ subsets show an increase during the daytime, whereas counts of T cells, B cells, $\alpha\beta$ T cells, and CD4$^+$ subset increase during the night [98].

Physical activity is another important cause for the variation of lymphocyte counts in peripheral blood. Only seconds after exercise, leukocytosis can be observed, with the number of leukocytes in blood more than doubling. An increased lymph flow is considered to be the reason for this phenomenon. NK cells, which play an important role in the response to virus-infected cells and tumor cells, display the greatest increase of 150–400% during physical activity. However, following intensive and prolonged exercise, the NK cell activity declines to a level of 40–60% for at least 6 h [99]. Shek et al. [100] found the NK cell count reduced to 40% for as long as 7 days after the cessation of exhaustive endurance exercise. The count of other leukocytes such as granulocytes, monocytes, and T lymphocytes also rises after initiation of physical exercise. Although the number of CD8$^+$ T lymphocytes increased by 50–100%, CD4$^+$ T lymphocyte and B lymphocyte counts remained almost constant. The resulting decline of CD4$^+$/CD8$^+$ ratio and the general decrease of lymphocytes down to 30–50% after prolonged, heavy exertion are assumed to be the reason for the so-called "open window" of impaired immunity that may last between 3 and 72 h. During this time frame, bacteria and viruses may easily cause infections, especially in the upper respiratory tract [99].

Some diseases and certain conditions influence the number of lymphocyte cells in the peripheral blood (Table 9.4). Special attention should be paid to diseases for which patients with immunosuppressive therapy are at greater risk, such as mononucleosis, non-Hodgkin lymphoma, and influenza infection. Mononucleosis is a widespread viral disease most commonly caused by the Epstein–Barr virus (EBV). Approximately 95% of adults are infected with EBV by the age of 30 years. Usually after infection, the virus becomes latent and persists in lymphocytes in the peripheral blood for a lifetime, normally with no health consequences. Babcock et al. [101] reported an increase of latently infected cells in the blood circulation of immunosuppressed patients. If EBV begins to multiply (reactivate) in patients with low immune system, a wide spectrum of malignancies can result. These include epithelial and mesenchymal tumors and lymphoid malignancies such as Hodgkin's lymphoma, which in turn can explain low lymphocyte counts in the patient's peripheral blood.

Table 9.4 Diseases and Conditions That Alter Amount of Lymphocytes in the Peripheral Blood [103,104]

Lymphocytosis (More Than 4000 Cells/μL Blood in Adults)	Lymphocytopenia (Less Than 1000 resp. 1500 Cells/μL Blood in Adults)
• Viral infections (e.g., infectious mononucleosis) • Bacterial and parasitic infections (e.g., toxoplasmosis, typhus abdominalis, brucellosis, pertussis) • Acute and chronic lymphocytic leukemia • Non-Hodgkin lymphoma	• Congenital immunodeficiency (e.g., severe combined immunodeficiency or telangiectasia) • HIV infection (selectively elimination of CD4$^+$ T cells) • Chemotherapy and radiation therapy or radiation exposure • Systemic lupus erythematosus • Tuberculosis (strong reduction in CD4$^+$ T-cell count) • Recent influenza infection • Sepsis • Steroid use • Others (e.g., sarcoidosis, uremia, Cushing's disease, inflammatory bowel disease or skin burns)

Data from Thomas [103] and Ng et al. [104].

Furthermore, EBV-related lymphoproliferative disorders and lymphomas are especially abundant in immunocompromised patients [102].

The immunosuppressants' mechanism of action can lead to lymphocytopenia in transplanted patients. For example, corticosteroids are known to reduce the number of peripheral lymphocytes due to impairment of proliferation (especially in T lymphocyte proliferation) and trigger redistribution of circulating lymphocytes to the bone marrow.

In summary, many influences lead to variations in lymphocyte count and subtype composition in the peripheral blood. Therefore, PBMCs isolated from venous blood may also vary widely in yield and cell type composition. A very low PBMC yield due to lymphocytopenia can present a major analytical challenge, making the availability of a highly sensitive yet robust method indispensable for determining drug concentrations. However, the extent of drug diffusion into lymphocytes should remain constant despite varying lymphocyte counts. Most immunosuppressants (CNIs and PSIs, but not MPA) are largely distributed in erythrocytes or are bound to plasma proteins. Lymphocytes only account for less than 0.1% of blood cells. Consequently, an increase or decrease of the lymphocyte count should be negligible on drug distribution characteristics.

Nevertheless, the variation of cell type and subtype composition can compromise the informative value of the analytical result. Optimally, the cell mixture should be characterized by flow cytometry analysis. In order to minimize the circadian lymphocyte subtype shift, the patients' blood should always be drawn at the same time of the day. Other influences, such as physical activity, diseases, and immunosuppressant regiments, should also be taken into account to interpret measured intracellular drug concentrations.

The amount of drug molecules entering the lymphocytes depends on their total availability in the peripheral blood. Due to the recirculation of lymphocytes, only a small portion is located in the blood, which is permanently replaced and mixed with lymphocytes returning from other compartments. To provide a maximum time span for partitioning equilibration of immunosuppressant drugs in the lymphocytes after drug absorption and distribution, it may be useful to draw blood from patients at trough levels, just before the next drug intake. Indeed, through-level monitoring (C_0) of whole blood drug concentrations is very common in transplant patients. Hence, the simultaneous collection of extra blood for study purposes should be practicable.

9.6 **CONCLUSIONS**

Intracellular monitoring of immunosuppressive agents at their site of action inside lymphocytes is an interesting approach with considerable potential for improving clinical outcome after transplantation. A number of studies have indicated the potential use of such techniques, especially based on a lack of association between whole blood and intracellular concentrations. However, low numbers of patients included with limited statistical power, rare incidence of unwanted events such as acute rejection, limited follow up, the use of a wide variety of different combination thera-pies and comedication, and, in particular, varying results make it difficult to come to a clear conclusion.

New, reliable, and highly sensitive methods have made such studies only possible in the past several years and continue to develop further. However, there are still a number of shortcomings that have to be addressed in future studies. Current methods for intracellular analysis are still very laborious. For potential regular clinical use, more automation will be urgently required in order to provide results in a timely and repro-ducible manner. Studies need to assess both the early and the later phase after transplan-tation when steady state is achieved. Also, assays for simultaneous drug quantifications are needed because combination therapies are standard after transplantation. Free drug fraction monitoring and the regular collection of other relevant biomarkers may help to better understand the results of studies. Comedication, in particular, with influence on P-gp activity, has to be controlled. Genetic influences, particularly enzymes of the CYP3A family and P-gp, must be considered. Despite ongoing research in the field, the consequences of *ABCB1* polymorphisms for immunosuppressive therapy are still not clear. Whether and how such tests could be incorporated into clinical routine along with intracellular concentration measurements is an open question and requires further research. Another field with potential to obscure results is the lack of standardized cell separation techniques. The characterization of PBMC cell numbers and types should be targeted, as well as uncontrolled physiological and other influences on lymphocyte blood counts. All these factors make comparisons of studies difficult.

In summary, the measurement of drug concentrations inside the target cell is very attractive in immunosuppressive therapy after transplantation. It is of particular inter-est because the target cells, the lymphocytes, are easily accessible by blood sampling compared to other tissues, lending them to regular monitoring. Such measurements may have the potential to individualize immunosuppressive drug therapy and con-siderably improve clinical outcome. However, currently, no recommendation can be given to pursue this in clinical practice due to a lack of convincing evidence. More and well-planned studies are needed along with further improvement and standardi-zation of analytical techniques.

REFERENCES

[1] Boudjema K, Camus C, Saliba F, Calmus Y, et al. Reduced-dose tacrolimus with mycophe-nolate mofetil vs. standard-dose tacrolimus in liver transplantation: a randomized study. Am J Transplant 2011;11:965–76.

[2] Wallemacq P, Armstrong VW, Brunet M, Haufroid V, et al. Opportunities to optimize tacrolimus therapy in solid organ transplantation: report of the European consensus con-ference. Ther Drug Monit 2009;31:139–52.

[3] Meaden ER, Hoggard PG, Newton P, Tjia JF, et al. P-glycoprotein and MRP1 expres-sion and reduced ritonavir and saquinavir accumulation in HIV-infected individuals. J Antimicrob Chemother 2002;50:583–8.

[4] Rouzes A, Berthoin K, Xuereb F, Djabarouti S, et al. Simultaneous determination of the antiretroviral agents: amprenavir, lopinavir, ritonavir, saquinavir and efavirenz in human peripheral blood mononuclear cells by high-performance liquid chromatography-mass spectrometry. J Chromatogr B Analyt Technol Biomed Life Sci 2004;813:209–16.

[5] Ehrhardt M, Möck M, Haefeli WE, Mikus G, et al. Monitoring of lopinavir and ritonavir in peripheral blood mononuclear cells, plasma, and ultrafiltrate using a selective and highly sensitive LC/MS/MS assay. J Chromatogr B Analyt Technol Biomed Life Sci 2007;850:249–58.

[6] Elens L, Veriter S, Yombi JC, Di Fazio V, et al. Validation and clinical application of a high performance liquid chromatography tandem mass spectrometry (LC-MS/MS) method for the quantitative determination of 10 anti-retrovirals in human peripheral blood mononuclear cells. J Chromatogr B 2009;877:1805–14.

[7] Masri MA, Barbari A, Stephan A, Rizk S, et al. Measurement of lymphocyte cyclosporine levels in transplant patients. Transplant Proc 1998;30:3561–2.

[8] Saumet A, Musuamba Tshinanu F, Capron A, Nguyen Thi MT, et al. P279 comparison of three methods for peripheral blood mononuclear cells separation. In: 12th international congress of therapeutic drug monitoring and clinical toxicology; 2011. p. 554.

[9] Capron A, Musuamba F, Latinne D, Mourad M, et al. Validation of a liquid chromatography-mass spectrometric assay for tacrolimus in peripheral blood mononuclear cells. Ther Drug Monit 2009;31:178–86.

[10] Falck P, Guldseth H, Asberg A, Midtvedt K, et al. Determination of ciclosporin A and its six main metabolites in isolated T-lymphocytes and whole blood using liquid chromatography-tandem mass spectrometry. J Chromatogr B Analyt Technol Biomed Life Sci 2007;852:345–52.

[11] Goldberg H, Ling V, Wong PY, Skorecki K. Reduced cyclosporin accumulation in multidrug-resistant cells. Biomed Biophys Res Commun 1988;152:552–8.

[12] Patil AG, D'Souza R, Dixit N, Damre A. Validation of quinidine as a probe substrate for the *in vitro* P-gp inhibition assay in Caco-2 cell monolayer. Eur J Drug Metab Pharmacokinet 2011;36:115–9.

[13] Ulmer AJ, Flad H-D. Discontinuous density gradient separation of human mononuclear leucocytes using Percoll as gradient medium. J Immunol Methods 1979;30:1–10.

[14] Plebanksi M. Preparation of lymphocytes and identification of lymphocyte subpopulations Rowland-Jones SL, McMichael A, editors. Lymphocytes: a practical approach. 2nd ed. : Oxford; 1999. p. 376.

[15] Rubinstien E, Ballow M. Isolation of monocyte-depleted and monocyte-rich fractions from human mononuclear cells. J Clin Lab Immunol 1989;30:35–9.

[16] Hata K, Zhang XR, Iwatsuki S, Van Thiel DH, et al. Isolation, phenotyping, and functional analysis of lymphocytes from human liver. Clin Immunol Immunopathol 1990;56:401–19.

[17] Falck P, Asberg A, Guldseth H, Bremer S, et al. Declining intracellular T-lymphocyte concentration of cyclosporine a precedes acute rejection in kidney transplant recipients. Transplantation 2008;85:179–84.

[18] Falck P, Asberg A, Byberg K-T, Bremer S, et al. Reduced elimination of cyclosporine A in elderly (>65 years) kidney transplant recipients. Transplantation 2008;86:1379–83.

[19] Masri M, Rizk S, Barbari A, Stephan A, et al. An assay for the determination of sirolimus levels in the lymphocyte of transplant patients. Transplant Proc 2007;39:1204–6.

[20] Roullet-Renoleau F, Lemaitre F, Antignac M, Zahr N, et al. Everolimus quantification in peripheral blood mononuclear cells using ultra high performance liquid chromatography tandem mass spectrometry. J Pharm Biomed Anal 2012;66:278–81.

[21] Lepage JM, Lelong-Boulouard V, Lecouf A, Debruyne D, et al. Cyclosporine monitoring in peripheral blood mononuclear cells: feasibility and interest. A prospective study on 20 renal transplant recipients. Transplant Proc 2007;39:3109–10.

[22] Ansermot N, Fathi M, Veuthey J-L, Desmeules J, et al. Quantification of cyclosporine A in peripheral blood mononuclear cells by liquid chromatography-electrospray mass spectrometry using a column-switching approach. J Chromatogr B Analyt Technol Biomed Life Sci 2007;857:92–9.

[23] Pitt JJ. Principles and applications of liquid chromatography-mass spectrometry in clinical biochemistry. Clin Biochem Rev 2009;30:19–34.

[24] Atkinson K, Britton K, Biggs J. Distribution and concentration of cyclosporin in human blood. J Clin Pathol 1984;37:1167–71.

[25] Akhlaghi F, Trull AK. Distribution of cyclosporin in organ transplant recipients. Clin Pharmacokinet 2002;41:615–37.

[26] Barbari A, Masri MA, Stephan A, Mokhbat J, et al. Cyclosporine lymphocyte versus whole blood pharmacokinetic monitoring: correlation with histological findings. Transplant Proc 2001;33:2782–5.

[27] Barbari A, Stephan A, Masri M, Mourad N, et al. Cyclosporine lymphocyte level and lymphocyte count: new guidelines for tailoring immunosuppressive therapy. Transplant Proc 2003;35:2742–4.

[28] Barbari AG, Masri MA, Stephan AG, Mourad N, et al. Cyclosporine lymphocyte maximum level: a new alternative for cyclosporine monitoring in kidney transplantation. Exp Clin Transplant 2005;3:293–300.

[29] Barbari AG, Masri MA, Stephan AG, El Ghoul B, et al. Cyclosporine lymphocyte maximum level monitoring in *de novo* kidney transplant patients: a prospective study. Exp Clin Transplant 2006;4:400–5.

[30] Barbari A, Masri M, Stephan A, Rizk S, et al. A novel approach in clinical immunosuppression monitoring: drug lymphocyte level. Exp Clin Transplant 2007;5:643–8.

[31] Crettol S, Venetz J-P, Fontana M, Aubert J-D, et al. Influence of ABCB1 genetic polymorphisms on cyclosporine intracellular concentration in transplant recipients. Pharmacogenet Genomics 2008;18:307–15.

[32] Ansermot N, Rebsamen M, Chabert J, Fathi M, et al. Influence of *ABCB1* gene polymorphisms and P-glycoprotein activity on cyclosporine pharmacokinetics in peripheral blood mononuclear cells in healthy volunteers. Drug Metab Lett 2008;2:76–82.

[33] Robertsen I, Falck P, Andreassen AK, Næss NK, et al. Endomyocardial, intralymphocyte, and whole blood concentrations of ciclosporin A in heart transplant recipients. Transplant Res 2013:1–8.

[34] Lindholm A, Henricsson S. Intra- and interindividual variability in the free fraction of cyclosporine in plasma in recipients of renal transplants. Ther. Drug Monit 1989;11:623–30.

[35] Venkataramanan R, Swaminathan A, Prasad T, Jain A, et al. Clinical pharmacokinetics of tacrolimus. Clin Pharmacokinet 1995;29:404–30.

[36] Kahan BD, Keown P, Levy GA, Johnston A. Therapeutic drug monitoring of immunosuppressant drugs in clinical practice. Clin Ther 2002;24:330–50.

[37] Zahir H, McCaughan G, Gleeson M, Nand RA, et al. Factors affecting variability in distribution of tacrolimus in liver transplant recipients. Br J Clin Pharmacol 2003;57:298–309.

[38] Zahir H, Nand RA, Brown KF, Tattam BN, et al. Validation of methods to study the distribution and protein binding of tacrolimus in human blood. J Pharmacol Toxicol Methods 2001;46:27–35.

[39] Capron A, Mourad M, De Meyer M, De Pauw L, et al. CYP3A5 and ABCB1 polymorphisms influence tacrolimus concentrations in peripheral blood mononuclear cells after renal transplantation. Pharmacogenomics 2010;11:703–14.

[40] Capron A, Lerut J, Latinne D, Rahier J, et al. Correlation of tacrolimus levels in peripheral blood mononuclear cells with histological staging of rejection after liver transplantation: preliminary results of a prospective study. Transpl Int 2012;25:41–7.

[41] Lemaitre F, Antignac M, Fernandez C. Monitoring of tacrolimus concentrations in peripheral blood mononuclear cells: application to cardiac transplant recipients. Clin Biochem 2013;46:1538–41.

[42] Lemaitre F, Blanchet B, Latournerie M, Antignac M, et al. Pharmacokinetics and pharmacodynamics of tacrolimus in liver transplant recipients: inside the white blood cells. Clin Biochem 2015 [Epub ahead of print].

[43] Haug C, Schmid-Kotsas A, Linder T, Bachem MG, et al. Influence of hepatocyte growth factor, epidermal growth factor, and mycophenolic acid on endothelin-1 synthesis in human endothelial cells. Nephrol Dial Transplant 2001;16:2310–6.

[44] Sollinger HW, Belzer FO, Deierhoi MH, Diethelm AG, et al. RS-61443 (mycophenolate mofetil). A multicenter study for refractory kidney transplant rejection. Ann Surg 1992;216:513–8 [discussion 518–519].

[45] Hesselink DA, van Hest RM, Mathot RAA, Bonthuis F, et al. Cyclosporine interacts with mycophenolic acid by inhibiting the multidrug resistance-associated protein 2. Am J Transplant 2005;5:987–94.

[46] Patel CG, Ogasawara K, Akhlaghi F. Mycophenolic acid glucuronide (MPAG) is transported by multidrug resistance-associated protein 2 (MRP2) and this transport is not inhibited by cyclosporine, tacrolimus or sirolimus. Xenobiotica 2013;43:229–35.

[47] Bénech H, Hascoët S, Furlan V, Pruvost A, et al. Development and validation of an LC/MS/MS assay for mycophenolic acid in human peripheral blood mononuclear cells. J Chromatogr B Analyt Technol Biomed Life Sci 2007;853:168–74.

[48] Nguyen Thi MT, Capron A, Mourad M, Wallemacq P. Mycophenolic acid quantification in human peripheral blood mononuclear cells using liquid chromatography-tandem mass spectrometry. Clin Biochem 2013;46:1909–11.

[49] Augustine JJ, Hricik DE. Experience with everolimus. Transplant Proc 2004;36:500S–3S.

[50] Kahan BD, Napoli KL, Kelly PA, Podbielski J, et al. Therapeutic drug monitoring of sirolimus: correlations with efficacy and toxicity. Clin Transplant 2000;14:97–109.

[51] Mabasa VH, Ensom MHH. The role of therapeutic monitoring of everolimus in solid organ transplantation. Ther Drug Monit 2005;27:666–76.

[52] Tedesco-Silva H, Medina-Pestana JO. Impact of everolimus: update on immunosuppressive therapy strategies and patient outcomes after renal transplantation. Transpl Res Risk Manag 2011;3:9–29.

[53] Robertsen I, Vethe NT, Midtvedt K, Falck P, et al. Closer to the site of action; everolimus concentrations in peripheral blood mononuclear cells correlate well with whole blood concentrations. Ther Drug Monit 2015 [Epub ahead of print].

[54] Vethe NT, Gjerdalen LC, Bergan S. Determination of cyclosporine, tacrolimus, sirolimus and everolimus by liquid chromatography coupled to electrospray ionization and tandem mass spectrometry: assessment of matrix effects and assay performance. Scand J Clin Lab Invest 2010;70:583–91.

[55] MacDonald A, Scarola J, Burke JT, Zimmerman JJ. Clinical pharmacokinetics and therapeutic drug monitoring of sirolimus. Clin Ther 2000;22(Suppl. B):B101–21.

[56] Cascorbi I, Haenisch S. Pharmacogenetics of ATP-binding cassette transporters and clinical implications. Methods Mol Biol 2010;596:95–121.

[57] Fukuda T, Goebel J, Cox S, Maseck D, et al. UGT1A9, UGT2B7 and MRP2 genotypes can predict mycophenolic acid pharmacokinetic variability in pediatric kidney transplant recipients. Ther Drug Monit 2013;34:671–9.

[58] Wang J, Figurski M, Shaw LM, Burckart GJ. The impact of P-glycoprotein and MRP2 on mycophenolic acid levels in mice. Transpl Immunol 2008;19:192–6.

[59] Takekuma Y, Kakiuchi H, Yamazaki K, Miyauchi S, et al. Difference between pharmacokinetics of mycophenolic acid (MPA) in rats and that in humans is caused by different affinities of MRP2 to a glucuronized form. J Pharm Pharm Sci 2007;10:71–85.

[60] Naesens M, Kuypers DRJ, Verbeke K, Vanrenterghem Y. Multidrug resistance protein 2 genetic polymorphisms influence mycophenolic acid exposure in renal allograft recipients. Transplantation 2006;82:1074–84.

[61] Westley IS, Brogan LR, Morris RG, Evans AM, et al. Role of MRP2 in the hepatic disposition of mycophenolic acid and its glucuronide metabolites: effect of cyclosporine. Drug Metab Dispos 2006;34:261–6.

[62] Kobayashi MM, Saitoh H, Kobayashi MM, Tadano K, et al. Cyclosporin A, but not tacrolimus, inhibits the biliary excretion of mycophenolic acid glucuronide possibly mediated by multidrug resistance-associated protein 2 in rats. J Pharmacol Exp Ther 2004;309:1029–35.

[63] Lin JH, Yamazaki M. Role of P-glycoprotein in pharmacokinetics: clinical implications. Clin Pharmacokinet 2003;42:59–98.

[64] Klimecki WT, Futscher BW, Grogan TM, Dalton WS. P-glycoprotein expression and function in circulating blood cells from normal volunteers. Blood 1994;83:2451–8.

[65] Von Richter O, Burk O, Fromm MF, Thon KP, et al. Cytochrome P450 3A4 and P-glycoprotein expression in human small intestinal enterocytes and hepatocytes: a comparative analysis in paired tissue specimens. Clin Pharmacol Ther 2004;75:172–83.

[66] Ufer M, Dilger K, Leschhorn L, Daufresne L, et al. Influence of CYP3A4, CYP3A5, and ABCB1 genotype and expression on budesonide pharmacokinetics: a possible role of intestinal CYP3A4 expression. Clin Pharmacol Ther 2008;84:43–6.

[67] Geick A, Eichelbaum M, Burk O. Nuclear receptor response elements mediate induction of intestinal MDR1 by Rifampin. J Biol Chem 2001;276:14581–7.

[68] Tirona RG, Lee W, Leake BF, Lan L-B, et al. The orphan nuclear receptor HNF4alpha determines PXR- and CAR-mediated xenobiotic induction of CYP3A4. Nat Med 2003;9:220–4.

[69] Johne A, Brockmöller J, Bauer S, Maurer A, et al. Pharmacokinetic interaction of digoxin with an herbal extract from St John's wort (*Hypericum perforatum*). Clin Pharmacol Ther 1999;66:338–45.

[70] Cascorbi I. P-glycoprotein: tissue distribution, substrates, and functional consequences of genetic variations. Handb Exp Pharmacol 2011:261–83.

[71] Janneh O, Jones E, Chandler B, Owen A, et al. Inhibition of P-glycoprotein and multidrug resistance-associated proteins modulates the intracellular concentration of lopinavir in cultured CD4 T cells and primary human lymphocytes. J Antimicrob Chemother 2007;60:987–93.

[72] Lucia MB, Rutella S, Leone G, Vella S, et al. HIV-protease inhibitors contribute to P-glycoprotein efflux function defect in peripheral blood lymphocytes from HIV-positive patients receiving HAART. J Acquir Immune Defic Syndr 2001;27:321–30.

[73] Ufer M, Häsler R, Jacobs G, Haenisch S, et al. Decreased sigmoidal ABCB1 (P-glycoprotein) expression in ulcerative colitis is associated with disease activity. Pharmacogenomics 2009;10:1941–53.

[74] Stein U, Walther W, Wunderlich V. Point mutations in the mdr1 promoter of human osteosarcomas are associated with *in vitro* responsiveness to multidrug resistance relevant drugs. Eur J Cancer 1994;30A:1541–5.

[75] Marzolini C, Paus E, Buclin T, Kim RB. Polymorphisms in human MDR1 (P-glycoprotein): recent advances and clinical relevance. Clin Pharmacol Ther 2004;75:13–33.

[76] Cascorbi I. Role of pharmacogenetics of ATP-binding cassette transporters in the pharmacokinetics of drugs. Pharmacol Ther 2006;112:457–73.

[77] Jiang Z-P, Wang Y-R, Xu P, Liu R-R, et al. Meta-analysis of the effect of MDR1 C3435T polymorphism on cyclosporine pharmacokinetics. Basic Clin Pharmacol Toxicol 2008;103:433–44.

[78] Renders L, Frisman M, Ufer M, Mosyagin I, et al. CYP3A5 genotype markedly influences the pharmacokinetics of tacrolimus and sirolimus in kidney transplant recipients. Clin Pharmacol Ther 2007;81:228–34.

[79] Yanagimachi M, Naruto T, Tanoshima R, Kato H, et al. Influence of CYP3A5 and *ABCB1* gene polymorphisms on calcineurin inhibitor-related neurotoxicity after hematopoietic stem cell transplantation. Clin Transplant 2010;24:855–61.

[80] Cattaneo D, Ruggenenti P, Baldelli S, Motterlini N, et al. ABCB1 genotypes predict cyclosporine-related adverse events and kidney allograft outcome. J Am Soc Nephrol 2009;20:1404–15.

[81] Tapirdamaz Ö, Hesselink DA, el Bouazzaoui S, Azimpour M, et al. Genetic variance in ABCB1 and CYP3A5 does not contribute toward the development of chronic kidney disease after liver transplantation. Pharmacogenet Genomics 2014;24:427–35.

[82] Vafadari R, Bouamar R, Hesselink DA, Kraaijeveld R, et al. Genetic polymorphisms in ABCB1 influence the pharmacodynamics of tacrolimus. Ther Drug Monit 2013;35:459–65.

[83] Anglicheau D, Le Corre D, Lechaton S, Laurent-Puig P, et al. Consequences of genetic polymorphisms for sirolimus requirements after renal transplant in patients on primary sirolimus therapy. Am J Transplant 2005;5:595–603.

[84] Miao L-Y, Huang C-R, Hou J-Q, Qian M-Y. Association study of *ABCB1* and *CYP3A5* gene polymorph-isms with sirolimus trough concentration and dose requirements in Chinese renal transplant recipients. Biopharm Drug Dispos 2008;29:1–5.

[85] Mourad M, Mourad G, Wallemacq P, Garrigue V, et al. Sirolimus and tacrolimus trough concentrations and dose requirements after kidney transplantation in relation to CYP3A5 and MDR1 polymorphisms and steroids. Transplantation 2005;80:977–84.

[86] Elens L, Capron A, Kerckhove VV, Lerut J, et al. 1199G > A and 2677G > T/A polymorphisms of ABCB1 independently affect tacrolimus concentration in hepatic tissue after liver transplantation. Pharmacogenet Genomics 2007;17:873–83.

[87] Dessilly G, Elens L, Panin N, Capron A, et al. ABCB1 1199G > A genetic polymorphism (Rs2229109) influences the intracellular accumulation of tacrolimus in HEK293 and K562 recombinant cell lines. PLoS One 2014;9:e91555.

[88] Shuker N, Bouamar R, Weimar W, van Schaik RHN, et al. ATP-binding cassette transporters as pharmacogenetic biomarkers for kidney transplantation. Clin Chim Acta 2012;413:1326–37.

[89] Kung L, Halloran P. Immunophilins may limit calcineurin inhibition by cyclosporine and tacrolimus at high drug concentrations. Transplantation 2000;70:327–35.

[90] Du S, Hiramatsu N, Hayakawa K, Kasai A, et al. Suppression of NF-kappaB by cyclosporin a and tacrolimus (FK506) via induction of the C/EBP family: implication for unfolded protein response. J Immunol 2009;182:7201–11.

[91] Weiwad M, Edlich F, Kilka S, Erdmann F, et al. Comparative analysis of calcineurin inhibition by complexes of immunosuppressive drugs with human FK506 binding proteins. Biochemistry 2006;45:15776–84.

[92] Bram RJ, Hung DT, Martin PK, Schreiber SL, et al. Identification of the immunophilins capable of mediating inhibition of signal transduction by cyclosporin A and FK506: roles of calcineurin binding and cellular location. Mol Cell Biol 1993;13:4760–9.

[93] Davis DL, Soldin SJ. Protein ubiquitin is an immunophilin. Ther Drug Monit 2002;24:32–5.

[94] Blanchet B, Hulin A, Ghaleh B, Giraudier S, et al. Distribution of calcineurin activity in blood cell fractions and impact of tacrolimus inhibition. Fundam Clin Pharmacol 2006;20:137–44.

[95] Brini AT, Harel-Bellan A, Farrar WL. Cyclosporin A inhibits induction of IL-2 receptor alpha chain expression by affecting activation of NF-kB-like factor(s) in cultured human T lymphocytes. Eur Cyctokine Netw 1990;1:131–9.

[96] Westermann J, Pabst R. Distribution of lymphocyte subsets and natural killer cells in the human body. Clin Investig 1992;70:539–44.

[97] Kanabrocki EL, Sothern RB, Scheving LE, Vesely DL, et al. Reference values for circadian rhythms of 98 variables in clinically healthy men in the fifth decade of life. Chronobiol Int 1990;7:445–61.

[98] Suzuki S, Toyabe S, Moroda T, Tada T, et al. Circadian rhythm of leucocytes and lymphocytes subsets and its possible correlation with the function of the autonomic nervous system. Clin Exp Immunol 1997;110:500–8.

[99] Nieman DC. Exercise effects on systemic immunity. Immunol Cell Biol 2000;78:496–501.

[100] Shek P, Sabiston B, Buguet A, Radomski M. Strenuous exercise and immunological changes. Int J Sports Med 1995;16:466–74.

[101] Babcock GJ, Decker LL, Freeman RB, Thorley-Lawson DA. Epstein–Barr virus-infected resting memory B cells, not proliferating lymphoblasts, accumulate in the peripheral blood of immunosuppressed patients. J Exp Med 1999;190:567–76.

[102] Maeda E, Akahane M, Kiryu S, Kato N, et al. Spectrum of Epstein–Barr virus-related diseases: a pictorial review. Jpn J Radiol 2009;27:4–19.

[103] Thomas L. Labor und diagnose. 8th ed. Frankfurt/Main: 4 TH-Books Verlagsgesellschaft; 2012.

[104] Ng WL, Chu CM, Wu AK, Cheng VC, et al. Lymphopenia at presentation is associated with increased risk of infections in patients with systemic lupus erythematosus. QJM 2006;99:37–47.

Markers of lymphocyte activation and proliferation

10

Eberhard Wieland

Central Institute for Clinical Chemistry and Laboratory Medicine,
Klinikum Stuttgart, Stuttgart, Germany

10.1 INTRODUCTION

Organ transplantation is an established therapy to replace the function of vital organs if their function is irreversibly lost due to chronic or acute tissue destruction. The main obstacle to a successful transplantation is the genetic difference between donor and recipient tissue. This is due to the unique major histocompatibility complex (MHC), also called human leukocyte antigen (HLA), pattern of every individual, which is recognized by the immune system as foreign if exposed to a genetically different environment. The development of modern immunosuppressive therapies in conjunction with sophisticated surgical techniques has paved the way for solid organ transplantation to become a standard therapy for end-stage organ failure. However, drug-related toxicities and chronic immune-mediated injuries continue to challenge long-term patient and graft survival. Therefore, a desirable goal is to tailor immunosuppressive therapy to achieve the required effect while minimizing toxicity. Therapeutic drug monitoring (TDM) is one way to adjust drug doses for achieving therapeutic ranges that have been established prospectively in controlled studies or retrospectively by observation. These therapeutic reference ranges are statistically derived averages from data collected in a population of many individuals. Therefore, they are not necessarily the optimal therapeutic window for an individual patient. Biomarkers that complement TDM are therefore investigated in order to obtain better information on drug-specific pharmacodynamic effects or the general effect on the immune system of the organ recipient. Such complementary biomarkers should allow a better personalization of the immunosuppressive therapy. This chapter focuses on immune monitoring mainly based on the assessment of T-cell activation and proliferation in isolated lymphocytes, whole blood, plasma, or serum.

M. Oellerich & A. Dasgupta (Eds): Personalized Immunosuppression in Transplantation.
DOI: http://dx.doi.org/10.1016/B978-0-12-800885-0.00010-2

10.2 LYMPHOCYTE PROLIFERATION AND ACTIVATION IN ALLOGRAFT REJECTION

The immune system's main role is to protect the body against infections by distinguishing between self (host) and non-self. When allogeneic cells or tissues from individuals belonging to the same species but genetically dissimilar are transplanted, they are also recognized as non-self by the immune system of the host. The first response is an immediate inflammatory reaction that involves the innate immune system [1].

The innate immune system is non-antigen specific and depends on phagocytes and cytokines that are activated by conserved patterns of pathogens also present on tissues. In contrast, the adaptive immune response is antigen specific and mainly represented by T and B lymphocytes.

Organ rejection can be categorized as hyperacute, acute, and chronic rejection [2]. Hyperacute rejection occurs immediately after the blood flow is established to a transplanted organ and is caused by preformed anti-donor antibodies against HLA molecules, which induce complement activation, thrombosis, and tissue destruction. Acute rejection occurs within the first weeks after organ transplantation and is predominantly caused by a T-lymphocyte-mediated immune response against the allogeneic tissue. Chronic rejection occurs later and is less well defined. Multiple factors are involved, including memory T lymphocytes (T cells), B lymphocytes (B cells), and the complement system [2].

T cells, which are characterized by the expression of the CD3 (CD = cluster of differentiation) receptor on their surface, play a central role in the cellular lymphocyte-mediated process of acute graft rejection. Classically, they can be subdivided in two major subclasses, CD4$^+$ helper and cytotoxic CD8$^+$ T cells, although it is known that the opportunities for helper diversity are far greater than just these two alternatives. Currently, Th17, Th9, and Th22, follicular helper T (Th) cells as well as different types of regulatory T cells can be distinguished. However, after engrafting of the transplant, T cells located in draining lymph nodes of the transplant recipient are faced with non-self-peptides presented on MHC molecules of antigen presenting cells (APCs) and become activated depending on the environment in which T-cell recognition of the alloantigens occurs [3]. Activation of T cells can be divided into three phases: the induction phase, the expansion phase, and the effector phase [4]. Activation leads to increased ATP synthesis, RNA synthesis, DNA replication, cytokine production, and expression of proteins on the cell surface.

In the induction phase, the first interaction with APC is mediated by adhesion molecules such as LFA, ICAM-1, and CD2 [4]. This nonspecific contact enables specific binding to donor antigens mediated by the T cell receptor (TCR). Antigens presented by APC on MHC class II molecules primarily interact with CD4$^+$ cells, whereas MHC class I molecules mainly interact with CD8$^+$ T cells [5]. MHC class I molecules are found on all nucleated cells, whereas MHC class II molecules are restricted to professional APCs such as dendritic cells, activated macrophages, and B cells [5]. Evidence suggests that T cells are also activated in a nonspecific manner by cytokines in the very early reperfusion phase after transplantation before they bind to a specific antigen [6].

Activated T cells proliferate in the recipient's lymph nodes and become competent to respond to subsequent signals. During this expansion phase, proliferating T cells divide rapidly and secrete interferon-γ (IFN-γ), interleukin 2 (IL-2), and a variety of other cytokines. CD4$^+$ helper cells (Th) further differentiate into subtypes, such as Th1 and Th2. Th1 cells produce IFN-γ, IL-2, and tumor necrosis factor-β (TNF-β), which activate macrophages and are mainly responsible for cell-mediated immunity. By contrast, Th2 cells produce IL-4, IL-5, IL-10, and IL-13, which are involved in humoral immunity, supporting B-cell activation and maturation [7].

In the effector phase, alloactivated CD8$^+$ T cells interact with their cognate antigens on target cells, causing cytotoxicity, cell destruction, and apoptosis. These effects are mediated by perforin, granzyme B, granulolysins, and CD95L (FAS ligand). Next, the effector T cells are eliminated through apoptosis, except for a small portion, which become memory T cells. The importance of memory T cells in transplant rejection is increasingly recognized, and they may be responsible for preventing the development of tolerance and for inducing and maintaining chronic rejection [8].

An allograft carries a number of donor APCs, also called "passenger cells," in the form of interstitial dendritic cells or B cells, which can directly stimulate the recipient's T cells. In addition, T cells can be activated by indirect mechanisms if the alloantigens are presented as processed peptides by HLA molecules on self-APCs found in the graft recipient. The direct pathway is therefore characterized by the recognition of unchanged donor HLA alloantigens on donor cells, whereas the indirect pathway relies on processing of alloantigens and presentation as peptides on HLA molecules of recipient cells [9]. It is considered that both pathways for T-cell activation persist after organ transplantation [10]. In addition, a semidirect pathway has been proposed, which is characterized by presentation of the intact alloantigen by the recipient APC after internalization but without processing [11,12].

Three signals are required to achieve complete T-cell activation: (i) the interaction of the TCR–CD3 complex with the alloantigens presented by MHC molecules; (ii) a costimulatory receptor–ligand interaction between the T cell and the APC, such as CD28 on the T-cell surface with CD80/CD86 on the APC; and (iii) inflammatory cytokines that directly act on naive CD4$^+$ and CD8$^+$ T cells [13].

T-cell-derived cytokines such as TNF-α and chemokines (e.g., CCL2, CCL5, and CX3CL1) are involved in the effector phase, promoting intense macrophage infiltration into the allograft. In addition, endothelial cells are also activated in the graft by T-cell-derived cytokines, leading to an upregulation of MHC, adhesion, and costimulatory molecules, thereby recruiting more T cells into the graft and amplifying the rejection process [4,7]. Furthermore, activated T cells express chemokine receptors such as CXCR3 and are attracted to inflamed tissues in a rejecting allograft by chemokines such as CXCL10, which is secreted by several cell types, including immune cells and non-immune cells [14]. In summary, T-cell activation is the first and crucial step of the host to defend non-self-antigens, and activated T cells acquire a variety of features that differentiate them from naive T cells.

10.3 EFFECT OF IMMUNOSUPPRESSANTS ON LYMPHOCYTE PROLIFERATION AND ACTIVATION

Most pharmacological immunosuppressants are directed against activation and proliferation of both T and B lymphocytes [15]. Silencing or depleting effector T cells is particularly important to prevent acute rejection. The calcineurin inhibitors cyclosporine (CsA) and tacrolimus are inhibitors of transcription by blocking calcineurin phosphatase activity and thereby cytokine-driven T-lymphocyte proliferation and activation. Mycophenolates (mycophenolate mofetil (MMF) and mycophenolate sodium (MPS)) inhibit cell proliferation of T and B cells by blocking production of guanine nucleotides. Sirolimus and everolimus block the response of T and B cells to activation by cytokines, thereby preventing cell cycle progression and proliferation. Corticosteroids inhibit lymphocyte proliferation and cell-mediated immune responses. Antibodies used for induction or anti-rejection therapy either block IL-2-driven cell proliferation by binding to the IL-2 receptor α-chain (CD25 antigen) on activated T cells (basiliximab and daclizumab) or completely deplete T cells (antithymocyte globulin and muromonab-CD3). Against this background, it is obvious that monitoring of T-cell activation and proliferation may have potential to serve as a non-drug-specific biomarker to assess the net state of immunosuppression, particularly with synergistic immunosuppressive treatment regimens. There are various methods to assess lymphocyte activation and proliferation.

10.3.1 CELL FUNCTION TESTS AND T-CELL ACTIVATION IN WHOLE BLOOD

Throughout the years, several approaches have evolved to assess lymphocyte activation and proliferation that can be roughly divided into indirect cell function tests and the direct assessment of cell activation markers. Cell function tests are either performed in vitro using isolated cells or whole blood from healthy blood donors or ex vivo using isolated cells or whole blood from transplant patients. Cell function tests require in vitro stimulation of isolated lymphocytes or whole blood containing T cells. When the cells are from immunosuppressed transplant patients, the stimulation is called ex vivo. This stimulation can be either allospecific or non-allospecific. Allospecific assays have the advantages that the immune response against a specific donor antigen can be monitored and patients with donor-specific hyporesponsiveness as an indicator of graft tolerance can be detected [16]. However, stimulation of only alloantigen-specific T-cell clones precludes the monitoring of interindividual sensitivity of different subjects to various immunosuppressants. In addition, if the organ is from a deceased donor, it can be difficult to store and preserve donor-specific antigens for long-term monitoring after transplantation [17]. To mimic the situation in vivo, donor and recipient peripheral blood mononuclear lymphocyte (PBMNL) cells are combined and incubated in mixed leukocyte reaction (MLR) or a limiting dilution assay (LDA). Alternatively, third-party cells with HLA mismatches can be used as surrogate [18]. In addition to these approaches, which reflect direct allorecognition,

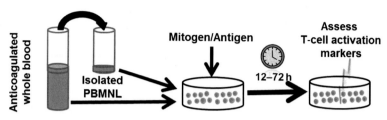

FIGURE 10.1 T-cell function tests.

Leukocytes contained in anticoagulated whole blood or isolated peripheral blood mononuclear lymphocytes (PBMNL) are stimulated by antigens or mitogens for 12–72h. T-cell activation is assessed by various markers as a readout.

the indirect pathway can be mimicked by adding processed HLA peptides to third-party cells [19].

However, to study the effect of immunosuppressants on T-cell activation, whole blood assays seem to be superior to incubations with isolated cells because the immunosuppressants present in the blood sample are not washed out during cell isolation, thereby preserving the equilibrium between drugs bound to plasma proteins and their distribution into blood cells. Furthermore, whole blood assays require less blood and prevent the selective loss of immune cells, which better reflects physiological conditions [20]. A general disadvantage of all cell function tests is that they require incubation times up to 72h, which usually precludes same-day reporting of results to the clinicians. The principle of cell function tests in shown in Figure 10.1.

Non-allospecific stimulation can be performed by using third-party cells, stimulating antibodies against surface receptors, antibody-coated beads, bacterial and viral toxins—for example, lipopolysaccharide (LPS), staphylococcal enterotoxin B (SEB), and cytomegalovirus protein 65 (CMCpp65)—or mitogens such as concanavalin A (CON A), pokeweed mitogen (PWM), phorbol 12-myristate 13-acetate (PMA), and phytohemagglutinin (PHA) [21]. A selection of stimuli is summarized in Table 10.1. A more straightforward approach is the direct assessment of in vivo activated T cells in anticoagulated whole blood without cell isolation and ex vivo stimulation.

10.3.2 ANALYTICAL TECHNIQUES TO ASSESS LYMPHOCYTE ACTIVATION AND PROLIFERATION

In both the indirect cell function test and the direct monitoring of activated T cells, a variety of cell proliferation and activation markers can be followed as the readout. These comprise the assessment of DNA replication, the detection of receptors and ligands upregulated on the cell surface (surface markers), the quantification of intracellular ATP (iATP) or cytokines, and expression analysis of single genes or gene expression profiles. If molecules upregulated upon activation are released, they can be assessed in the incubation medium or the circulation using immunoassays, or they

Table 10.1 Stimuli Used for Lymphocyte Activation

Kind of Stimulus	Stimuli
Allospecific	• Donor APC • Other donor cells (e.g., fibroblasts) • HLA mismatched third-party cells as surrogate • Donor peptides plus third-party cells

Non-allospecific	• Third-party cells
	• Antibodies (e.g., anti-CD3, anti-CD28)
	• Antibody-coated beads (e.g., anti-CD28 plus anti-CD3/TCR)
	• Mitogens
	  • Phorbol 12-myristate 13-acetate (PMA)
	  • Ionomycin (ION)
	  • Concanavalin A (CON A)
	  • Phytohemagglutinin (PHA)
	  • Pokeweed mitogen (PMW)
	• Viral peptides (e.g., CMVpp65)
	• Bacterial toxins
	  • Lipopolysaccharide (LPS)
	  • Staphylococcal enterotoxin B (SEB)

can be captured by enzyme-linked antibodies immobilized on a membrane, forming spots. In renal transplantation, urine is an alternative fluid in which ongoing T-cell activation within the kidney can be indirectly monitored by measuring soluble markers or by searching for activated lymphocytes. The most commonly applied analytical techniques to follow cell activation in cell function tests and the direct assessment of activation markers are flow cytometry for both intracellular molecules and surface markers, enzyme-linked immunosorbent assay (ELISA) performed in a single or multiplex manner using beads, enzyme-linked immunospot (ELISPOT) assays, gene expression studies using array technologies and/or quantitative PCR (qPCR). The assessment of iATP is based on the ATP-dependent firefly luciferase assay [22]. Cell proliferation can also be followed by using labeled DNA precursors and dyes.

10.3.2.1 T-cell activation markers

Frequently a combination of different markers has been used in clinical investigations to assess T-cell activation. In the following paragraphs the single markers or marker groups are presented separately but where useful associations between different markers are mentioned.

10.3.2.2 Proliferation markers

Proliferation and division of eukaryotic cells is characterized by DNA synthesis. If labeled DNA precursors such as radioactive thymidine (^{3}H-thymidine) or the thymidine analog 5-bromo-2′-deoxyuridine (BrdU) are added, they are incorporated into the newly synthesized DNA strands. Radiolabeled ^{3}H-thymidine can be detected by a scintillation counter, and BrdU can be detected by a quantitative enzyme

Table 10.2 Proliferation Markers

Marker	Readout
• 5-Bromo-2′-deoxyuridine (BrdU)	ELISA, flow cytometry
• ^{3}H-thymidine	Isotope
• Carboxy-fluorescein diacetate (CFSE)	Flow cytometry
• 3-(4,5-Dimethylthiazol-2-yl)-2,5-diphenyl-tetrazolium bromide; thiazolyl blue (MTT)	Photometry
• PCNA protein	Flow cytometry
• PCNA mRNA	qPCR

immunoassay using monoclonal antibodies [23,24]. Cell division and growth need energy, and metabolic activity assays are based on this premise. The cells are incubated with a colorimetric substrate such as the tetrazolium salt MTT (3-(4,5-dimethylthiazol-2-yl)-2,5-diphenyl-tetrazolium bromide; thiazolyl blue), which is reduced by mitochondrial succinate dehydrogenase [25]. In addition, a number of other markers have been developed to study cell proliferation, such as the succinimidyl ester of carboxy fluorescein diacetate (CFSE), which irreversibly binds to proteins both on the cell surface and intracellular by reaction with lysine and other amine groups. During cell division, CFSE labeling is distributed equally between the daughter cells, thereby losing fluorescence, which can be followed by flow cytometry [26]. Proliferating cell nuclear antigen (PCNA) is a DNA clamp that is essential for cell replication. Therefore, PCNA expression is an indicator of proliferation and can be accessed on the protein level by flow cytometry, or PCNA mRNA expression can be followed by real-time qPCR [27,28]. Whereas PCNA protein expression needs approximately 72 h to become reliably measurable, PCNA mRNA expression can be assessed 24 h after the onset of stimulation. Proliferation markers are summarized in Table 10.2.

Proliferation markers have been predominately studied in vitro and ex vivo with isolated PBMNL. The antiproliferative effect of immunosuppressants became evident when the drugs were added to the cell incubation media during stimulation of PBMNL of healthy volunteers [17,29]. However, proliferation of PBMNL isolated from transplant patients under immunosuppression and stimulated ex vivo was also inhibited. Lymphocytes from kidney transplant patients under therapy with prednisone, MMF, and CsA showed a reduced cell proliferation compared to healthy controls using PCNA protein and ^{3}H-thymidine incorporation as markers [29]. Interestingly, PCNA expression was related to mycophenolic acid (MPA) plasma concentrations and inhibition of inosine monophosphate dehydrogenase activity, which is the pharmacodynamic target of MPA [30]. A study with conversion from MMF to MPS showed increased cell proliferation using PCNA expression, possibly indicating a weaker immunosuppressive effect of MPS [31]. The effect of everolimus on lymphocyte proliferation was investigated by Böhler et al. using the MTT assay with PBMNL isolated from stable kidney transplant recipients and stimulated with an anti-CD3 antibody for 72 h. Adding everolimus to an immunosuppressive therapy based on CsA and prednisolone, they observed a proliferation inhibition of 45% after 21 days of therapy compared to baseline values and that of patients who received a placebo. After cessation of the everolimus therapy, values returned to baseline after 21 days [32]. The strong effect of everolimus was seen as a synergistic action of CsA and everolimus. In general, all experiments in which immunosuppressants were added in vitro and ex vivo to cell function assays have shown that the effect of the drugs becomes evident by inhibiting cell proliferation. The next question, of course, is whether this observation translates into clinical events or can be used to personalize immunosuppression.

Using the proliferation marker CFSE in an allospecific ex vivo MLR with living donor liver transplantation patients, the stimulation index of $CD4^+$ T cells in the anti-self-reaction was increased in recurrent cases of autoimmune hepatitis [33]. The authors conclude that optimization of the immunosuppressant agents based on the CSFE–MLR assay may be promising in patients after liver transplantation. ^{3}H-thymidine incorporation has also been used to follow the combined effect of calcineurin inhibitors and Sir in PHA-activated lymphocytes in vitro [34] and in an ex vivo model with isolated PBMNL from transplant patients in a so-called immune status assay. In this assay, PBMNL were stimulated with graft-derived fibroblasts as a source of alloantigens in the presence and absence of IL-2. Forming a score depending on IL-2 allowed the prediction of rejections with a sensitivity of 82% and a specificity of 81% [35]. Cell proliferation of PBMNL was investigated in a donor-specific ex vivo assay in children treated with tacrolimus and experiencing rejection episodes 60 days after liver transplantation. CSFE-positive cells were increased in rejecters after incubation in an MLR for 3 days. However, T-cell activation was better reflected by the cell surface marker CD154 [18]. In an own study with BrdU incorporation into proliferating PBMNL stimulated ex vivo with PHA for 72 h, a weak association between a suppressed cell proliferation and leukopenia was observed in kidney transplant patients as a possible indication of over-immunosuppression [36].

Some studies have used whole blood samples to assess cell proliferation in recipients of solid organ transplants. In a study with stable liver transplant patients undergoing weaning of immunosuppression, T-cell proliferation in whole blood stimulated with CON A (72 h) as assessed by PCNA and flow cytometry was increased after drug minimization. In addition, patients with rejection had an increased proliferation of $CD8^+$ cells [37]. PCNA mRNA expression has been used in an immune stimulation assay based on the ratio between stimulated (PMA + ION) and nonstimulated whole blood in de novo renal transplant patients, and inhibition of cell proliferation has been associated with over-immunosuppression indicated by more reactivation of viral infections [28]. Although a straightforward proof of principle approach to assess the immunosuppressive effect of different drugs on T cells, proliferation markers have not been widely used in clinical trials or under routine conditions. One reason may be that assay protocols require extended incubation times, precluding a reasonable turnaround time (TAT), which is mandatory for clinical decision making. This could also explain why no trials have been conducted to determine whether immunosuppression can be tailored based on proliferation markers.

10.3.2.3 Intracellular ATP

As mentioned previously, cell activation and proliferation depend on the provision of energy, and it is a logical approach to follow the rise of the iATP as a tool to asses T-cell activation. ATP can be very sensitively measured using the firefly lucif-erase system [22]. An assay for the bioluminescent monitoring of iATP in CD4$^+$ cells (ImmuKnow) has been developed by Cylex, Inc. (Columbia, MD), and it has been approved by the US Food and Drug Administration (FDA) for the detection of cell-mediated immune response in populations undergoing immunosuppressive therapy following organ transplantation. The assay is exclusively offered by a central labora-tory in the United States (Viracor-IBT Laboratories, Lee's Summit, MO). Mitogenic stimulation of whole blood is achieved by an overnight incubation (15–18h) of the patient's whole blood sample with PHA. Blood samples are stable for 30h at room temperature. CD4$^+$ cells are selected by magnetic separation, and after cell lysis iATP is measured in a luminometer [38]. This assay is much more standardized and advanced to assess T-cell activation than the approaches mentioned previously that are based on cell proliferation. Therefore, many studies have been performed with this commercially available test system during the past several years. High iATP concen-trations are suggested to indicate a strong T-cell activation, whereas low values reflect inhibition. Clinical trials were mainly focused on predicting rejection indicating inad-equate immunosuppression and infections as a result of over-immunosuppression.

In many studies, high CD4$^+$ T-cell iATP concentrations were associated with an increased risk of acute rejection in recipients of kidney, liver, heart, and small bowel transplants, whereas low CD4$^+$ T-cell iATP concentrations were linked to a higher risk of infections [39–42]. From a meta-analysis, a target immunological response zone between 25 and 700ng/mL ATP was defined, which was suggested to better allow discriminating the relative risks of infection and rejection than individually measured values [38]. A concentration of 280ng/mL ATP was associated with the lowest risk for infection and rejection. At this cutoff concentration, the assay dem-onstrated a negative predictive value of greater than 96%. In a study of 50 renal and 34 liver transplant patients, Millan et al. observed that iATP seems to be more effec-tive in identifying over-immunosuppression than a high risk of rejection [43]. Other studies support this assumption by showing a significant relationship between low ImmuKnow test results and occurrence of infections [44–46].

Although no association between iATP and clinical events was observed in a recent retrospective trial with stable renal transplant recipients, it was found that the strength of immunosuppression was associated with iATP concentrations. In proto-cols using azathioprine, iATP was significantly higher compared to that of therapies with other immunosuppressants ($P < 0.01$). Tac therapy was associated with lower values than CsA therapy, possibly indicating a weaker immunosuppression of the latter [47]. In another study, the association between immune response and short-term mortality risk was shown [48]. The study comprised 362 patients with differ-ent allografts and 1031 iATP measurements. Patients with at least one iATP assay result less than 175ng/mL died more frequently (14.4%) compared to those with all ImmuKnow concentrations greater than 175ng/mL (5.2%).

However, the significance of iATP measurement in CD4$^+$ cells is currently inconclusive because contradictory results have been published regarding the prediction of acute rejection and infection. A published meta-analysis incorporating multiple organ transplants [49] concluded that the current evidence suggests that monitoring iATP is not suitable to identify individuals at risk of rejection or infection.

In the meantime, more single-center studies have been performed in different organ transplant patients to establish the value of the iATP assay as a predictor of allograft rejection and infection in kidney transplantation [50,51], liver transplantation [52], and intestinal transplantation [53]. These studies reconfirm statistically significant differences in iATP concentrations in transplant recipients with infection or rejection compared to patients free of these complications and to healthy controls. However, from these investigations, it is not clear whether it is possible to prospectively predict which individuals are at high risk of infection or transplantation rejection. Furthermore, no evidence has been generated that individualization of the immunosuppressive therapy based on the results of iATP determinations is associated with improved clinical outcomes in solid organ transplant recipients.

A potential explanation for the inconclusive findings with the ImmuKnow assay may be that most studies are retrospective and many use only single time point measurements or have small patient numbers. In addition, results may not be comparable between transplant populations because clinical event risks substantially differ between graft types. Target ranges for iATP adjusted to different organs and patient populations may be required. Furthermore, with respect to the prediction of acute rejection, it should also be taken into consideration that the assay is not donor specific and rather reflects the general immune status of CD4$^+$ cells than the specific T cell response toward the allograft. In general, serial longitudinal measurements appear to provide a diagnostic tool for identifying over-immunosuppression in the individual patient and may indicate an increased risk of short-term mortality. However, more evidence must be generated from clinical trials to support appropriate interpretation of the test results. A drawback from the analytical standpoint is that the assay is a time-consuming indirect cell function test requiring stimulation and a cell isolation step. Furthermore, pre-analytics are critical because blood samples have to be stimulated within 30 h. Advantageous is the standardized assay procedure.

10.3.2.4 Cell surface markers

Proteins expressed on the surface of a cell can reflect the activation status of the respective cell. A published review summarized the evidence with respect to T-cell activation in solid organ transplantation up to the year 2012 [54]. Such surface markers indicating an activated state are found on most activated lymphocytes, including T cells, B cells, NK cells, dendritic cells, and cells of the myeloid lineage (neutrophils, monocytes, macrophages, and eosinophils). On T cells, receptor proteins, costimulatory molecules, adhesion molecules, chemokine receptors, and MHC class II molecules can be found upregulated. In general, these surface markers possess a number within the CD used for immunophenotyping of leukocytes. A variety of receptor proteins, such as CD25 (IL-2 receptor), CD69 (early activation antigen),

CD70 (ki24 antigen), CD71 (transferrin receptor), or CD95 (Fas receptor), have been investigated [55–59]. Costimulatory molecules either belong to the IgG superfamily, the TNF–TNF receptor family, or the TIM family (type 1 transmembrane glycoprotein). Typical proteins of the IgG superfamily are CD28, CD152, CD152 or CTLA-4, ICOS, and PD-I. The TNF–TNF receptor family members are CD27, CD30, CD154 or CD40L, CD134 (OX40), CD137 (4-IBB), GITR, and HVEM. Representatives of the TIM family are TIM1 and TIM2 [60]. Dipeptidyl peptidase IV (CD26), a member of the S9B protein family, is also expressed on activated T cells [61]. It is a multifunctional protein that has adenosine binding properties and enzymatic activity [62]. Adhesion molecules belong to either the integrins or the immunoglobulins. Lymphocyte function-associated antigen 1 (LFA-1) or CD11a and VLA-4 (dimer of CD49d and CD29) are members of the integrins. Intercellular adhesion molecule 1 (ICAM-1), also termed CD54 and CD2, is a member of the immunoglobulin family [63]. Chemokine receptors such as CXCR3 and CCR5 are strongly induced in activated T cells and involved in transplant rejection [64]. Donor-specific T cells upregulate peripheral chemokine receptors that enable them to enter the transplanted allograft [65]. Furthermore, all isotypes of MHC class II molecules (HLA-DR, HLA-DQ, and HLA-DP) can be found on activated T cells [66]. These surface markers can be monitored by flow cytometry using monoclonal antibodies labeled with fluorescent dyes. Surface markers of T-cell activation are summarized in Table 10.3.

Various in vitro experiments using cell function tests and flow cytometry have shown that immunosuppressants have an effect on surface marker expression as it has been reported previously for cell proliferation. For example, CD25 and CD71 expression has been shown to be inhibited in mitogen-stimulated whole blood (72 h) dose dependently by CsA, tacrolimus, MPA, and methylprednisolone [17]. However, for clinical purposes, blood samples or cells from transplant patients are of interest. Therefore, several groups have investigated ex vivo stimulated cells or whole blood from organ recipients treated with different immunosuppressive protocols with respect to surface marker expression and tried to correlate these effects to the immunosuppressive therapy or clinical events. Older investigations showed that in renal transplant patients on an immunosuppressive drug regimen with CsA, MMF, and prednisone, expression of different surface activation antigens on T cells was reduced compared to that of healthy volunteers when whole blood was stimulated ex vivo

Table 10.3 Cell Surface Markers

Molecule	Markers
Receptor proteins	CD25, CD69, CD71, CD95
Costimulatory molecules	CD26, CD27, CD28, CD30, CD134, CD137, CD152 (CTLA-4), CD154, CD279, ICOS, TIM1, TIM2
Adhesion molecules	CD2 (LFA-2), CD11a (LFA-1), CD154 (ICAM-1)
Chemokine receptors	CXCR3, CCR5
MHC molecules	Class II: HLA-DR, HLA-DQ, HLA-DP

with PMA. Most affected were CD11a and CD154, followed by CD71, CD25, and CD95 [67]. A different effect of CsA and tacrolimus has been shown in renal transplant recipients [68]. The authors reported a stronger effect of tacrolimus on CD154, CD28, and CD54 expression compared to CsA. The direct effect of a single dose of MPA had a dramatic but transient effect within 1 h after intake on CD25 and CD71 expression on CD3$^+$ cells in diluted whole blood from kidney transplant recipients stimulated with CON A for 2 days [69]. In stable renal graft recipients, CD25 and CD71 expression showed a trend to increase in undiluted whole blood stimulated by PMA and ION for 30 min after conversion from MMF to enteric-coated MPS in kidney allograft recipients [31]. This was accompanied by a slightly enhanced cell proliferation. In heart and lung graft transplantation, a switch from CsA to tacrolimus was not reflected in CD25 expression on CD3$^+$ cells monitored after stimulation of diluted whole blood with PMA [27]. In general, ex vivo investigations comparing the immunosuppressive effect of different drugs showed a trend to a more efficient inhibition of surface marker expression with tacrolimus compared to CsA. However, note that cell function tests to assess the immunosuppressant effect of different drugs or drug combinations are mainly based on non-allospecific cell stimulation using mitogens. A common finding was that there is no close correlation between whole blood concentrations of immunosuppressant drugs and nonspecific pharmacodynamic effects observed with surface marker expression. This raises the question whether surface markers can be used to individually predict clinical events associated with over- or under-immunosuppression.

Investigations addressing this question are not always conclusive. Using ex vivo stimulation of isolated PBMNL from kidney transplant recipients treated with calcineurin inhibitor (CNI) showed that CD25 expression on CD3$^+$ and CD4$^+$ cells could not be used to distinguished rejection or infection but clearly distinguished episodes of CsA nephrotoxicity and allograft dysfunction [70]. A lower CD25 and CD71 expression on CD3$^+$ T cells after mitogenic stimulation of PBMNL may be a sign of over-immunosuppression in patients with cardiac allograft dysfunction [71]. CD25 was also used as a ratio before and after liver transplantation to assess the risk of rejection [72]. In pediatric liver transplant patients, an increased expression of CD154 on cytotoxic T memory cells (TcM) before transplantation was associated with a significant risk of rejection in these patients. The results were better if allospecific stimulation was applied in the ex vivo MLR using the so-called surrogate donor cells compared to third-party cells [18]. These donor-like cells are PBMNL from normal human subjects, which are HLA matched to the donor. Calculating an immune response ratio (IR) by using the ratio of allospecific versus non-allospecific stimulation, a value greater than 1.23 was correlated with the histological grade and clinical severity of acute cellular rejection in children after intestine transplantation [73]. The assay has been FDA approved and is commercially available under the name Pleximmune. It is currently restricted to patients younger than age 21 years with liver or small bowel transplantation and performed in a central laboratory of the company Plexision (Pittsburgh, PA), which guarantees reproducibility. The test needs isolated PBMNL from the graft recipient and HLA typing of the donor. It is worth mentioning that activated memory T cells are most meaningful in this test, and this may be related to the understanding that these cells are most likely responsible for chronic cell-mediated rejection [8]. CD154 expression, together with CD69, is also used as a readout in a commercially available test kit to monitor the function of regulatory T cells (FastImmune Human Regulatory T Cell Function Kit, BD Bioscience, San Jose, CA). Although promising, the Pleximmune test requires cell isolation, shipment to a central laboratory, and ex vivo stimulation, making it inconvenient for routine application. In addition, no laboratory outside the United States currently offers the test.

CD69 also acts as a costimulatory molecule and is rapidly detectable within a few hours after T-cell stimulation [74]. In an MLR with donor B cells, expression of CD69 was increased on CD3$^+$ cells in heart transplant patients with acute rejection compared to those without rejection. Furthermore, CD69 expression was increased in a subgroup of patients in response to donor peptides [75]. As mentioned previously, CD69 is together with CD154 used as an activation marker on T cells in a commercially available test kit to assess the function of regulatory T cells (FastImmune Human Regulatory T Cell Function Kit).

A more direct approach is to monitor activated T cells in whole blood without ex vivo stimulation. In such a direct approach, Beik et al. found, as already mentioned, that an increased expression of CD25 on CD3$^+$, CD4$^+$, and CD8$^+$ cells was associated with acute rejection episodes and cytomegalovirus (CMV) infection but not with CsA nephrotoxicity in 28 kidney graft recipients [70]. In long-term liver transplant patients, an association between CD28 expression on CD8$^+$ cells and malignancies as well as CD28 expression on CD3$^+$ cells and rejection has been reported by Boleslawski et al. A higher CD28 expression on CD3$^+$ cells was seen in rejecting patients, whereas a lower expression was noted in patients with malignancies, suggesting under- and over-immunosuppression, respectively [76,77]. However, because CD28 is constitutively expressed on CD3 cells, these findings can also be considered as a T-cell subset, indicating the activation of the immune system. In liver transplantation, the combined determination of CD95 and CD28 on CD4$^+$ cells was able to segregate patients with hepatitis C virus (HCV) infection from those with rejection. Whereas CD95 was upregulated in both patients with HCV infection and rejection CD28 was not higher in viral infection but associated with rejection [78]. The ONE Study consortium has proposed a T-cell activation panel that is based on the expression of CD57 or HLA-DR and, surprisingly, loss of CD27 or CD28 on both CD4$^+$ and CD8 T cells [79].

The chemokine receptors CXCR3, CCR2, and CCR5 have been followed on T-cell subsets directly in peripheral whole blood in small studies with kidney transplant patients that revealed partly contradictory results. One study found increased expression of CXCR3 on the surface of CD4$^+$ T cells in patients developing allograft rejection. CXCR3 on CD8$^+$ T cells and CCR5 on CD4$^+$ and CD8$^+$ cells remained stable throughout the study [80]. The expression of the chemokine receptors CXCR3, CCR2, and CCR5 has also been studied on CD4$^+$ and CD8$^+$ T cells in the peripheral blood of kidney transplant recipients in another study, and a higher frequency of the chemokine receptors CCR5$^+$ and CCR2$^+$ but not of CXCR3 was observed on both

CD4$^+$ and CD8$^+$ T cells in patients with biopsy-proven rejections [81]. Although analytically promising and comparably straightforward as well as simple to perform, there are currently only single-center reports on the direct assessment of T-cell surface activation markers in peripheral blood of solid organ recipients.

Currently, CD154 expression on memory T cells stimulated in an allospecific manner seems to be the most advanced approach for immune monitoring using T-cell surface markers. Standardization or harmonization of assay protocols as well as a robust cross-validation in different laboratories are missing, as is an answer to the question whether whole blood samples can be stabilized for longer periods of time in order to enable shipment to specialized laboratories for centers without flow cytometry available on site. These are prerequisites for performing large multi-center studies and ultimately adoption for routine diagnostic use. Except for CD154 (Pleximmune), there is currently no evidence from prospective clinical trials that T-cell surface markers can support clinical decision making.

10.3.3 SOLUBLE LYMPHOCYTE SURFACE MOLECULES IN PLASMA OR SERUM

Lymphocyte surface molecules can be cleaved off the cell surface upon activation, and the determination in cell culture supernatants or in the circulation becomes possible. After the release, they are termed soluble markers such as sCD25, sCD26, sCD30, or sCD44. A major advantage of monitoring soluble T-cell activation markers in peripheral blood is that although not really standardized, commercially available ELISA formats are available. In addition, a fluorescent microsphere immunoassay (Luminex technology) has been developed that allows multiplex determination along with other molecules in the same sample and opens new analytical perspectives [82].

A considerable number of studies have been published particularly on the utility of sCD30 as a tool for immune monitoring in transplantation both pre-transplant and post-transplantation. It has been shown that allo-stimulation causes upregulation and release of CD30 particularly from CD4$^+$ as well as CD8$^+$ memory T cells by an IFN-γ and IL-2 regulated process [83]. CD30 is cleaved off by zinc metalloproteinases and released into the bloodstream [84–86]. It is therefore assumed that the serum concentration of sCD30 reflects the activation state of the immune system.

A considerable number of outcome studies with sCD30 have been published for kidney transplantation. Pre-transplant concentrations (>100 U/mL) in sera of 3899 cadaver kidney recipients from the Collaborative Transplant Study were significantly associated with the occurrence of acute allograft rejection, need of anti-rejection treatment in the first year post-transplantation, as well as risk of graft loss during the 5-year follow-up [87]. Combining sCD30 with other immunological markers such as panel reactive antibodies (PRAs) showed that patients with both PRA and high pre-transplant sCD30 had a particularly poor graft outcome [87]. Furthermore, for kidney graft recipients with high pre-transplant sCD30, HLA matching was particularly advantageous [88]. However, a meta-analysis by Chen et al. revealed that there is not sufficient evidence that pre-transplantation sCD30 is able to identify patients at risk for acute rejection [89]. As shown by Altermann et al. [90], there is considerable intraindividual variation of the sCD30 concentrations in approximately 20% of patients on the waiting list; thus, the measurement of sCD30 at one single time point is probably not useful, and sequential monitoring (e.g., quarterly) might be advantageous. An open question is whether sCD30 clearance is dependent on kidney function.

However, pre-transplant sCD30 concentrations that remained high early after kidney transplantation were associated with acute rejection [91]. In a multicenter study involving more than 2000 kidney transplant recipients, it was noted that a low concentration was reached on day 30, and values greater than 40 U/mL were related to a significantly inferior graft survival rate [92]. With patients on either tacrolimus or CsA therapy in combination with azathioprine or MMF, there were no significant differences in sCD30 concentration, depending on the immunosuppressive therapy [93].

The marker has been investigated not only in kidney transplantation but also as predictor of outcome of non-renal transplantation (e.g., heart, lung, islet, and liver) [94–98]. Unfortunately, these studies were small, and their results are sometimes contradictory. As for kidney transplantation, unresolved issues are the optimal time point for sCD30 determination as well as the appropriate cutoffs. Moreover, studies investigating the effects of different immunosuppressive drugs or drug combinations on sCD30 are unfortunately lacking.

Other soluble surface markers have not been sufficiently considered as markers of immune activation. There is one small investigation in which the soluble forms of CD25, CD30, and CD44 were determined in parallel with other markers of immune activation, such as lymphocyte subsets and mixed lymphocyte cultures. Renal transplant recipients with acute rejection after living donor kidney transplantation showed the highest pre-transplant serum concentrations of sCD25, sCD30, and sCD44. Multivariate logistic regression yielded a prognostic score for prediction of rejection with 75.0% sensitivity and 69.2% specificity [99].

10.3.4 CYTOKINES

Another approach to assess the state of T-cell activation is to examine the upregulation of cytokines. $CD4^+$ Th1 cells are the primary source for the pro-inflammatory cytokines IFN-γ, IL-2, and TNF-β, whereas IL-4, IL-5, IL-9, IL-10, IL-13, and IL-25 are produced by $CD4^+$ Th2 cells [100]. Activated $CD8^+$ effector and memory T cells also produce IL-2, IL-10, TNF-α, and IFN-γ [101]. Cytokines can be monitored inside activated T cells or the release of cytokines from stimulated T cells can be followed. For the detection of intracellular cytokines, flow cytometry is commonly used. Cytokine release into cell culture supernatants or the bloodstream of patients is commonly monitored by ELISAs. Alternatively, antibody-coated beads and flow cytometry can be applied (e.g., Human Th1/Th2 Cytokine CBA Kit, Becton Dickinson). Cytokines released by single cells can be followed using the ELISPOT assay technique [102,103]. Cytokines of interests are summarized in Table 10.4. However, most data have been generated with IL-2, IFN-γ, and TNF-α.

Table 10.4 Cytokines Used to Asses T-cell Activation

Principle	Cytokine	Methods
Intracellular cytokines in activated T cell	IL-1β, IL-2, IFN-γ, TNF-α	Flow Cytometry
Cytokines released by activated T cells		
• Cell function assays	IL-2, IL-4, IL-6, IL-10, IL-13, IFN-γ, TNF-α, GM-CSF, RANTES and TGF-βIL-4, IL-6, IL-10, IFN-γ, TNF-α	Immunoassay (ELISA, Multiplex)
• Cytokines in serum/plasma	IL-4, IL-6, IL-10, IFN-γ, TNF-α	Immunoassay (ELISA, Multiplex)
• Single cells	IFN-γ	ELISPOT

10.3.4.1 Intracellular cytokines

An advantage of intracellular cytokine monitoring in cell function assays is the relatively short response time (2–5 h) compared to that of cell surface expression or iATP production, which require much longer stimulation times. In vitro experiments with PBMNL showed that immunosuppressive drugs such as Tac were able to suppress TNF-α and IL-1β production in PBMNL stimulated by an anti-CD3/CD28 antibody in a dose-dependent manner [104]. Böhler et al. studied in vitro the intracellular expression of IL-2 and TNF-α by T cells in PMA/ION stimulated whole blood cultures from healthy volunteers to which CsA, tacrolimus, sirolimus, MPA, and prednisolone were added in various concentrations. Whereas there was a dose-dependent inhibition by CsA and tacrolimus on both IL-2 and TNF-α expression, sirolimus and MPA had no, and prednisolone only a slight, effect [17]. These experiments show that cytokine production can be used as a readout of T-cell activation and may serve as a tool for pharmacodynamic monitoring of immunosuppression in transplant patients. Stalder et al. reported that the production of intracellular cytokines (IL-2, IFN-γ, and TNF-α) was significantly lower in T cells from kidney transplant recipients treated with CsA and MMF than in healthy control subjects using ex vivo mitogen-stimulated whole blood cultures [67].

Millán et al. studied intracellular IFN-γ in whole blood of stable liver transplant patients in vivo undergoing drug weaning. The percentage of CD8$^+$ IFN-γ$^+$ and CD4$^+$ IFN-γ$^+$ cells was significantly higher in patients who rejected than in those who did not [37]. Intracellular expression of IFN-γ and IL-2 before and after liver transplantation and clinical outcome were investigated by the same group. The authors showed that patients with a significant increase of intracellular T-cell IFN-γ in CD4$^+$ and CD8$^+$ early after transplantation had a high association with the incidence of acute rejection [105]. A further study of 79 kidney and 63 liver transplant patients reconfirmed the potential benefit of intracellular cytokine monitoring in this small prospective trial by showing that intracellular %IFN-γ in CD4$^+$CD69$^+$ and %IFN-γ in CD8$^+$CD69$^+$ was associated with a higher risk of acute rejection. This was also true for %IL-2 in CD8$^+$CD69$^+$ cells in kidney patients [106]. In a larger cohort of 407 stable kidney recipients, the percentage of CD8$^+$ cells with increased IL-2 was greater in patients who had experienced a rejection, and the relative occurrence of IL-2-positive cells in this retrospective observation depended on the number of rejection events [107]. The latter study used isolated PBMNL to follow intracellular cytokines. However, results observed from analysis of whole blood compared to isolated cells may have an impact on the overall results [108]. In a study of de novo liver transplant recipients treated with CsA or tacrolimus, Boleslawski et al. observed that intracellular IL-2 production in CD8$^+$ T cells before transplantation was closely related to the onset of acute rejection, particularly in patients under tacrolimus therapy [109].

10.3.4.2 Released cytokines

Cytokines released from activated cells can be determined in supernatants of in vitro or ex vivo cell function assays, in whole blood, or using the ELISPOT method. Using irradiated donor cells, van Besouw et al. reported for kidney transplant patients that the TH1 cytokines IFN-γ and TNF-α were positively related with the presence of donor-specific T-lymphocyte precursors in a LDA [110]. In kidney transplant patients, the effect of immunosuppression on cytokine production could be shown in a whole blood stimulation assay using PMA and following IL-2 and IFN-γ production. A stronger immunosuppressive exposure was reflected by lower IL-2 concentrations, whereas IFN-γ was unaffected [111]. A model to study the effect of immunosuppressants on the release of a whole panel of cytokines released from mitogen-stimulated rat whole blood using a multiplex platform for the parallel determination of 10 cytokines has been published [112].

Cytokines in plasma have also been investigated as a biomarker to predict outcome after transplantation. In stable kidney transplant patients, increased plasma IFN-γ and decreased plasma IL-4 late after transplantation were associated with good long-term graft outcome [113]. In liver transplantation, Azarpira et al. reported in a small prospective study that higher IL-6 and TNF-α plasma concentrations in donors before organ procurement were associated with more postoperative complications in liver graft recipients [114]. However, data on serum or plasma cytokine concentrations are not conclusive because there are also reports that have shown no association of IL-2, IFN-γ, IL-4, and IL-10 concentrations and rejection at least in kidney transplantation [115]. To date, serum or plasma cytokines have not been used to tailor immunosuppression under clinical conditions, and prospective outcome studies are lacking. This is understandable because circulating cytokine concentrations can be influenced by many factors in vivo and cannot be specifically traced to T-cell activation.

However, a very elegant and much more specific way to follow T-cell activation is the cytokine release measured by the ELISPOT technique, in which cells are incubated on top of a membrane that is coated with a primary antibody for the cytokine of interest. The ELISPOT plates are then incubated for 18–24h with antigens such as peptides, proteins, or whole APC, which allows responding cells to recognize their specific antigens and to release their cytokines. The cytokine of interest is then directly bound in close vicinity to its source of secretion. The captured cytokine is detected by an enzyme-linked second antibody, which recognizes an epitope on the cytokine distinct from that recognized by the primary antibody. Spots at the site of the cytokine secretion are then stained with a chromogenic substrate for the antibody-linked enzyme. Each spot corresponds to a single cell, and the readout is the number of secreting cells per number of cells plated. Naive T cells do not produce interferon within the 18- to 24-h time period, and therefore it can be assumed that IFN-γ ELISPOT assay is measuring activation of either cytotoxic or memory T cells. With proteins or peptides as stimulators, the assay represents the effects of indirect antigen presentation due to APC contained within the population of plated peripheral PBMNL. In contrast, the use of donor cells reflects direct antigen presentation. The method has been extensively used to assess IFN-γ release by T cells, but it can also be applied to B cells and other cytokines. It has recently also been employed to follow donor-specific IgG secretion by B cells [116]. The ELISPOT technique can be standardized, which is facilitated by the development of image analysis hardware and software. Consortia both in Europe (Reprogramming the Immune System for Establishment of Tolerance (RISET)) and in the United States (Clinical Trials in Organ Transplantation (CTOT)) have implemented a rigorous approach to validate this assay, enabling its highly standardized use in multiple laboratories [117–119]. Recently, an external proficiency testing scheme was developed to fulfill the requirements of the good clinical laboratory practice guidelines for laboratories performing endpoint IFN-γ ELISPOT assay for clinical trials [117].

The IFN-γ ELISPOT has been shown to be useful for both pre-transplant immune risk assessment and post-transplant monitoring [120,121]. It has been demonstrated that pre-transplant donor-specific IFN-γ ELISPOT testing was predictive of acute immunologic damage after transplantation. Conversely, low or negative IFN-γ ELISPOT testing prior to transplantation appeared to be a particularly good indicator of low immunological risk. A retrospective study with 130 kidney transplant recipients suggested that antibody induction therapy was particularly beneficial for transplant candidates with strong pre-transplant donor-reactive cellular immunity, and pre-transplant ELISPOT assessments could permit individualized use of induction therapy [122]. After kidney transplantation, the IFN-γ ELISPOT assay was predictive of poor long-term graft function in a cohort of 55 primary kidney transplant recipients because it correlated significantly with the serum creatinine concentration at both 6 and 12 months following transplantation [121]. Bestard et al. reported a prospective study with 120 de novo renal transplant patients in which the use of a donor-specific INF-γ ELISPOT assay before and after kidney transplantation allowed decisions on both CNI-free or CNI-based initial therapy after transplantation and on therapy optimization including mycophenolate or corticosteroid weaning as well as CNI minimization at 6–12 months thereafter [123]. Kim et al. observed that donor-specific IFN-γ spots correlated highly with rejection in living donor kidney graft recipients using third-party cells as stimulators, suggesting that some patients were already broadly sensitized against HLA antigens [124]. Paralleling the concept of PRAs, the detection of IFN-γ spots against a panel of stimulators has been referred to as a "panel of reactive T cells" or "PRT" [103]. Although the ELISPOT assay is very much advanced to monitor T-cell activation in solid organ transplantation, a drawback for the introduction of this technique in the clinic remains its complexity, labor and time intensity, as well as high costs.

10.3.4.3 Gene expression studies to asses T-cell activation

T-cell activation is accompanied by upregulation of genes such as those coding for cell division, cytokines, adhesion molecules, or cytotoxic peptides. These genes can be followed individually by qPCR. In addition, gene signatures have been described using DNA microarrays. Many publications are available on gene expression in tissue samples; however, the current summary focuses on studies performed with blood or urine samples and does not consider reports with organ biopsies. As a proof of principle, it has been shown that immunosuppressive drugs can inhibit gene expression in vitro in mitogen-stimulated PBMNL from healthy blood donors. Briggs et al. observed that CsA was more suppressive on IL-2 mRNA expression than glucocorticoids, with a variable effect in cells from different donors [125]. By using a cDNA microarray, it was demonstrated that gene expression profiles clustered in drug-specific groups in a model of PBMNL stimulated in the presence of CsA, tacrolimus, MPA, everolimus, and sirolimus or drug combinations [126]. Kern et al. showed that mRNA expression of IL-1β, IL-2, IL-4, IL-8, IL-10, TNF-α, and IFN-γ was upregulated in PBMNL and T-cell subsets of kidney transplant recipients with CMV infection compared to healthy controls and patients with rejection but without CMV infection [127]. This finding addresses a general dilemma with lymphocyte activation markers because most assays cannot distinguish between cell activation due to alloantigens and that due to other causes such as infection. The authors have achieved some separation by examining T-cell subsets and mRNA expression of the toxic molecule granzyme A. The nonspecific pharmacodynamic effect of sirolimus has been followed in vitro in healthy individuals and ex vivo in three kidney transplant patients using antibody (anti-CD3/CD28)-stimulated whole blood samples and monitoring cytokine mRNA expression by qPCR. It was reported that IL-2 and IL-4 mRNA was reduced by sirolimus both in vitro and ex vivo; however, there was remarkable interindividual variation at the same sirolimus concentrations [128]. An ex vivo cell function assay for pharmacodynamic monitoring of calcineurin inhibitors is based on the assessment genes expressed under the control of nuclear factor of activated T lymphocytes (NFAT) in mitogen-stimulated peripheral blood by qPCR [129].

The association between acute rejection and expression of perforin, granzyme B, or Fas ligand (FasL) in nonstimulated PBMNL has been investigated in transplant patients by several authors. In kidney transplantation, the mRNA upregulation of two or more of these molecules correlated with acute rejection [130,131]. The cytotoxic T-cell genes granzyme B and perforin, as well as HLA-DRA, were elevated in PBMNL isolated from patients with allograft rejection compared to cases without rejection as assessed by qPCR [132]. The authors point to the favorable TAT because mRNA was extracted from isolated PBMNL without in vitro stimulation. In another investigation, it was shown that perforin, granzyme B, and FasL gene expressions were significantly associated with acute rejection in kidney transplant recipients in biopsies, PBMNL, and urinary cells. The diagnosis of acute rejection was also possible in patients with delayed graft function [133]. Interestingly, serial monitoring of perforin and granzyme B expression in whole blood was able to predict acute kidney graft rejection approximately 1 week in advance [134,135]; however, this finding was not confirmed in another study [136]. Gene expression profiling in PBMNL of renal transplant recipients has been performed by Flechner et al. [137]. The authors identified a gene expression profile in acute rejection that was different from that of patients without rejection and from healthy volunteers. Genes could be clustered into those involved in cell growth regulation, inflammation, signaling, protein synthesis, and transcription factors. However, when these expression profiles were compared to the gene expression pattern in kidney biopsies, they had very little in common. A recent report from the same group showed that peripheral blood gene expression profiling can be used as a minimally invasive tool to accurately reveal acute kidney transplant rejection, particularly against the background of confounding diagnoses such as acute dysfunction with no rejection [138]. The activation marker tribbles 1 (TRIB1) was found to be significantly upregulated in PBMNL of kidney patients with deteriorating graft function and antibody-mediated rejection [139]. In heart transplantation, 39 genes were followed in PBMNL using qPCR, and 8 were significantly different between rejecting and non-rejecting patients [140]. A large multicenter gene expression profiling study, the Cardiac Allograft Rejection Gene Expression Observation (CARGO) study, revealed 20 gene classifiers discriminating rejection from non-rejection in which the T-cell activation marker PDCD1 is included [141]. Longitudinal observation of this profile showed an association between baseline expression and rejection as well as an effect of anti-rejection therapy [142]. This gene expression pattern is commercially available from a reference laboratory (CareDx, Brisbane, CA) under the name AlloMap, and it received FDA clearance in 2008. Recently, Sarwal and Sigdel reported a set of 10 genes in blood to identify kidney and heart recipients at high risk for graft dysfunction that preceded biopsy-proven rejection [143].

In kidney transplantation, urine represents an alternative matrix for noninvasive monitoring of T-cell activation of the graft. mRNA expression profiling for gene-encoding T-cell activation (perforin and granzyme B), inflammation, cytokines, chemokines, and their receptors could be linked to organ rejection [144–148]. The CTOT consortium has launched an initiative to standardize gene expression profiling in blood and urine [149]. Genes investigated and methods used to follow gene expression are summarized in Table 10.5.

10.3.5 ASSAY PERFORMANCE

A general problem of all markers used to assess lymphocyte activation and proliferation is that the analytical performance of the assays is sometimes not firmly established, and intralaboratory and interlaboratory reproducibility has frequently not been investigated. Furthermore, many reports are single-center experiences with

Table 10.5 Genes and Methods Used to Asses T-Cell Activation in Blood and Urine

Principle	Genes	Method
Gene expression in blood leukocytes (pharmacodynamic cell function assay for CNI)	NFAT regulated genes (IL-2, IFN-γ, GCMSF)	qPCR
Single genes in blood leukocytes	e.g. Perforin, granzyme B, FasL, PCNA	qPCR
Gene expression profiling in blood leukocytes	e.g. TRIB1, PDCD1	Array
Single genes in urine cells	e.g. Perforin, granzyme B, IL-8, CXL19, CXCL10	qPCR

a limited number of patients and events. Standardization and cross-validation of assay protocols in different laboratories are frequently lacking. This precludes comparability and repeatability of results. This is partly due to the critical pre-analytical steps for cell function assays, which hamper sample distribution between laboratories. However, efforts for standardization have increased in recent years. Three lymphocyte activation monitoring assays have received FDA clearance, all of which are performed in a central laboratory. These are the AlloMap gene expression panel to predict rejection in heart transplantation, the ImmuKnow assay to monitor iATP (Viracor-IBT Laboratories), and the Pleximmune assay offered by Plexison to predict rejection in children with liver or small bowel transplantation. Standardization efforts have been launched, particularly by the CTOT consortium, for the promising ELISPOT assay to assess IFN-γ release from memory T cells and gene expression profiling [119,149]. Simultaneously in Europe, the RISET consortium has also started efforts to standardize ELISPOT results [118]. For the assessment of T-cell surface markers by flow cytometry, the ONE study consortium has published standardized protocols for whole blood [79]. The authors report that staining samples must be performed within 4 h after blood collection for reliable results. Efforts have been undertaken to stabilize whole blood to enable extended storage at room temperature before cytometry or to freeze samples after staining. Commercial products such as Cyto-Chex BCT blood collection tubes (Streck, Omaha, NE) enable storage of whole blood up to 7 days for some surface markers. However, the T-cell antigens CD25 and HLA-DR seem to be stable for only 72 and 48 h, respectively [17]. For lymphocyte proliferation assays, blood samples should not be stored beyond 24 h at room temperature [20]. For gene expression studies, pre-analytical storage is also important. Stabilization can be achieved by using the PAXgene system (PreAnalytiX GmbH, Hombrechtikon, Switzerland) [150]. Furthermore, gene expression arrays are expensive, and results are complex and require biostatistical expertise to be interpreted properly. Compared to qPCR, they are less sensitive to detect small changes in gene expression due to background noise and a limited dynamic range. Cross-validation in separate laboratories is usually lacking.

Using standardized assay protocols, intra- and interassay variability can be reduced to coefficients of variation (CVs) between 10% and 20% for IFN-γ using the ELISPOT [151], flow cytometry of intracellular cytokines, and surface markers [17,79]. For the Pleximmune assay, a prespecified threshold for the CVs was set to less than 20%. For other assays to follow T-cell activation, such as the iATP determination in CD4 cells, CVs less than 25% are also achievable with fresh samples according to the manufacturer. sCD30 can be determined by a commercially available ELISA sold by different vendors, and according to the assay's manual, the intra-assay and inter-assay CVs are 9.2% and 12.9%, respectively. The Luminex version of the sCD30 assay is more precise, with intra-assay and inter-assay CVs of 7% and 8%, respectively [82].

Another issue is the diagnostic sensitivity and specificity of T-cell activation or lymphocyte proliferation assays. In clinical investigations, most T-cell activation and lymphocyte proliferation assays have a high diagnostic specificity and negative predictive values, but the diagnostic sensitivity and the resulting positive predictive values for rejection are commonly compromised by the fact that T-cell activation is not exclusively triggered by transplant rejection and by the low number of clinical events in most single-center studies. Therefore, although a statistically significant association between organ rejection and T-cell activation is frequently noted, a diagnostic cutoff to distinguish rejection from other immune-activating events is difficult and requires large prospective clinical trials.

10.4 CONCLUSIONS

Noninvasive monitoring of immune activation using T-cell activation markers is intriguing because T-cell activation is a key event after organ transplantation and immunosuppressive regimens are aimed at inhibiting recipients' T cells from attacking the donor organ. This pharmacological breakthrough has definitively contributed to making transplantation a standard therapy for irreversible loss of organ function. Many approaches have been pursued to use T-cell activation monitoring as a complementary tool to TDM for adjusting the immunosuppressive therapy to the individual needs. However, to date, only very few approaches have made it into multicenter clinical trials, and none has yet been established in clinical routine monitoring of transplant patients. One drawback is the use of time-consuming cell function assays, which sometimes require cell isolation and always require incubation and stimulation steps. An unresolved issue is the decision of which stimulus is most suitable. Is a donor-specific approach more advantageous than a nonspecific stimulation with mitogens, antigens, or third-party cells? Both approaches have advantages as well as disadvantages. In the first case, the individual response against a certain antigen is monitored, but the general effect of immunosuppressants on the immune system may be missed. Nonspecific stimulation allows comparisons of the interindividual sensitivity of various subjects to various immunosuppressants and to assess the individual immune activation status before transplantation. However, this approach may miss patients with donor-specific hyporesponsiveness, which is a sign of graft tolerance [16]. A common observation irrespective of the readout of such cell function approaches is that the currently used immunosuppressant drugs are all able to show their effect on T-cell activation. Many in vitro experiments have reported an interindividual variation in the inhibitory effect of comparable drug concentrations. This supports the notion that drug concentrations within the therapeutic range are not necessarily tailored to the individual transplant patient. This is supported by the observation that ex vivo cell function assays with cells or blood from immunosuppressed organ recipients also show interindividual variation. However, an open issue is whether it is better to isolate cells or stimulate lymphocytes in whole blood. The latter approach has the advantage that immunosuppressive drugs and certain cell populations are not lost during the cell isolation step.

In summary, the discussed biomarkers are potential complementary tools in addition to TDM. Such biomarkers may be useful to identify patients who are candidates for a minimization of immunosuppressive therapy, may identify patients at risk for acute rejection or infection, and may be useful to manage the timing and rate of immunosuppressant weaning. Serial longitudinal immune monitoring may allow maintenance of an individualized immunosuppressive regimen. Progress has been made in assay standardization, which will lead to more comparable reports from international multicenter trials that are eagerly awaited.

REFERENCES

[1] Asgari E, Farrar CA, Sacks SH. Control of innate immunological mechanisms as a route to drug minimization. Curr Opin Organ Transplant 2014;19:342–7.
[2] Moreau A, Varey E, Anegon I, Cuturi M. Effector mechanisms of rejection. Cold Spring Harb Perspect Med 2013;3.
[3] Hirahara K, Poholek A, Vahedi G, Laurence A, et al. Mechanisms underlying helper T-cell plasticity: implications for immune-mediated disease. J Allergy Clin Immunol 2013;131:1276–87.
[4] Barrett AJ, Rezvani K, Solomon S, Dickinson AM, et al. New developments in allotransplant immunology. Hematology Am Soc Hematol Educ Program 2003:350–7.
[5] Bharat A, Mohanakumar T. Allopeptides and the alloimmune response. Cell Immunol 2007;248:31–43.
[6] Otterbein LE, Fan Z, Koulmanda M, Thronley T, et al. Innate immunity for better or worse govern the allograft response. Curr Opin Organ Transplant 2015;20:8–12.
[7] Nankivell BJ, Alexander SI. Rejection of the kidney allograft. N Engl J Med 2010;363:1451–62.
[8] Li XC, Kloc M, Ghobrial RM. Memory T cells in transplantation—progress and challenges. Curr Opin Organ Transplant 2013;18:387–92.
[9] Lechler RI, Lombardi G, Batchelor JR, Reinsmoen N, et al. The molecular basis of alloreactivity. Immunol Today 1990;11:83–8.
[10] Bestard O, Nickel P, Cruzado JM, Schoenemann C, et al. Circulating alloreactive T cells correlate with graft function in longstanding renal transplant recipients. J Am Soc Nephrol 2008;19:1419–29.

[11] Caballero A, Fernandez N, Lavado R, Bravo MJ, et al. Tolerogenic response: allorecognition pathways. Transpl Immunol 2006;17:3–6.

[12] Geneugelijk K, Thus KA, Spierings E. Predicting alloreactivity in transplantation. J Immunol Res 2014;2014:159479.

[13] Curtsinger JM, Mescher MF. Inflammatory cytokines as a third signal for T cell activation. Curr Opin Immunol 2010;22:333–40.

[14] Romagnani P, Crescioli C. CXCL10: a candidate biomarker in transplantation. Clin Chim Acta 2012;413:1364–73.

[15] Halloran PF. Immunosuppressive drugs for kidney transplantation. N Engl J Med 2004;351:2715–29.

[16] Babel N, Reinke P, Volk H. Lymphocyte markers and prediction of long-term renal allograft acceptance. Curr Opin Nephrol Hypertens 2009;18:489–94.

[17] Böhler T, Nolting J, Kamar N, Gurragchaa P, et al. Validation of immunological biomarkers for the pharmacodynamic monitoring of immunosuppressive drugs in humans. Ther Drug Monit 2007;29:77–86.

[18] Ashokkumar C, Talukdar A, Sun Q, Higgs BW, et al. Allospecific CD154+ T cells associate with rejection risk after pediatric liver transplantation. Am J Transplant 2009;9:179–91.

[19] Stegmann S, Muller A, Zavazava N. Synthetic HLA-A2 derived peptides are recognized and presented in renal graft recipients. Hum Immunol 2000;61:1363–9.

[20] Dambrin C, Klupp J, Morris RE. Pharmacodynamics of immunosuppressive drugs. Curr Opin Immunol 2000;12:557–62.

[21] Barten MJ, Gummert JF, van Gelder T, Shorthouse R, et al. Flow cytometric quantitation of calcium-dependent and -independent mitogen-stimulation of T cell functions in whole blood: inhibition by immunosuppressive drugs *in vitro*. J Immunol Methods 2001;253:95–112.

[22] McElroy WD, DeLuca MA. Firefly and bacterial luminescence: basic science and applications. J Appl Biochem 1983;5:197–209.

[23] Wu J, Palladino MA, Figari IS, Morris RE. Comparative immunoregulatory effects of rapamycin, FK 506 and cyclosporine on mitogen-induced cytokine production and lymphoproliferation. Transplant Proc 1991;23:238–40.

[24] Shipkova M, Wieland E, Schütz E, Wiese C, et al. The acyl glucuronide metabolite of mycophenolic acid inhibits the proliferation of human mononuclear leukocytes. Transplant Proc 2001;33:1080–1.

[25] Böhler T, Waiser J, Budde K, Lichter S, et al. The in vivo effect of rapamycin derivative SDZ RAD on lymphocyte proliferation. Transplant Proc 1998;30:2195–7.

[26] Lyons AB, Parish CR. Determination of lymphocyte division by flow cytometry. J Immunol Methods 1994;171:131–7.

[27] Barten MJ, Tarnok A, Garbade J, Bittner HB, et al. Pharmacodynamics of T-cell function for monitoring immunosuppression. Cell Prolif 2007;40:50–63.

[28] Niwa M, Miwa Y, Kuzuya T, Iwasaki K, et al. Stimulation index for PCNA mRNA in peripheral blood as immune function monitoring after renal transplantation. Transplantation 2009;87:1411–4.

[29] Barten MJ, Dhein S, Chang H, Bittner HB, et al. Assessment of immunosuppressive drug interactions: inhibition of lymphocyte function in peripheral human blood. J Immunol Methods 2003;283:99–114.

[30] Premaud A, Rousseau A, Johnson G, Canivet C, et al. Inhibition of T-cell activation and proliferation by mycophenolic acid in patients awaiting liver transplantation: PK/PD relationships. Pharmacol Res 2011;63:432–8.

[31] Böhler T, Canivet C, Galvani S, Therville N, et al. Pharmacodynamic monitoring of the conversion from mycophenolate mofetil to enteric-coated mycophenolate sodium in stable kidney-allograft recipients. Int Immunopharmacol 2008;8:769–73.

[32] Böhler T, Waiser J, Lichter S, Schumann B, et al. Pharmacodynamic effects of everolimus on anti-CD3 antibody-stimulated T-lymphocyte proliferation and interleukin-10 synthesis in stable kidney-transplant patients. Cytokine 2008;42:306–11.

[33] Sakai H, Ishiyama K, Tanaka Y, Ide K, et al. Potential benefit of mixed lymphocyte reaction assay-based immune monitoring after living donor liver transplantation for recipients with autoimmune hepatitis. Transplant Proc 2014;46:785–9.

[34] Khanna AK. Mechanism of the combination immunosuppressive effects of rapamycin with either cyclosporine or tacrolimus. Transplantation 2000;70:690–4.

[35] Fernandez LA, Tsuchida M, Manthei E, Fechner JH, et al. Immune status assay (ISA): a noninvasive procedure for studying allograft rejection. Transpl Immunol 2004;13:147–54.

[36] Wieland E, Shipkova M, Martius Y, Hasche G, et al. Association between pharmacodynamic biomarkers and clinical events in the early phase after kidney transplantation: a single-center pilot study. Ther Drug Monit 2011;33:341–9.

[37] Millán O, Benitez C, Guillen D, Lopez A, et al. Biomarkers of immunoregulatory status in stable liver transplant recipients undergoing weaning of immunosuppressive therapy. Clin Immunol 2010;137:337–46.

[38] Kowalski RJ, Post DR, Mannon RB, Sebastian A, et al. Assessing relative risks of infection and rejection: a meta-analysis using an immune function assay. Transplantation 2006;82:663–8.

[39] Israeli M, Yussim A, Mor E, Sredni B, et al. Preceding the rejection: in search for a comprehensive post-transplant immune monitoring platform. Transpl Immunol 2007;18:7–12.

[40] Israeli M, Ben-Gal T, Yaari V, Valdman A, et al. Individualized immune monitoring of cardiac transplant recipients by noninvasive longitudinal cellular immunity tests. Transplantation 2010;89:968–76.

[41] Cabrera R, Ararat M, Soldevila-Pico C, Dixon L, et al. Using an immune functional assay to differentiate acute cellular rejection from recurrent hepatitis C in liver transplant patients. Liver Transpl 2009;15:216–22.

[42] Schulz-Juergensen S, Burdelski MM, Oellerich M, Brandhorst G. Intracellular ATP production in CD4+ T cells as a predictor for infection and allograft rejection in trough-level guided pediatric liver transplant recipients under calcineurin-inhibitor therapy. Ther Drug Monit 2012;34:4–10.

[43] Millán O, Sanchez-Fueyo A, Rimola A, Guillen D, et al. Is the intracellular ATP concentration of CD4+ T-cells a predictive biomarker of immune status in stable transplant recipients? Transplantation 2009;88:S78–84.

[44] Israeli M, Klein T, Brandhorst G, Oellerich M. Confronting the challenge: individualized immune monitoring after organ transplantation using the cellular immune function assay. Clin Chim Acta 2012;413:1374–8.

[45] Sanchez-Velasco P, Rodrigo E, Valero R, Ruiz JC, et al. Intracellular ATP concentrations of CD4 cells in kidney transplant patients with and without infection. Clin Transplant 2008;22:55–60.

[46] Kobashigawa JA, Kiyosaki KK, Patel JK, Kittleson MM, et al. Benefit of immune monitoring in heart transplant patients using ATP production in activated lymphocytes. J Heart Lung Transplant 2010;29:504–8.

[47] Vittoraki AG, Boletis JN, Darema MN, Kostakis AJ, et al. Adenosine triphosphate production by peripheral blood CD4(+)T cells in clinically stable renal transplant recipients. Transplant Proc 2014;46:108–14.

[48] Berglund D, Bengtsson M, Biglarnia A, Berglund E, et al. Screening of mortality in transplant patients using an assay for immune function. Transpl Immunol 2011;24:246–50.

[49] Ling X, Xiong J, Liang W, Schroder PM, et al. Can immune cell function assay identify patients at risk of infection or rejection? A meta-analysis. Transplantation 2012;93:737–43.

[50] He J, Li Y, Zhang H, Wei X, et al. Immune function assay (ImmuKnow) as a predictor of allograft rejection and infection in kidney transplantation. Clin Transplant 2013;27:E351–8.

[51] Martinez-Flores JA, Serrano M, Morales P, Paz-Artal E, et al. Comparison of several functional methods to evaluate the immune response on stable kidney transplant patients. J Immunol Methods 2014;403:62–5.

[52] Mizuno S, Muraki Y, Nakatani K, Tanemura A, et al. Immunological aspects in late phase of living donor liver transplant patients: usefulness of monitoring peripheral blood CD4+ adenosine triphosphate activity. Clin Dev Immunol 2013;2013:982163.

[53] Wozniak LJ, Venick RS, Gordon Burroughs S, Ngo KD, et al. Utility of an immune cell function assay to differentiate rejection from infectious enteritis in pediatric intestinal transplant recipients. Clin Transplant 2014;28:229–35.

[54] Shipkova M, Wieland E. Surface markers of lymphocyte activation and markers of cell proliferation. Clin Chim Acta 2012;413:1338–49.

[55] Schlegel PG. The role of adhesion and costimulation molecules in graft-versus-host disease. Acta Haematol 1997;97:105–17.

[56] Testi R, Phillips JH, Lanier LL. T cell activation via Leu-23 (CD69). J Immunol 1989;143:1123–8.

[57] Hintzen RQ, Lens SM, Lammers K, Kuiper H, et al. Engagement of CD27 with its ligand CD70 provides a second signal for T cell activation. J Immunol 1995;154:2612–23.

[58] Schuurman HJ, van Wichen D, de Weger RA. Expression of activation antigens on thymocytes in the 'common thymocyte' stage of differentiation. Thymus 1989;14:43–53.

[59] Miyawaki T, Uehara T, Nibu R, Tsuji T, et al. Differential expression of apoptosis-related Fas antigen on lymphocyte subpopulations in human peripheral blood. J Immunol 1992;149:3753–8.

[60] Li XC, Rothstein DM, Sayegh MH. Costimulatory pathways in transplantation: challenges and new developments. Immunol Rev 2009;229:271–93.

[61] Ohnuma K, Takahashi N, Yamochi T, Hosono O, et al. Role of CD26/dipeptidyl peptidase IV in human T cell activation and function. Front Biosci 2008;13:2299–310.

[62] Ohnuma K, Dang NH, Morimoto C. Revisiting an old acquaintance: CD26 and its molecular mechanisms in T cell function. Trends Immunol 2008;29:295–301.

[63] Heemann UW, Tullius SG, Azuma H, Kupiec-Weglinsky J, et al. Adhesion molecules and transplantation. Ann Surg 1994;219:4–12.

[64] Tan J, Zhou G. Chemokine receptors and transplantation. Cell Mol Immunol 2005;2:343–9.

[65] Sallusto F, Baggiolini M. Chemokines and leukocyte traffic. Nat Immunol 2008;9:949–52.

[66] Holling TM, Schooten E, van Den Elsen PJ. Function and regulation of MHC class II molecules in T-lymphocytes: of mice and men. Hum Immunol 2004;65:282–90.

[67] Stalder M, Birsan T, Holm B, Haririfar M, et al. Quantification of immunosuppression by flow cytometry in stable renal transplant recipients. Ther Drug Monit 2003;25:22–7.

[68] Weimer R, Melk A, Daniel V, Friemann S, et al. Switch from cyclosporine A to tacrolimus in renal transplant recipients: impact on Th1, Th2, and monokine responses. Hum Immunol 2000;61:884–97.

[69] Kamar N, Glander P, Nolting J, Bohler T, et al. Pharmacodynamic evaluation of the first dose of mycophenolate mofetil before kidney transplantation. Clin J Am Soc Nephrol 2009;4:936–42.

[70] Beik AI, Morris AG, Higgins RM, Lam FT. Serial flow cytometric analysis of T-cell surface markers can be useful in differential diagnosis of renal allograft dysfunction. Clin Transplant 1998;12:24–9.

[71] Deng MC, Erren M, Roeder N, Dreimann V, et al. T-cell and monocyte subsets, inflammatory molecules, rejection, and hemodynamics early after cardiac transplantation. Transplantation 1998;65:1255–61.

[72] Lun A, Cho MY, Muller C, Staffa G, et al. Diagnostic value of peripheral blood T-cell activation and soluble IL-2 receptor for acute rejection in liver transplantation. Clin Chim Acta 2002;320:69–78.

[73] Sindhi R, Ashokkumar C, Higgs BW, Gilbert PB, et al. Allospecific CD154 + T-cytotoxic memory cells as potential surrogate for rejection risk in pediatric intestine transplantation. Pediatr Transplant 2012;16:83–91.

[74] Ziegler SF, Ramsdell F, Alderson MR. The activation antigen CD69. Stem Cells 1994;12:456–65.

[75] Tugulea S, Ciubotariu R, Colovai AI, Liu Z, et al. New strategies for early diagnosis of heart allograft rejection. Transplantation 1997;64:842–7.

[76] Boleslawski E, BenOthman S, Grabar S, Correia L, et al. CD25, CD28 and CD38 expression in peripheral blood lymphocytes as a tool to predict acute rejection after liver transplantation. Clin Transplant 2008;22:494–501.

[77] Boleslawski E, Othman SB, Aoudjehane L, Chouzenoux S, et al. CD28 expression by peripheral blood lymphocytes as a potential predictor of the development of *de novo* malignancies in long-term survivors after liver transplantation. Liver Transpl 2011;17:299–305.

[78] Minguela A, Miras M, Bermejo J, Sanchez-Bueno F, et al. HBV and HCV infections and acute rejection differentially modulate CD95 and CD28 expression on peripheral blood lymphocytes after liver transplantation. Hum Immunol 2006;67:884–93.

[79] Streitz M, Miloud T, Kapinsky M, Reed MR, et al. Standardization of whole blood immune phenotype monitoring for clinical trials: panels and methods from the ONE study. Transplant Res 2013;2:17.

[80] Inston N, Drayson M, Ready A, Cockwell P. Serial changes in the expression of CXCR3 and CCR5 on peripheral blood lymphocytes following human renal transplantation. Exp Clin Transplant 2007;5:638–42.

[81] Saxena A, Panigrahi A, Gupta S, Dinda AK, et al. Frequency of T cell expressing Th1 and Th2 associated chemokine receptor in patients with renal allograft dysfunction. Transplant Proc 2012;44:290–5.

[82] Pavlov I, Martins TB, Delgado JC. Development and validation of a fluorescent microsphere immunoassay for soluble CD30 testing. Clin Vaccine Immunol 2009;16:1327–31.

[83] Velasquez SY, Garcia LF, Opelz G, Alvarez CM, et al. Release of soluble CD30 after allogeneic stimulation is mediated by memory T cells and regulated by IFN-gamma and IL-2. Transplantation 2013;96:154–61.

[84] Eichenauer DA, Simhadri VL, von Strandmann EP, Ludwig A, et al. ADAM10 inhibition of human CD30 shedding increases specificity of targeted immunotherapy in vitro. Cancer Res 2007;67:332–8.

[85] Hansen HP, Dietrich S, Kisseleva T, Mokros T, et al. CD30 shedding from Karpas 299 lymphoma cells is mediated by TNF-alpha-converting enzyme. J Immunol 2000;165:6703–9.

[86] Tarkowski M. Expression and a role of CD30 in regulation of T-cell activity. Curr Opin Hematol 2003;10:267–71.

[87] Süsal C, Pelzl S, Dohler B, Opelz G. Identification of highly responsive kidney transplant recipients using pretransplant soluble CD30. J Am Soc Nephrol 2002;13:1650–6.

[88] Süsal C, Pelzl S, Opelz G. Strong human leukocyte antigen matching effect in non-sensitized kidney recipients with high pretransplant soluble CD30. Transplantation 2003;76:1231–2.

[89] Chen Y, Tai Q, Hong S, Kong Y, et al. Pretransplantation soluble CD30 level as a predictor of acute rejection in kidney transplantation: a meta-analysis. Transplantation 2012;94:911–8.

[90] Altermann W, Schlaf G, Rothhoff A, Seliger B. High variation of individual soluble serum CD30 levels of pre-transplantation patients: sCD30 a feasible marker for prediction of kidney allograft rejection? Nephrol Dial Transplant 2007;22:2795–9.

[91] Pelzl S, Opelz G, Daniel V, Wiesel M, et al. Evaluation of posttransplantation soluble CD30 for diagnosis of acute renal allograft rejection. Transplantation 2003;75:421–3.

[92] Süsal C, Dohler B, Sadeghi M, Salmela KT, et al. Posttransplant sCD30 as a predictor of kidney graft outcome. Transplantation 2011;91:1364–9.

[93] Sengul S, Keven K, Gormez U, Kutlay S, et al. Identification of patients at risk of acute rejection by pretransplantation and posttransplantation monitoring of soluble CD30 levels in kidney transplantation. Transplantation 2006;81:1216–9.

[94] Nikaein A, Spiridon C, Hunt J, Rosenthal J, et al. Pre-transplant level of soluble CD30 is associated with infection after heart transplantation. Clin Transplant 2007;21:744–7.

[95] Shah AS, Leffell MS, Lucas D, Zachary AA. Elevated pretransplantation soluble CD30 is associated with decreased early allograft function after human lung transplantation. Hum Immunol 2009;70:101–3.

[96] Ypsilantis E, Key T, Bradley JA, Morgan CH, et al. Soluble CD30 levels in recipients undergoing heart transplantation do not predict post-transplant outcome. J Heart Lung Transplant 2009;28:1206–10.

[97] Hire K, Hering B, Bansal-Pakala P. Relative reductions in soluble CD30 levels post-transplant predict acute graft function in islet allograft recipients receiving three different immunosuppression protocols. Transpl Immunol 2010;23:209–14.

[98] Kim KH, Oh E, Jung E, Park Y, et al. Evaluation of pre- and posttransplantation serum interferon-gamma and soluble CD30 for predicting liver allograft rejection. Transplant Proc 2006;38:1429–31.

[99] Vondran FW, Timrott K, Kollrich S, Steinhoff AK, et al. Pre-transplant immune state defined by serum markers and alloreactivity predicts acute rejection after living donor kidney transplantation. Clin Transplant 2014;28:968–79.

[100] Zhu J, Paul WE. CD4 T cells: fates, functions, and faults. Blood 2008;112:1557–69.

[101] Zhang N, Bevan MJ. CD8(+) T cells: foot soldiers of the immune system. Immunity 2011;35:161–8.

[102] Brunet M. Cytokines as predictive biomarkers of alloreactivity. Clin Chim Acta 2012;413:1354–8.

[103] Augustine JJ, Hricik DE. T-cell immune monitoring by the ELISPOT assay for interferon gamma. Clin Chim Acta 2012;413:1359–63.

[104] Sakuma S, Kato Y, Nishigaki F, Sasakawa T, et al. FK506 potently inhibits T cell activation induced TNF-alpha and IL-1beta production in vitro by human peripheral blood mononuclear cells. Br J Pharmacol 2000;130:1655–63.

[105] Millán O, Rafael-Valdivia L, Torrademe E, Lopez A, et al. Intracellular IFN-gamma and IL-2 expression monitoring as surrogate markers of the risk of acute rejection and personal drug response in *de novo* liver transplant recipients. Cytokine 2013;61:556–64.

[106] Millán O, Rafael-Valdivia L, San Segundo D, Boix F, et al. Should IFN-gamma, IL-17 and IL-2 be considered predictive biomarkers of acute rejection in liver and kidney transplant? Results of a multicentric study. Clin Immunol 2014;154:141–54.

[107] Akoglu B, Lafferton B, Kalb S, Yosuf SE, et al. Rejection quantity in kidney transplant recipients is associated with increasing intracellular interleukin-2 in CD8+ T-cells. Transpl Immunol 2014;31:17–21.

[108] Ahmed M, Venkataraman R, Logar AJ, Rao AS, et al. Quantitation of immunosuppression by tacrolimus using flow cytometric analysis of interleukin-2 and interferon-gamma inhibition in CD8(−) and CD8(+) peripheral blood T cells. Ther Drug Monit 2001;23:354–62.

[109] Boleslawski E, Conti F, Sanquer S, Podevin P, et al. Defective inhibition of peripheral CD8+ T cell IL-2 production by anti-calcineurin drugs during acute liver allograft rejection. Transplantation 2004;77:1815–20.

[110] van Besouw NM, de Kuiper R, van der Mast BJ, van de Wetering J, et al. Deficient TNF-alpha and IFN-gamma production correlates with nondetectable donor-specific cytotoxicity after clinical kidney transplantation. Transplantation 2009;87:1451–4.

[111] Millán O, Brunet M, Campistol JM, Faura A, et al. Pharmacodynamic approach to immunosuppressive therapies using calcineurin inhibitors and mycophenolate mofetil. Clin Chem 2003;49:1891–9.

[112] Ai W, Li H, Song N, Li L, et al. Optimal method to stimulate cytokine production and its use in immunotoxicity assessment. Int J Environ Res Public Health 2013;10:3834–42.

[113] Sadeghi M, Daniel V, Naujokat C, Schmidt J, et al. Evidence for IFN-gamma up- and IL-4 downregulation late post-transplant in patients with good kidney graft outcome. Clin Transplant 2007;21:449–59.

[114] Azarpira N, Nikeghbalian S, Kazemi K, Geramizadeh B, et al. Association of increased plasma interleukin-6 and TNF-alpha levels in donors with the complication rates in liver transplant recipients. Int J Organ Transplant Med 2013;4:9–14.

[115] Ghafari A, Makhdoomi K, Ahmadpour P, Afshari AT, et al. Serum T-lymphocyte cytokines cannot predict early acute rejection in renal transplantation. Transplant Proc 2007;39:958–61.

[116] Lynch RJ, Silva IA, Chen BJ, Punch JD, et al. Cryptic B cell response to renal transplantation. Am J Transplant 2013;13:1713–23.

[117] Sanchez AM, Rountree W, Berrong M, Garcia A, et al. The external quality assurance oversight laboratory (EQAPOL) proficiency program for IFN-gamma enzyme-linked immunospot (IFN-gamma ELISpot) assay. J Immunol Methods 2014;409:31–43.

[118] Bestard O, Crespo E, Stein M, Lucia M, et al. Cross-validation of IFN-gamma Elispot assay for measuring alloreactive memory/effector T cell responses in renal transplant recipients. Am J Transplant 2013;13:1880–90.

[119] Ashoor I, Najafian N, Korin Y, Reed EF, et al. Standardization and cross validation of alloreactive IFNgamma ELISPOT assays within the clinical trials in organ transplantation consortium. Am J Transplant 2013;13:1871–9.

[120] Hricik DE, Poggio ED, Woodside KJ, Sarabu N, et al. Effects of cellular sensitization and donor age on acute rejection and graft function after deceased-donor kidney transplantation. Transplantation 2013;95:1254–8.

[121] Hricik DE, Rodriguez V, Riley J, Bryan K, et al. Enzyme linked immunosorbent spot (ELISPOT) assay for interferon-gamma independently predicts renal function in kidney transplant recipients. Am J Transplant 2003;3:878–84.

[122] Augustine JJ, Poggio ED, Heeger PS, Hricik DE. Preferential benefit of antibody induction therapy in kidney recipients with high pretransplant frequencies of donor-reactive interferon-gamma enzyme-linked immunosorbent spots. Transplantation 2008;86:529–34.

[123] Bestard O, Cruzado JM, Lucia M, Crespo E, et al. Prospective assessment of antidonor cellular alloreactivity is a tool for guidance of immunosuppression in kidney transplantation. Kidney Int 2013;84:1226–36.

[124] Kim SH, Oh EJ, Kim MJ, Park YK, et al. Pretransplant donor-specific interferon-gamma ELISPOT assay predicts acute rejection episodes in renal transplant recipients. Transplant Proc 2007;39:3057–60.

[125] Briggs WA, Han SH, Miyakawa H, Burdick JF, et al. Effects of glucocorticoids and cyclosporine on IL-2 and I kappa B alpha mRNA expression in human peripheral blood mononuclear cells. J Clin Pharmacol 1999;39:119–24.

[126] Rumberger B, Kreutz C, Nickel C, Klein M, et al. Combination of immunosuppressive drugs leaves specific "fingerprint" on gene expression *in vitro*. Immunopharmacol Immunotoxicol 2009;31:283–92.

[127] Kern F, Ode-Hakim S, Nugel H, Vogt K, et al. Peripheral T cell activation in long-term renal transplant patients: concordant upregulation of adhesion molecules and cytokine gene transcription. J Am Soc Nephrol 1996;7:2476–82.

[128] Müller-Steinhardt M, Wortmeier K, Fricke L, Ebel B, et al. The pharmacodynamic effect of sirolimus: individual variation of cytokine mRNA expression profiles in human whole blood samples. Immunobiology 2009;214:17–26.

[129] Giese T, Zeier M, Meuer S. Analysis of NFAT-regulated gene expression *in vivo*: a novel perspective for optimal individualized doses of calcineurin inhibitors. Nephrol Dial Transplant 2004;19(Suppl. 4) iv55–60.

[130] Vasconcellos LM, Schachter AD, Zheng XX, Vasconcellos LH, et al. Cytotoxic lymphocyte gene expression in peripheral blood leukocytes correlates with rejecting renal allografts. Transplantation 1998;66:562–6.

[131] Dugre FJ, Gaudreau S, Belles-Isles M, Houde I, et al. Cytokine and cytotoxic molecule gene expression determined in peripheral blood mononuclear cells in the diagnosis of acute renal rejection. Transplantation 2000;70:1074–80.

[132] Sabek O, Dorak MT, Kotb M, Gaber AO, et al. Quantitative detection of T-cell activation markers by real-time PCR in renal transplant rejection and correlation with histopathologic evaluation. Transplantation 2002;74:701–7.

[133] Aquino-Dias EC, Joelsons G, da Silva DM, Berdichewski RH, et al. Non-invasive diagnosis of acute rejection in kidney transplants with delayed graft function. Kidney Int 2008;73:877–84.

[134] Simon T, Opelz G, Wiesel M, Ott RC, et al. Serial peripheral blood perforin and granzyme B gene expression measurements for prediction of acute rejection in kidney graft recipients. Am J Transplant 2003;3:1121–7.

[135] Veale JL, Liang LW, Zhang Q, Gjertson GW, et al. Noninvasive diagnosis of cellular and antibody-mediated rejection by perforin and granzyme B in renal allografts. Hum Immunol 2006;67:777–86.

[136] Shin G, Kim S, Lee T, Oh C, et al. Gene expression of perforin by peripheral blood lymphocytes as a marker of acute rejection. Nephron Clin Pract 2005;100:c63–70.

[137] Flechner SM, Kurian SM, Head SR, Sharp SM, et al. Kidney transplant rejection and tissue injury by gene profiling of biopsies and peripheral blood lymphocytes. Am J Transplant 2004;4:1475–89.

[138] Kurian SM, Williams AN, Gelbart T, Campbell D, et al. Molecular classifiers for acute kidney transplant rejection in peripheral blood by whole genome gene expression profiling. Am J Transplant 2014;14:1164–72.

[139] Ashton-Chess J, Giral M, Mengel M, Renaudin K, et al. Tribbles-1 as a novel biomarker of chronic antibody-mediated rejection. J Am Soc Nephrol 2008;19:1116–27.

[140] Schoels M, Dengler TJ, Richter R, Meuer SC, et al. Detection of cardiac allograft rejection by real-time PCR analysis of circulating mononuclear cells. Clin Transplant 2004;18:513–7.

[141] Deng MC, Eisen HJ, Mehra MR, Billingham M, et al. Noninvasive discrimination of rejection in cardiac allograft recipients using gene expression profiling. Am J Transplant 2006;6:150–60.

[142] Mehra MR, Kobashigawa JA, Deng MC, Fang KC, et al. Transcriptional signals of T-cell and corticosteroid-sensitive genes are associated with future acute cellular rejection in cardiac allografts. J Heart Lung Transplant 2007;26:1255–63.

[143] Sarwal M, Sigdel T. A common blood gene assay predates clinical and histological rejection in kidney and heart allografts. Clin Transplant 2013:241–7.

[144] Kotsch K, Mashreghi MF, Bold G, Tretow P, et al. Enhanced granulysin mRNA expression in urinary sediment in early and delayed acute renal allograft rejection. Transplantation 2004;77:1866–75.

[145] Li B, Hartono C, Ding R, Sharma VK, et al. Noninvasive diagnosis of renal-allograft rejection by measurement of messenger RNA for perforin and granzyme B in urine. N Engl J Med 2001;344:947–54.

[146] Yannaraki M, Rebibou J, Ducloux D, Saas P, et al. Urinary cytotoxic molecular markers for a noninvasive diagnosis in acute renal transplant rejection. Transpl Int 2006;19:759–68.

[147] Matz M, Beyer J, Wunsch D, Mashreghi MF, et al. Early post-transplant urinary IP-10 expression after kidney transplantation is predictive of short- and long-term graft function. Kidney Int 2006;69:1683–90.

[148] Tatapudi RR, Muthukumar T, Dadhania D, Ding R, et al. Noninvasive detection of renal allograft inflammation by measurements of mRNA for IP-10 and CXCR3 in urine. Kidney Int 2004;65:2390–7.

[149] Keslar KS, Lin M, Zmijewska AA, Sigdel TK, et al. Multicenter evaluation of a standardized protocol for noninvasive gene expression profiling. Am J Transplant 2013;13:1891–7.

[150] Chai V, Vassilakos A, Lee Y, Wright JA, et al. Optimization of the PAXgene blood RNA extraction system for gene expression analysis of clinical samples. J Clin Lab Anal 2005;19:182–8.

[151] Zhang W, Caspell R, Karulin AY, Ahmad M, et al. ELISPOT assays provide reproducible results among different laboratories for T-cell immune monitoring—even in hands of ELISPOT-inexperienced investigators. J Immunotoxicol 2009;6:227–34.

Monitoring calcineurin inhibitors response based on NFAT-regulated gene expression

11

Sara Bremer[1], Nils Tore Vethe[2], and Stein Bergan[2,3]

[1]Department of Medical Biochemistry, Oslo University Hospital, Oslo, Norway;
[2]Department of Pharmacology, Oslo University Hospital, Oslo, Norway;
[3]School of Pharmacy, University of Oslo, Oslo, Norway

11.1 INTRODUCTION

During the last 30 years, the pharmacological principle of inhibiting the calcineurin phosphatase activity in T cells has been applied to prevent rejection following solid organ transplantation. Cyclosporine A (CsA) was introduced into clinical practice in the early 1980s, followed by tacrolimus approximately 10 years later. In the capacity of being calcineurin inhibitors (CNIs), these two immunosuppressive agents primarily reduce the production of proinflammatory cytokines in activated T cells [1]. Immunosuppressive drug regimens with CsA or tacrolimus have proven to be successful in improving short-term outcome after transplantation. However, the long-term outcome is apparently negatively affected by adverse effects such as nephrotoxicity, hyperlipidemia, hypertension, neurotoxicity, infections, and malignancy. The balancing between acute rejection and adverse effects in renal transplant recipients has been most successful with drug regimens including low-dose tacrolimus, mycophenolate, and glucocorticoids [2].

The CNIs are usually administered twice daily in oral formulations. Also, a once-daily extended-release formulation of tacrolimus (Advagraf) is available in some countries. The absorption of CsA and tacrolimus is highly variable, and the drugs are substrates of cytochrome P450 (CYP) 3A and P-glycoprotein (P-gp). Thus, the pharmacokinetics of CsA and tacrolimus varies considerably between and within individuals, and monitoring of whole blood trough (C_0) levels is routinely performed to achieve drug exposure within narrow therapeutic ranges (see Chapter 1). However, acute rejection episodes and adverse effects may occur in individual patients despite apparent therapeutic exposure. Such observations indicate that CNI concentrations do not accurately predict the drug effects, and it has motivated the development

M. Oellerich & A. Dasgupta (Eds): Personalized Immunosuppression in Transplantation.
DOI: http://dx.doi.org/10.1016/B978-0-12-800885-0.00011-4

of pharmacodynamic biomarkers that reflect the molecular response of the drugs. Hereby, both the pharmacokinetic and the pharmacodynamic variability are taken into account [3]. A promising biomarker of the clinical response to CNIs is the calcineurin/nuclear factor of activated T cells (NFAT)-dependent gene expression of certain cytokines in ex vivo stimulated T cells [4]. The rationale for this monitoring strategy as well as methodological aspects and correlations to clinical outcome are discussed in detail in the following sections.

11.2 MECHANISM OF ACTION OF CNIs

The immunosuppressive effect of CNIs is primarily caused by inhibition of the calcineurin–NFAT signaling pathway in T helper cells.

11.2.1 ACTIVATION OF THE CALCINEURIN–NFAT SIGNALING IN T CELLS

Immunogenic activation of the T-cell receptor (TCR) together with the CD4 and CD28 co-receptors results in the release of intracellular calcium (Ca^{2+}) stores. Calcineurin is a calmodulin-dependent serine/threonine phosphatase comprising a catalytic A subunit and a regulatory B subunit; the latter senses intracellular Ca^{2+} levels and regulates the activation of the catalytic A subunit. The increase in cytosolic Ca^{2+} activates calcineurin, which in turn dephosphorylates the cytoplasmic NFAT. Consequently, NFAT is translocated into the nucleus, where it binds to DNA response elements and induces transcription of genes essential for T-cell activation and proliferation (Figure 11.1). This includes cytokines such as interleukin-2 (IL-2), IL-3, IL-4, IL-5, IL-13, interferon-γ (IFN-γ), tumor necrosis factor-α (TNF-α), and granulocyte–macrophage colony-stimulating factor (GM-CSF), as well as membrane-bound proteins including CD40 ligand, Fas ligand, and cytotoxic T-lymphocyte-associated antigen-4 (CTLA4) [5]. Further details of the NFAT-regulated cytokines are presented in Table 11.1.

In addition to NFAT, the transcription of the NFAT-regulated cytokines requires cooperative binding of additional transcription factors, including proteins of the inducible activator protein-1 (AP-1) family and nuclear factor κ light-chain enhancer of activated B cells (NF-κB) [5].

11.2.2 CNI EFFECTS IN IMMUNE CELLS

Despite different molecular structures, CsA and tacrolimus have similar mechanisms of action. Both drugs bind with high affinity to immunophilins. CsA binds cyclophilins and tacrolimus binds FK-506 binding protein (FKBP12), forming complexes that inhibit calcineurin. This prevents the dephosphorylation and subsequent translocation of NFAT into the nucleus, leading to reduced transcription of cytokines required for T-cell activation and proliferation (Figure 11.1). Of the downstream responses, inhibition of IL-2 is probably the best described immunosuppressive mechanism of CNIs.

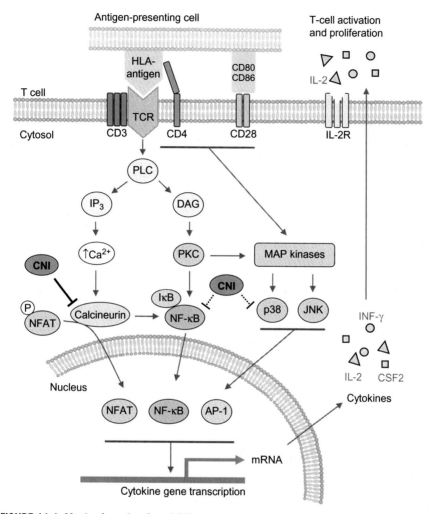

FIGURE 11.1 Mechanism of action of CNIs.

Antigen presentation to T cells results in the activation of several interacting signaling pathways essential for T-cell activation, proliferation, and differentiation. The immunosuppressive action of CNIs is mainly due to inhibition of calcineurin. This prevents the dephosphorylation of NFAT and consequently the transcription of NFAT-regulated cytokines. In addition, CNIs mediate immunosuppressive effects by calcineurin-independent inhibition of NF-κB and MAP kinase (p38 and JNK) signaling. AP-1, activator protein 1; CNIs, calcineurin inhibitors; CSF2, colony-stimulating factor 2; DAG, diacylglycerol; HLA, human leukocyte antigen; IL-2, interleukin-2; IL-2R, IL-2 receptor; INF-γ, interferon-γ; IP$_3$, inositol triphosphate; JNK, c-Jun N-terminal kinases; MAP, RAS-mitogen-activated protein; NFAT, nuclear factor of activated T cells; NF-κB, nuclear factor κ light-chain enhancer of activated B cells; PKC, protein kinase C; PLC, phospholipase C; TCR, T cell receptor.

Table 11.1 NFAT-Regulated Cytokines

Cytokine	Major Immune Cell Source	Function
GM-CSF (CSF2)	– Th1 cells – Macrophages	– Hematopoietic growth factor – Activation and differentiation of granulocytes, eosinophils, and monocytes/macrophages – Promotes Th1-biased immune responses
IFN-γ	– Th1 cells – Tc cells – NK cells	– Induction of Th1 cell responses – Activation of macrophages – Upregulation of HLA I and II expression
IL-2	– Th0 and Th1 cells – Some Tc cells	– Activation and differentiation of Th cells, Tc cells, NK cells, B cells, and monocytes/macrophages – Driver of Th1 cell responses
IL-3	– Th1 and Th2 cells	– Stimulation of hematopoietic stem cells and myeloid cell linages
IL-4	– Th2 cells	– Driver of Th2 responses – Proliferation and differentiation of B cells – Regulation of IgE- and eosinophil-mediated immune reactions
IL-5	– Th2 cells	– Growth and activation of eosinophils and B cells
IL-10	– Macrophages – Th2 cells	– Suppression of innate and Th1-mediated immune responses – Reduction of proinflammatory cytokines and effector T-cell function – Inhibition of antigen presentation – Stimulation of B cells
IL-13	– Th0, Th1, and Th2 cells – Tc cells – Mast cells – Eosinophils	– Differentiation of B cells and monocytes – Induction of IgE class switching – Downregulation of macrophage activity
IL-17	– Th 17 cells	– Induction of proinflammatory cytokines and chemokines
TNF-α	– Macrophages – Th1 cells	– Cytotoxicity – Upregulation of chemokines and adhesion molecules – Recruitment of macrophages and neutrophils – Stimulation of lymphoid cells

HLA, human leukocyte antigen; NK, natural killer; Tc, cytotoxic T cells; GM-CSF, granulocyte–macrophage colony-stimulating factor; IL, interleukin; Th0, naive T helper cells; Th1, T helper cell type 1; Th2, T helper cell type 2; Th 17, IL-17-producing T helper cells; TNF, tumor necrosis factor.

The inhibition of calcineurin also interferes with NF-κB-mediated immune responses. Calcineurin activates NF-κB indirectly by inducing the degradation of the inhibitory protein IκB. Studies have shown that both tacrolimus and CsA prevent IκB degradation by attenuating the assembly of the CBM (Carma1–Bcl10–Malt1) complex [6,7].

In addition to their potent immunosuppressive effect by inhibiting calcineurin, CNIs mediate immunosuppressive effects by interfering with other signaling pathways. Both CsA and tacrolimus suppress mitogen-activated protein kinase p38 (MAPK14) and c-Jun N-terminal kinase (JNK; MAPK8) signaling [8,9]. The inhibition is probably calcineurin independent, but the exact mechanisms are not known [8]. Signaling through p38 and JNK is induced by stimulation of the TCR–CD28 molecules and in response to cytokines. The pathways are involved in the regulation of transcription factors, including AP-1 and NF-κB, and mediate the production of cytokines essential for T-cell activation and proliferation (Figure 11.1) [9,10].

Transforming growth factor-β (TGF-β) demonstrates immunosuppressive and fibrogenic effects. Both CsA and tacrolimus have been shown to increase TGF-β expression, and this may contribute to the immunosuppressive effect, as well as the nephrotoxicity, of these drugs [11,12]. However, the results are not consistent between studies, and further investigations are needed to determine the mechanism and clinical relevance of the TGF-β induction [13].

In addition to the inhibition of T helper cells, CNIs also have direct and indirect effects on other immune cells, such as CD8$^+$ T cells, granulocytes, macrophages, monocytes, natural killer (NK) cells, and B cells [14]. Activation of B cells depends on T-cell help, and both tacrolimus and CsA are reported to inhibit B cells indirectly by reducing the expression of T-cell costimulatory ligands (CD154 and CD278) and decreasing the levels of B-cell stimulatory cytokines in T cells (Table 11.1) [15]. Furthermore, CNIs have been shown to reduce IFN-γ production and degranulation of NK cells [16] and to inhibit IgE-dependent histamine and serotonin release from basophils and mast cells [17]. In addition to the effects on adaptive immune responses, recent studies have reported that NFAT signaling plays an important role in the regulation of the innate immune system [18].

11.2.3 EFFECTS OF CNI ON NON-IMMUNE CELLS

The inhibition of the calcineurin–NFAT pathway by CNIs is not immune cell specific. Calcineurin is widely distributed in different cells and tissues, and it mediates intracellular signaling involved in the regulation of numerous homeostatic processes. The inhibitory action of CsA and tacrolimus on substrates such as IκB, Na-K-ATPase, and nitric oxide synthase (NOS) may explain some of the adverse effects observed with these drugs [1]. The suppression of inducible NOS and subsequent reduction of nitric oxide has been associated with hypertension and nephrotoxicity [19]. Furthermore, the calcineurin–NFAT pathway is involved in the regulation of cyclooxygenase-2 (COX-2). CNIs reduce COX-2 expression and consequently the levels of prostaglandin E2. This may explain some of the renal effects of CNIs, including vasoconstriction and reduced glomerular filtration rate (GFR) [20,21]. The increased intragraft TGF-β levels associated with CNI therapy may be involved in the development of allograft fibrosis [11,12]. Furthermore, MAPK inhibition decreases apoptosis in vascular cells, cardiomyocytes and fibroblasts, which in turn may contribute to cardiovascular remodeling and vasculopathy [22].

11.2.4 DIFFERENCES BETWEEN CYCLOSPORINE AND TACROLIMUS

Tacrolimus is 10–100 times more potent than CsA in inhibiting cytokines and T-cell proliferation in vitro and in vivo [23,24]. However, in vitro studies demonstrated that calcineurin was only partly inhibited by high tacrolimus concentrations ($C_0 > 20\,\mu g/L$), whereas the inhibition by CsA ($C_0 > 700\,\mu g/L$) was almost complete [24]. Tacrolimus has also been associated with less calcineurin inhibition than CsA in vivo [25,26]. Importantly, the lower degree of inhibition with tacrolimus does not appear to compromise the immunosuppressive efficacy [26]. Furthermore, tacrolimus has been reported to be more effective in inhibiting ongoing acute rejection [27,28]. This may be explained by differences in additional immunosuppressive mechanisms.

Tacrolimus and CsA have been associated with different patterns of cytokine inhibition, especially of IL-4, IL-6, and IL-10 [29]. Tacrolimus also suppresses the expression of cytokine receptors, thereby inhibiting the effect of cytokines on target cells [30]. Animal studies have shown lower levels of $CD8^+$ T cell and NK cell infiltration with tacrolimus compared to CsA [31]. At high CNI exposure, the degree of calcineurin inhibition may be limited by the concentration of immunophilins. The levels of cyclophilin and FKBP12 vary between cell types, and this might contribute to the distinct toxicity profiles of CsA and tacrolimus [32].

11.3 STRATEGIES FOR PHARMACODYNAMIC MONITORING OF CNIs

Various strategies have been investigated to monitor the pharmacodynamic response of CNIs, involving measurement of general immune status parameters or more drug-specific biomarkers. General biomarkers reflect the overall immunosuppression and include lymphocyte subset numbers and measurement of lymphocyte activation and proliferation [33]. In theory, general biomarkers might be advantageous considering immunosuppressive combination regimens. However, currently, there are only limited and conflicting data relating general biomarkers and clinical outcome after transplantation [33]. Drug-selective biomarkers of CNI response include calcineurin phosphatase activity, translocation of NFAT into the nucleus, and NFAT-regulated cytokine levels [34–36]. This chapter focuses primarily on CNI-specific markers and NFAT-regulated gene expression.

11.3.1 CALCINEURIN PHOSPHATASE ACTIVITY

The phosphatase activity of calcineurin in peripheral blood mononuclear cells (PBMCs) could be a potential biomarker of CNI immunosuppressive efficacy and toxicity. Two isoforms (α and β) of the calcineurin subunit A are expressed in lymphocytes. The Aβ isoform appears to have predominant importance for the immune function, and the level of calcineurin Aβ in complex with calmodulin in PBMC has been associated with immunosuppression and the incidence of acute rejection following renal transplantation [37]. CsA and tacrolimus inhibit the phosphatase activity of both the calcineurin Aα and Aβ isoforms [38]. In addition, the two isoforms share the substrates that are used in calcineurin activity assays in vitro. This implies that the catalytic activity and inhibition of Aα as well as Aβ will be included when such assays are applied to investigate the pharmacodynamics of CsA and tacrolimus in clinical samples.

In one 2-year longitudinal study in lung transplant recipients using CsA, the authors showed significant relationships between pre-dose calcineurin activity in PBMC and clinical outcome. The risk of acute rejection was elevated in patients with very high or low calcineurin activity, and the risks of malignancies and viral infections were increased when the calcineurin activity was below a certain threshold level [34]. In a study of liver transplant recipients on tacrolimus, significantly higher calcineurin activity was observed in patients developing rejection episodes, whereas those experiencing nephrotoxicity had decreased enzyme activity during the early postoperative period [24].

So far, the clinical benefit of adjusting CNI doses according to calcineurin activity has not been investigated. Although the calcineurin activity in PBMC may be an indicator of immune activation and CNI-mediated immunosuppression, it remains to be elucidated whether well-defined cutoff values may be established for this biomarker in distinct patient populations. It represents a direct approach to selectively quantify the CNI target activity, but it does not take into account potential variability of downstream effectors and drug effects that may be independent of calcineurin.

11.3.2 NUCLEAR TRANSLOCATION OF NFAT

The NFAT family consists of five proteins, where NFAT1, NFAT2, and NFAT4 mediate immune regulation downstream of calcineurin in T cells [39]. Maguire et al. described a rapid, quantitative, flow cytometry-based assay for the measurement of nuclear translocation of NFAT1 [35]. Following stimulation with mitogens, tacrolimus inhibited the translocation of NFAT1 in a dose-dependent manner in vitro. Furthermore, the pharmacodynamic response differed considerably between individuals [35]. Although a promising marker, there is need for further studies investigating the association between NFAT1 translocation and clinical outcome.

11.3.3 CYTOKINE RESPONSES

Measurement of NFAT-regulated cytokines is reported to represent a relatively drug-specific biomarker of CNI response downstream of calcineurin and NFAT [36]. Compared to calcineurin or NFAT measurements, the cytokine response may also include CNI effects on other signaling pathways, thereby allowing better prediction of the immunosuppressive effect. Furthermore, cytokine levels may to some degree also represent the effect of other immunosuppressive drugs, such as glucocorticoids and mycophenolate [40,41].

Several studies have quantified cytokine protein levels in plasma, whole blood, or specific cell populations using enzyme-linked immunosorbent assays, enzyme-linked immunospot assays, or flow cytometry [33]. Normally, the expression level of many NFAT-regulated cytokines is very low and often below the limit of quantification of assays. Thus, measurement of these cytokines requires ex vivo immune activation, which is usually performed by incubating the sample material with mitogens before analysis.

Different studies have demonstrated concentration-dependent inhibition of IL-2 or IFN-γ protein levels in transplanted patients following CNI exposure [42–44]. However, other studies did not observe any significant correlation between CNI concentration and inhibition of cytokines at the protein level [45–47].

Currently, there are only a limited number of reports relating cytokine protein levels during CNI therapy to clinical outcome after transplantation. Studies of liver transplant recipients have shown higher IL-2 levels in CD8$^+$ T cells among patients with acute rejection [48,49]. Furthermore, IL-2 levels were correlated with the grade of rejection [49]. Millán et al. reported that liver transplant patients with acute rejection during tacrolimus therapy had less than 40% inhibition of IL-2 and IFN-γ in CD8$^+$ T cells and that acute rejection could be predicted by IFN-γ expression levels before transplantation [50]. Another study showed that a high IFN-γ/IL-5 ratio, indicating a high proportion of Th1 versus Th2 cells, was associated with an increased risk of graft loss among renal transplant recipients [51]. Importantly, the studies did not observe any association between CNI levels and outcome, supporting the potential of cytokine measurement as an additional tool for individualizing CNI therapy [48,50].

Recently, several studies have focused on the quantification of cytokine mRNA levels. Changes in gene expression are more dynamic and precede changes at the protein levels. Furthermore, real-time polymerase chain reaction (PCR) allows fast, highly sensitive, and reproducible quantification of the gene expression of NFAT-regulated cytokines.

Zucker et al. described the first pharmacodynamic analysis of CsA response based on IL-2 (*IL2*) mRNA levels [52]. Other studies investigated the mRNA response of several cytokines. Härtel et al. demonstrated that CsA reduced the expression of the genes encoding IL-2 (*IL2*), IL-4 (*IL4*), and TNF-α (*TNF*) [53]. Later, Giese et al. reported that the strongest response to CsA was observed for the genes encoding IL-2 (*IL2*), IFN-γ (*IFNG*), and granulocyte–macrophage colony-stimulating factor (*CSF2*) [36,54]. The following section provides a detailed presentation of NFAT-regulated gene expression measurements.

11.4 MEASUREMENT OF NFAT-REGULATED GENE EXPRESSION

The procedure for measurement of NFAT-regulated gene expression involves ex vivo immune activation, RNA extraction, reverse transcription (RT), quantitative PCR (qPCR), and data analysis.

11.4.1 SPECIMEN

The pharmacodynamic response of CNIs has been investigated in isolated immune cell populations as well as in whole blood assays [52,54,55]. Halloran et al. demonstrated that the CsA-mediated inhibition of calcineurin was maintained after isolation of leukocytes [55]. In contrast, the washing steps during isolation of PBMCs reduced the inhibitory response of CNIs at the cytokine gene expression level, probably due to a washout of intracellular drug exposure [54]. Based on these observations, Giese et al. developed an immune stimulation protocol for whole blood samples [36]. Compared to procedures involving isolation of cellular subsets, direct addition of mitogens to whole blood provides a simpler and less time-consuming assay. Furthermore, this allows measurement of the pharmacodynamic effect in the in vivo environment where the response occurs and where the drug concentration is maintained.

11.4.2 SAMPLING TIME POINT

The pharmacodynamic response to CNIs is probably best reflected by repeated measurements throughout the dosing interval. However, the sampling scheme should be practical for routine monitoring, involving a minimal number of samples. The strongest suppression of cytokine expression occurs at the time of peak drug concentration, approximately 1.5 and 2 h after dosing of tacrolimus and CsA, respectively [54,56,57]. The subsequent decrease in drug concentration is followed by a rapid decline in cytokine inhibition, with a complete recovery of cytokines 6 h after CsA dosing [36]. Thus, the studies discussed in the following sections collected samples at 1.5 h post-dose for the analysis of tacrolimus responses and 2 h after dosing for investigations of CsA. In addition, samples were drawn before dosing to allow correction for differences in baseline cytokine expression levels [26,54,58].

11.4.3 EX VIVO STIMULATION WITH MITOGENS

Resting or nonactivated T cells usually show minimal or undetectable cytokine levels. Thus, measurement of NFAT-regulated cytokines requires ex vivo immune activation, which is usually performed by incubating heparinized blood or blood cell fractions with mitogens. Heparin is the generally recommended anticoagulant for T-cell assays, preserving cellular functions and viability [59].

Different immune activation strategies have been utilized to investigate cytokine gene expression in response to CNI exposure. The majority of studies have used stimulation with phorbol myristate acetate (PMA) and ionomycin [26,54,58]. Ionomycin increases intracellular Ca^{2+}, mimicking the effect of TCR-induced phospholipase C activation, whereas PMA activates protein kinase C (PKC). This results in polyclonal T-cell activation independent of accessory cells and TCR activation (Figure 11.1). Other studies have utilized anti-CD3/anti-CD28 monoclonal antibodies, which activate T cells by binding the TCR and the CD28 costimulatory molecule, or phytohemagglutinin (PHA), which interacts with CD2 molecules and the TCR [52,53,60,61].

Following immune activation, mRNA levels of early cytokines such as IL-2, IFN-γ, and TNF-α are reported to increase more than 25% within 1 h and reach maximum levels approximately 8 h after anti-CD3 or PHA stimulation [62]. Next, the cytokine expression declines rapidly. This is probably related to the presence of AU-rich elements in the 3′-untranslated regions of cytokine mRNA sequences, targeting the mRNA molecules for rapid degradation [63]. Giese et al. investigated cytokine mRNA levels in response to CsA at 2, 6, and 10 h after PMA/ionomycin stimulation [36]. The cytokine expression was strongly suppressed after 2 h, followed by a rapid recovery and lack of inhibition at 6 h [36]. This corresponds to the findings of Härtel et al. [60] showing a maximum inhibition of *IL2* mRNA at the earliest measurement time point 4 h after anti-CD3/anti-CD28 stimulation [60]. In later studies, ex vivo immune activation has generally been performed by 3-h stimulation with PMA/ionomycin at 37°C [54], allowing early detection of drug responses.

Sommerer et al. reported whole blood samples to be stable for 24 h at 20°C. However, although the relative gene expression remained stable, the absolute mRNA levels declined with time [4]. Importantly, the conservation of mRNA production upon stimulation and the mRNA stability may differ between target and reference genes, implying that further studies are needed to evaluate the stability of sample materials.

11.4.4 RT AND qPCR

RT followed by qPCR has become a powerful molecular biological tool. The method allows quantification over a large dynamic range (greater than eightfold) and represents one of the most sensitive techniques for the detection of low-copy-number molecules, with a theoretical lower limit of detection (LOD) of three copies per PCR [64]. However, the sensitivity and exponential nature of PCR also constitute the major challenges of this technique. Thus, RT-qPCR assays should be carefully designed and validated to ensure reliable results. The Minimum Information for Publication of Quantitative Real-Time PCR Experiments (MIQE) guidelines summarize the minimal information necessary for evaluating qPCR experiments [65].

11.4.5 EXTRACTION OF RNA AND RT

Sample collection, transportation, and processing may have significant impact on mRNA profiles, and rapid stabilization of mRNA is essential to obtain reliable RT-qPCR results. The reported NFAT-regulated gene expression assays have used a chaotropic buffer containing guanidinium thiocyanate (i.e., Lysis/Binding Buffer, Roche, Indianapolis, IN) and dithiothreitol to promote cell lysis and inactivation of ribonucleases before sample storage at −70°C [54]. Extraction of RNA has generally been performed using automated robotic systems [54,58]. This minimizes the manual workload, reduces the risk of contamination, and improves precision of the assay.

According to the MIQE guidelines, presentation of gene expression results must include data on RNA quality and quantity, as well as confirm the absence of PCR inhibitors [65]. However, to date, only limited data on the validation of the RNA quality, quantity, and purity have been reported for NFAT-regulated gene expression assays.

PCR inhibitors may originate from the sample or be introduced during sample preparation steps. Sample additives such as heparin and dithiothreitol have been reported to act as PCR inhibitors at certain concentrations [66,67]. The RT step contributes substantially to the variability of an RT-qPCR assay [65]. Most of the reported analyses so far have used the avian myeloblastosis virus reverse transcriptase (AMV-RT) and an oligo-(dT) priming strategy [54,58]. The cDNA synthesis efficiency may depend on the choice of priming strategy, RT enzyme, buffer, and temperature protocol. Thus, future studies should include a thorough evaluation of RT parameters.

11.4.6 REAL-TIME PCR

Real-time PCR implies monitoring amplicons as they are generated during PCR. This allows analysis of data from the exponential (log) phase of PCR, which is essential for the quantification of gene expression. To date, most studies of cytokine gene expression have utilized SYBR Green I for real-time detection of PCR products [36]. SYBR Green I binds to any double-stranded DNA, representing a nonspecific fluorescent reporter. Alternatively, the generation of amplicons can be monitored using sequence-specific probes, offering an extra level of specificity. However, probe-based detection formats are more expensive than SYBR Green I.

11.4.7 RELATIVE QUANTIFICATION OF GENE EXPRESSION

The kinetics of the exponential phase of PCR can be described by the following equation:

$$N_n = N_0 * (1+E)^n$$

where E is PCR efficiency, and N_0 and N_n are the number of template molecules after 0 (pre-PCR) and n cycles, respectively. The equation provides the basis for qPCR calculations including the variables E and quantification cycle (C_q), also known as crossing point. In theory, the number of amplicons doubles in each PCR cycle ($E = 1$). However, in practice the PCR efficiency is generally lower ($E < 1$) due to suboptimal reaction conditions and the presence of PCR inhibitors. Actual PCR efficiencies can be estimated by generating standard curves of serially diluted templates [65]. The C_q value is defined as the cycle where the fluorescent signal reaches a predefined threshold, thus reflecting a constant number of template copies. The C_q of each sample can be determined by different, more or less user-independent, methods (e.g., second derivative maximum vs. fit point).

Relative quantification of gene expression involves normalization of the target gene concentration to the concentration of one or more reference genes. Simplified, this can be expressed as follows:

$$\text{Relative gene expression} = \frac{\text{concentration of target gene(s)}}{\text{concentration of reference gene(s)}}$$

Studies of cytokine mRNA responses to CNIs have generally focused on the expression of one or more of the target genes *IL2*, *IL4*, *IL10*, *IFNG*, *TNF*, and *CSF2* [52–54,61]. Giese et al. suggested that the combined response of the three target genes *IL2*, *IFNG*, and *CSF2* provided a robust and relatively specific marker of the CNI effect [54], reducing the impact of divergent regulation of individual genes, for example, during disease processes. Consequently, most of the subsequent studies have investigated the combined gene expression response of these three cytokines [26,54,58]. The gene expression analysis is generally performed by quantification of target genes normalized to the expression of one or more reference genes.

The selection of appropriate reference genes is essential to obtain reliable gene expression results. Normalization of the target gene expression to the mRNA level of one or more reference genes compensates for differences in sample amount, RNA recovery, RNA integrity, cDNA synthesis efficiency, and differences in the overall transcriptional activity of the tissues and cells analyzed. Optimal reference genes show stable expression across cell populations, developmental phases, and are not regulated by the experimental treatment. However, no single gene can be defined as a universal reference, and different candidate genes should be validated to find an optimal combination of reference genes for each experimental system. The expression of target genes should be normalized to three reference genes, selected by at least three stability algorithms [68]. So far, the studies using a combination of reference genes have generally normalized the NFAT-dependent target gene expression to the arithmetic mean expression of the reference genes [54,58]. However, the geometric mean of reference genes probably represents a more robust measure, reducing the impact of outliers and compensating for differences in absolute expression levels of the reference genes [69].

The published assays for quantification of NFAT-regulated gene expression have normalized the target gene expression to glyceraldehyde phosphate dehydrogenase (*GAPDH*) [53,61], β-actin (*ACTB*) alone [60], or a combination of *ACTB* and cyclophilin B (*PPIB*) [36]. Giese et al. reported the gene expression of *ACTB* and *PPIB* to be relatively stable during the 3 h of ex vivo immune activation [36]. Importantly, several studies have demonstrated significant regulation of the commonly used reference genes *ACTB* and *GAPDH* in various experimental settings [70], and the selection of reference genes for the determination of NFAT-regulated gene expression should be validated in further studies.

11.4.8 RESIDUAL GENE EXPRESSION

The large interindividual variability in baseline gene expression of cytokines supports the use of an additional level of data normalization. Giese et al. reported results as the relative degree of suppression of the three target genes [36,54]:

$$\text{Relative inhibition} = 100 - \text{Exp}_{\text{peak}}/\text{Exp}_0 \times 100$$

where Exp_0 represents the gene expression pre-dose, and Exp_{peak} represents the gene expression at the maximum drug concentration. Sommerer et al. introduced the term residual gene expression (RGE), where the gene expression at 1.5 or 2 h for tacrolimus and CsA, respectively, is normalized to the level of gene expression before dose [58]:

$$RGE = Exp_{peak} / Exp_0 \times 100$$

The normalization of the gene expression measurements to pre-dose levels corrects for individual variability in baseline cytokine expression levels related to differences in parameters such as immune status, comorbidity, response to surgery, comedication, dialysis, and genetics [71]. Furthermore, the pre-dose normalization allows the establishment of target values independent of the technical platform for gene expression analysis.

11.4.9 ASSAY VALIDATION

RT and qPCR represent a highly sensitive technique. However, the performance depends on thorough assay design, optimization, and validation of all steps.

According to the MIQE guidelines, essential performance characteristics include determination of PCR efficiency, linear dynamic range, LOD, and imprecision [65]. The assay validation should focus on both technical (e.g., PCR replicates) and biological variability (e.g., two different samples from the same individual). The technical imprecision of qPCR depends on the initial template concentration and should therefore be determined over a range of relevant concentrations. Furthermore, information on the interassay imprecision (reproducibility) between laboratories and operators is essential to allow comparisons of gene expression data between study locations [65].

The performance characteristics of the cytokine expression assays reported so far are limited. Giese et al. reported only minor variability in the CsA-mediated gene expression response among eight adult transplant patients with repeated analysis within a 10-month period [36,54]. Sommerer et al. measured NFAT-regulated gene expression twice within an interval from 4 weeks to 12 months and reported an intraindividual variability of 9%, whereas the interindividual variability was 14% among transplant patients receiving CsA doses of 100 mg. The average technical variability (coefficient of variation) of the RT and qPCR steps was less than 11% [58]. Another study of pediatric transplant patients on stable CsA doses reported an intraindividual variability of 22% within a 3-month period [72]. Although the preliminary reports are promising, further studies should include a more comprehensive validation of NFAT-regulated gene expression assays to ensure reliable quantification of CNI responses.

11.4.10 ASSAY SPECIFICITY

The presented NFAT-regulated gene expression is relatively CNI specific and insensitive to the effects of glucocorticoids, mycophenolic acid (MPA), sirolimus, and azathioprine [36]. However, other studies have demonstrated reduced expression of IL-2 during therapy with glucocorticoids and MPA [40,41]. Glucocorticoids regulate a range of transcription factors and have been shown to suppress AP-1 and, to a less degree, NFAT activity [41]. Furthermore, MPA interferes with proinflammatory signaling, including the p38, JNK, and NF-κB pathways [73]. Considering other potential concomitantly used drugs, ciprofloxacin has been reported to increase the expression of *IL2* and counteract the inhibitory action of CsA [74]. The expression of NFAT-regulated cytokines is also influenced by factors such as surgery, therapy with antithymocyte globulin or muromonab-CD3 (brand name: OKT3), and ongoing infections [52]. However, the effect of these latter factors is probably relatively stable at the pre- and post-dose measurements and thereby compensated for by the pre-dose normalization.

The different findings regarding comedication may be related to the study design and different doses of, for example, glucocorticoids. Thus, further studies are needed to characterize the impact of glucocorticoids and other drugs.

11.5 MOLECULAR RESPONSE TO CNI EXPOSURE

To date, only a limited number of studies have characterized cytokine gene expression profiles within tacrolimus or CsA dosing intervals. Investigations in renal and liver transplant patients demonstrated significant inverse correlations between cytokine and CNI levels after dosing. The strongest suppression of cytokines was observed approximately 1.5 and 2h after administration of tacrolimus and CsA, respectively, before gene expression levels recovered rapidly and returned to baseline within 6h post-dose [36,56,57]. Furthermore, cytokine RGE at the time of maximum drug concentration was inversely correlated with CsA C_2 ($r^2 < 0.647$, $P < 0.01$) and tacrolimus $C_{1.5}$ ($r^2 < 0.487$, $P < 0.01$) in different transplant populations [56,72,75–77]. Similar correlations were also observed between RGE and the relative change in drug concentration after dosing (C_{peak}/C_0), whereas there was no correlation with C_0 levels [77]. Importantly, there is a considerable variability in cytokine expression responses between patients, especially in the lower range of drug concentrations [26,60]. Moreover, the correlations were weaker among de novo (rho = 0.487) versus long-term stable CsA-treated transplant patients (rho = 0.771) [71]. Konstandin et al. reported that the correlation between cytokine response and drug concentration was best described using a sigmoid graph, which could be approximated by using two linear regressions. Cardiac transplant recipients with CsA C_2 greater than 575 μg/L showed strong cytokine inhibition (RGE < 14%), whereas concentrations less than 575 μg/L were associated with highly variable gene expression responses (7.4–86.4%) [78]. Other studies reported that pediatric transplant patients with CsA C_2 levels greater than 400 μg/L presented RGE less than 25%, whereas patients with concentrations of 200–250 μg/L demonstrated RGE between 17% and 72% [72,77]. Regarding tacrolimus, an absolute increase in drug concentration ($C_{1.5}–C_0$) of 11.4 μg/L has been reported to differentiate patients with strong (RGE < 30%) versus limited cytokine inhibition [26]. However, the response among patients with low tacrolimus $C_{1.5}$ and increments less than 11.4 μg/L was highly variable (RGE of 0–138%) [26].

The highly variable cytokine responses in the lower range of CsA and tacrolimus concentration may be explained by interindividual differences in the sensitivity to the CNIs. Furthermore, the variability may be related to different sensitivities or exposure to other immunosuppressive drugs (e.g., glucocorticoids). The lack of additional inhibitory effect by increasing CNI levels in the higher concentration range suggests that there may be room for lowering the CNI exposure while still maintaining the immunosuppressive effect. Altogether, this supports the potential of cytokine expression measurements as a tool for further individualization of CNI therapy.

11.5.1 DIFFERENCES IN MOLECULAR RESPONSES OF TACROLIMUS AND CYCLOSPORINE

Patients treated with tacrolimus demonstrated significantly lower cytokine inhibition and higher RGE than patients treated with CsA [76,77]. Long-term stable pediatric liver transplant recipients presented median RGE of 43% (range, 11–88%) and 105% (range, 19–199%) during treatment with CsA and tacrolimus, respectively [77]. Similar findings were observed in adult liver transplant patients (43 ± 29% vs. 79 ± 27%) [76]. Furthermore, conversion from CsA to tacrolimus therapy has been associated with a rapid increase in NFAT-regulated gene expression and a median sevenfold higher RGE [26,52]. The lower inhibitory effect of tacrolimus versus CsA was also observed at the cytokine protein level and by measurement of calcineurin activity [26,79]. Importantly, this did not result in more frequent acute rejection episodes, and tacrolimus seems to provide effective immunosuppression despite limited inhibition of the investigated cytokines [26,76]. This may be related to differences in molar concentrations, binding to immunophilins, alterations of cytokine profiles, cytokine receptor blockade, or additional mechanisms of action.

So far, the studies on NFAT-regulated gene expression in response to tacrolimus have focused on patients treated with the conventional twice-daily tacrolimus formulation. Importantly, an increasing number of transplant patients are treated with the once-daily extended-release formulation of tacrolimus. Despite similar C_0, tacrolimus peak levels have been reported to be lower and time to reach C_{max} longer with the extended-release compared to the conventional formulation [80]. This emphasizes the need for further investigations of NFAT-regulated gene expression during treatment with the extended-release formulation.

11.5.2 INTERINDIVIDUAL VARIABILITY IN MOLECULAR CNI RESPONSES

The variability in cytokine expression levels between patients may be related to differences in the underlying disease, comorbidities, drug therapy, genetic factors, immune status, or the response to surgery. Liver transplant recipients have shown higher pre-dose cytokine levels than those of renal and cardiac transplant patients with similar CsA exposure [36]. This suggests an impact of the other immunosuppressive drugs used among the renal and cardiac transplant patients [36]. Furthermore, measurement of CNI concentrations in whole blood does not necessarily reflect the drug concentrations at the site of action. The relation between whole blood and intracellular concentrations may differ between patients due to drug interactions or genetics with functional impact on drug transporters, binding, or metabolism [81].

The CsA and tacrolimus concentrations have generally been determined by immunochemical assays or liquid chromatography–tandem mass spectrometry (Tables 11.2 and 11.3) [26,54,71]. Different assays present various degrees of cross-reactivity with active and inactive CNI metabolites, and this may be of importance regarding studies of drug exposure versus response.

Table 11.2 Cyclosporine Pharmacodynamics and Clinical Outcome After Transplantation

Authors	Materials and Methods[a]	Results
Giese et al. [36,54]	*Patients* 65 transplanted patients (25 renal, 26 cardiac, 14 liver) Long-term stable phase (2–201 months after transplantation) *Immunosuppression* CsA monotherapy, dual or triple regimens of CsA + glucocorticoids ± AZA/MPA *CsA measurement* EMIT	*Rejection* One patient with recurrent rejection episodes showed no suppression of *CSF2* and only 20% and 40% inhibition of *IL2* and *IFNG*, respectively.
Sommerer et al. [58]	*Patients* 133 adult renal transplant patients, >5 years post-transplant *Immunosuppression* Dual or triple regimens CsA + glucocorticoids ± MPA/AZA *CsA measurement* EMIT	*Infections* Stronger inhibition of cytokine expression among patients with infection versus without infections (13 (2–47)%) vs. 18 (2–50)%, $P = 0.004$) No difference in CsA C_0 and C_2 *Malignancies* Stronger inhibition of cytokines among patients with malignancies versus without: RGE of 11 (2–37)% versus 17 (2–50)%, $P = 0.006$. Patients with non-skin malignancy had lower RGE compared to patients with skin cancer: 4 (2–9)% versus 10 (4–37)%, $P = 0.02$. Higher C_2 among patients with cancer: 579 (341–1103) µg/L versus 507 (158–1228) µg/L, $P < 0.05$. No difference in CsA C_0 ROC curve analysis identified a critical cutoff for an increased risk of infectious and malignant complications at less than 15% RGE.

(Continued)

Authors	Materials and Methods[a]	Results
Konstandin et al. [78]	*Patients* 53 adult heart transplant patients, long-term stable (mean 90 months post-transplant) *Immunosuppression* Dual or triple regimens CsA + MPA/AZA ± glucocorticoids *Gene expression analysis* At the time of enrollment *CsA measurement* EMIT	*Infections* Lower RGE among patients with infections during follow-up (13 vs. 29%, $P < 0.05$) No association between infections and CsA exposure
Sommerer et al. [82]	*Patients* 20 renal transplant patients and 20 pair-matched controls, median greater than 4 years post-transplant *Immunosuppression* CsA + glucocorticoids Study group: cumulative CsA dose reduction of 28.5% *CsA measurement* EMIT *Gene expression analysis* At inclusion, regular intervals during follow-up and at the end of the study	*Rejection* One patient with acute rejection presented RGE of 47% prior to the rejection episode. Median RGE was 20 (7–32)% among patients without rejection. *Renal function* Stable renal function in the CsA-tapered group, while eGFR decreased from median 55 to 40 mL/min ($P < 0.05$) in the control group *Blood pressure* Lower mean arterial pressure in CsA-tapered group versus control group: 100 (77–110) mmHg versus 93 (77–110) mmHg, $P < 0.05$.
Sommerer et al. [89]	*Patients* 55 elderly (>60 years) long-term stable renal transplant patients (>36 months post-transplant) *Immunosuppression* Triple or dual regimens CsA + glucocorticoids ± MPA *CsA measurement* EMIT *Gene expression analysis* At the time of enrollment	*Malignancy* Lower RGE among patients with non-melanoma skin cancer versus patients without skin cancer: 4.9 (0.91–13)% versus 12 (3.3–41)%, $P < 0.001$

(Continued)

Table 11.2 (Continued)

Authors	Materials and Methods[a]	Results
Giese et al. [90]	*Patient* Case report of one patient with recurrent non-melanoma skin cancer 12 years post-transplant *Immunosuppression* CsA + glucocorticoids *CsA measurement* EMIT *Gene expression analysis* At three time points following dose reductions	*Malignancy* Prevention of new malignant lesions by immunosuppressive dose reductions during CsA and RGE monitoring
Billing et al. [72]	*Patients* 45 pediatric renal transplant patients (median 16 years, range 5.4–23 years), >18 months post-transplant *Immunosuppression* CsA + MMF or methylprednisolone *CsA measurement* EMIT	*Infections* Lower RGE among patients with recurrent infections: 18.2 (5.7–37.8)% versus 31.7 (3.6–62)%, $P = 0.012$ No difference in CsA concentrations ROC curve analysis: RGE cutoff of 23% discriminated between patients with and without infections (sensitivity, 71.1%; specificity, 65.4%). *Rejection* Two patients with RGE of 26% and 38% experienced acute rejection 1 month later.
Sommerer et al. [75]	*Patients* 36 renal allograft recipients ≥65 years, median 100 (12–269) months post-transplant Follow-up period: 12 months *Immunosuppression* CsA + glucocorticoids *CsA measurement* EMIT assay *Gene expression analysis* At the time of enrollment	*Infections* Lower RGE among patients with opportunistic infections: 4 (3–13)% versus 11 (3–37)%, $P < 0.05$. No difference in CsA concentrations. *Malignancies* Trend toward lower RGE among patients with malignancies: 7 (3–24)% versus 12 (3–37)%, $P = 0.1$ No difference in CsA concentrations

(Continued)

Authors	Materials and Methods[a]	Results
		Infections and malignancies Three patients with RGE of 3%, 4%, and 10% experienced both infections and malignancies.
		Lower RGE among patients with infections and/or malignancies: 7 (3–24)% versus 12 (3–37)%, $P < 0.05$ No difference in CsA concentration
		Rejection No acute rejection episodes
Herden et al. [71]	*Patients* 20 de novo (<3 months post-transplant) and 20 long-term stable liver transplant patients	*Infections (de novo group)* No significant association between RGE and the occurrence of infection ($P = 0.412$), but a weak correlation between RGE and C-reactive protein (rho = 0.275, $P < 0.01$) and leukocyte count (rho = 0.208, $P < 0.01$)
	Immunosuppression De novo patients Dual, triple, or quadruple regimens of: CsA + prednisolone + basiliximab/ everolimus/MMF Long-term stable patients CsA monotherapy or dual or triple regimens of CsA + MMF/ prednisolone/azathioprine	*Rejection (de novo group)* One patient with RGE of 47% on day 6 after transplantation experienced acute rejection on day 7.
	CsA measurement Liquid chromatography– tandem mass spectrometry	*Long-term group* No episodes of infection or rejection
Billing et al. [77]	*Patients* 33 pediatric liver transplant patients, median 41 (24–200) months post-transplant	*Infection (CsA group)* Lower RGE among patients with recurrent infection versus without: median 27% versus 50%, $P = 0.04$. No difference in CsA concentrations between patients with and without infections
	Immunosuppression CsA ($n = 20$) ± glucocorticoids or tacrolimus ($n = 13$) ± glucocorticoids	ROC curve analysis: RGE cutoff of 18% discriminated between patients with and without infections (sensitivity, 88%; specificity, 50%).
	CsA measurement EMIT	
	Gene expression analysis At the end of the study	

(Continued)

Table 11.2 (Continued)

Authors	Materials and Methods[a]	Results
Steinebrunner et al. [57]	*Patients* 22 de novo liver transplant patients (<12 months post-transplant) *Immunosuppression* CsA ($n = 13$) + glucocorticoids ± MPA or tacrolimus ($n = 9$) + glucocorticoids ± MPA 4 patients were switched from CsA to tacrolimus *Gene expression analysis* Approximately 1 month, 2–3 months, 4–7 months, and 8–12 months post-transplant (all patients) + gene expression profiles 0–12 h post-dose (six patients) *CsA/tacrolimus measurement* EMIT	*Rejection (CsA group)* Higher RGE among patients with rejection ($n = 2$): $39 \pm 0\%$ versus $11 \pm 5\%$, $P < 0.001$ Lower CsA C_2 levels, but no difference in CsA C_0
Steinebrunner et al. [88]	*Patients* 20 liver transplant patients with CMV infection, mean 12 months (1–115 months) post-transplant 40 healthy dose-matched liver transplant controls (see Zahn et al. [76]) *Immunosuppression* CMV group: CsA ($n = 10$) ± MPA or tacrolimus ± MPA ($n = 10$) *Gene expression analysis* Single measurement at the time of acute CMV infection *CsA/tacrolimus measurement*: EMIT	*CsA group* Numerically lower RGE among patients with CMV versus controls: $30 \pm 17\%$ versus $44 \pm 20\%$, $P = 0.067$ Significantly lower *IFNG* expression in patients with CMV versus controls: $26 \pm 17\%$ versus $43 \pm 17\%$, $P = 0.0125$ CsA dosage or concentrations were comparable between groups.

AZA, azathioprine; C_0, pre-dose concentration; C_2, concentration 2 h post-dose; CsA, cyclosporine; EMIT, enzyme multiplication immunoassay technique; MPA, mycophenolic acid; RGE, residual gene expression; ROC, receiver operating characteristic.
[a]Gene expression measurements were performed as described by Giese et al. and Sommerer et al. [54,58].

Table 11.3 Tacrolimus Pharmacodynamics and Clinical Outcome After Transplantation

Authors	Materials and Methods[a]	Results
Sommerer et al. [26]	*Patients* 262 renal transplant patients, 0–214 months post-transplant *Immunosuppression* Tacrolimus + MPA + glucocorticoids ($\leq$20 mg/day) *Gene expression analysis* Single measurement (all patients) + gene expression profiles 0–12 h post-dose (35 patients) *CsA/tacrolimus measurement* EMIT	*Rejection* Higher RGE among patients with rejection: 57 (5–99)% versus 21 (0–138)%, $P < 0.001$ Lower tacrolimus $C_{1.5}$ among patients with rejection: 10 (4–49) μg/L versus 18 (5–67) μg/L, $P < 0.001$ No difference in tacrolimus C_0 *Infections* Lower RGE among patients with infections: 12 (0–68)% versus 32 (3–138)%, $P < 0.001$ Higher tacrolimus $C_{1.5}$ among patients with infection: 22 (5–67) μg/L versus 16 (4–65) μg/L, $P < 0.001$ No difference in tacrolimus C_0 *Renal function* Better renal function among patients with RGE greater than or equal to 30% versus patients with RGE less than 30% (56 (27–113) mL/min vs. 43 (16–98) mL/min, $P < 0.001$)
Sommerer et al. [56]	*Patients* 73 long-term stable renal transplant patients (>6 months post-transplant) *Immunosuppression* Tacrolimus + MPA + glucocorticoids ($\leq$20 mg/day) *Gene expression analysis* Single measurement after enrollment (all patients) + gene expression profiles 0–12 h post-dose (10 patients) *Tacrolimus measurement* EMIT	*Rejection* Higher RGE among patients with rejection versus without rejection: 43 (23–59)% versus 21 (1–84)%, $P < 0.05$ Tacrolimus concentrations were similar among patients with and without infection/viremia or rejection. *Infection/viremia* Lower RGE among patients with CMV viremia: 13 (1–21)% versus 26 (1–84)%, $P = 0.02$

(Continued)

Table 11.3 (Continued)

Authors	Materials and Methods[a]	Results
Zahn et al. [76]	*Patients* 100 adult liver transplant patients, stable phase mean 71 months (12–248 months) post-transplant *Immunosuppression* CsA ($n = 45$) ± MPA or Tacrolimus ($n = 55$) ± MPA *CsA/tacrolimus measurement* EMIT	*Malignancies (tacrolimus group)* Two patients developed non-melanoma skin cancer. Both patients showed RGE below the mean RGE, despite the tacrolimus exposure being lower than the mean concentrations. *Infections* No significant associations between RGE or CNI concentrations and infections
Steinebrunner et al. [57]	*Patients* 22 de novo liver transplant patients (<12 months post-transplant) *Immunosuppression* CsA ($n = 13$) + glucocorticoids ± MPA or Tacrolimus ($n = 9$) + glucocorticoids ± MPA Four patients were switched from CsA to tacrolimus. *Gene expression analysis* At approximately 1 month, 2–3 months, 4–7 months, and 8–12 months post-transplant (all patients) + gene expression profiles 0–12h post-dose (six patients) *CsA/tacrolimus measurement* EMIT	*Rejection (tacrolimus group)* Higher RGE among patients with rejection ($n = 2$): 48 ± 12% versus 18 ± 10%, $P < 0.01$ No difference in tacrolimus concentrations between groups
Steinebrunner et al. [88]	*Patients* 20 liver transplant patients with CMV infection, mean 12 months (1–115 months) post-transplant 40 healthy dose-matched liver transplant controls (see Zahn et al. [76]) *Immunosuppression* CMV group: CsA ($n = 10$) ± MPA or tacrolimus ± MPA ($n = 10$) *Gene expression analysis* Single measurement at the time of acute CMV infection *CsA/tacrolimus measurement* EMIT	*Tacrolimus group* Numerically lower RGE among patients with CMV versus controls: 68 ± 25% versus 84 ± 22%, $P = 0.0769$ Significantly lower *IFNG* expression in patients with CMV versus controls: 61 ± 24% versus 88 ± 29%, $P = 0.0154$ Tacrolimus dosage and $C_{1.5}$ were similar between groups, whereas tacrolimus C_0 was higher among controls (4 vs. 6 µg/L, $P = 0.0276$).

CMV, cytomegalovirus; CsA, cyclosporine; EMIT, enzyme multiplication immunoassay technique; MPA, mycophenolic acid; RGE, residual gene expression.
[a]Gene expression measurements were performed as described by Giese et al. and Sommerer et al. [54,58].

11.5.3 INTRAINDIVIDUAL VARIABILITY IN MOLECULAR CNI RESPONSES

Repeated measurements of NFAT-regulated gene expression among patients with stable CsA doses demonstrated relatively unchanged cytokine responses with time after transplantation [36,58,82]. In contrast, Zahn et al. observed significantly higher RGE during CNI therapy in patients 2–5 years after liver transplantation compared to another cohort 1–2 years after transplantation ($68 \pm 31\%$ vs. $51 \pm 39\%$, $P < 0.05$) [76]. Moreover, the time since transplantation was longer among tacrolimus-treated renal transplant patients with RGE greater than 80%, suggesting reduced cytokine suppression with time after transplantation [26]. Similar findings were also observed among liver transplant recipients with stable CsA and tacrolimus exposure, demonstrating higher RGE levels 8–12 months post-transplant (CsA, $50 \pm 8\%$;tacrolimus, $79 \pm 40\%$) than after 1 month (CsA, $15 \pm 12\%$; tacrolimus, $25 \pm 16\%$) [57]. Herden et al. reported 10-fold higher absolute cytokine expression levels among long-term stable versus de novo liver transplant patients on CsA therapy, whereas the relative degree of cytokine inhibition was similar between the groups [71].

Similar changes in pharmacodynamic response have also been reported considering calcineurin activity. Tumlin et al. reported a significant positive correlation between basal calcineurin activity and time after transplantation among CsA- and tacrolimus-treated patients [83]. Another study investigated calcineurin inhibition during CsA therapy early after transplantation and 5 years later. Despite similar CsA pre-dose concentrations, post-dose levels were reduced and the suppression of calcineurin activity was minimal or absent after 5 years [84].

The change of CNI response with time may be related to alterations in CNI pharmacokinetics, comedication, immune status—or it might be the effect of homeostatic processes during long-term CNI exposure. The bioavailability of CsA and tacrolimus increases after transplantation while steady-state clearance decreases slowly [85,86]. Consequently, CNI dose requirements are generally reduced with time since transplantation. This may be related to the tapering of glucocorticoids, which have been shown to induce the expression of CYP3A enzymes and P-gp (ABCB1) and thereby reduce CNI exposure [86]. Furthermore, inflammation and cytokine levels may influence the CNI pharmacokinetics by regulating the expression of CYP3A enzymes and drug transporters such as P-gp [87].

Altogether, the findings argue for further investigations of NFAT-regulated gene expression in different patient populations, including different immunosuppressive regimens and phases after transplantation.

11.6 CNI PHARMACODYNAMICS AND CLINICAL OUTCOME

To determine the value of pharmacodynamic monitoring based on NFAT-regulated gene expression, the correlation between the cytokine response and clinical outcome needs to be characterized. To date, the majority of studies have investigated patients receiving CsA-based immunosuppression (Table 11.2) [4]. Studies in renal, heart, and liver transplant populations have shown stronger cytokine inhibition among CsA-treated patients with recurrent infections, and RGE cutoff values of 15–23% have been reported to discriminate patients with and without infection [58,72,75,77,78,88]. Importantly, the studies did not observe any associations between infection or viremia and CsA C_0 or C_2 levels [58,72,75,77,78,88]. Furthermore, strong cytokine suppression (RGE < 15%) and age have been reported to be independent risk factors for malignancies among renal transplant patients, and the lowest RGE levels were observed among patients with non-skin malignancies [58,75,89]. A case study of a 67-year-old patient with recurrent non-melanoma skin cancer demonstrated that the development of malignant lesions could be prevented by CsA and glucocorticoid dose reductions during CsA and RGE monitoring [90].

Similar associations have also been reported in tacrolimus-treated patients (Table 11.3). Renal transplant recipients with recurrent infections or CMV viremia demonstrated stronger cytokine inhibition and lower RGE than patients without infectious complication. In contrast, there was no consistent difference in tacrolimus concentrations [26,56,88]. Furthermore, two liver transplant patients with non-melanoma skin cancer demonstrated strong cytokine inhibition despite relatively low tacrolimus C_0 and $C_{1.5}$ levels [76], indicating that cytokine gene expression may be a better marker of over-immunosuppression than tacrolimus concentrations.

On the other hand, low cytokine inhibition has been associated with an increased risk of rejection (Tables 11.2 and 11.3). An early study by Giese et al. reported that a patient with recurrent rejection episodes showed no inhibition of *CSF2* and only minimal suppression of *IL2* and *IFNG* during CsA therapy [36]. Furthermore, studies in different CsA-treated patient populations described relatively low inhibition of NFAT-regulated cytokines (RGE > 26%) in individual patients with rejection (Table 11.2) [57,71,72,82]. Similar results were also reported among tacrolimus-treated renal and liver transplant patients, where the individuals experiencing rejection demonstrated significantly less cytokine suppression 1.5 h after tacrolimus dosing (Table 11.3). In contrast, there was no difference in tacrolimus C_0, and the results regarding tacrolimus $C_{1.5}$ were variable [26,56,57]. Importantly, the association between CNI response and clinical outcome is not consistent between studies, and several patients showed minimal or no inhibition of NFAT-regulated cytokines without developing acute rejection [26,76].

Cytokine responses during CNI therapy have also been associated with renal function and blood pressure. Renal transplant patients with CsA dose reductions, and a subsequent increase of RGE, demonstrated higher estimated GFR and lower blood pressure than did patients on stable CsA doses (Table 11.2) [82]. Similarly, tacrolimus-treated patients with RGE of 30% or greater demonstrated better renal function compared to patients with RGE less than 30% (Table 11.3) [26]. However, the association between NFAT-regulated gene expression and nephrotoxicity is not consistent between studies, suggesting that the development of nephrotoxicity may be related to calcineurin–NFAT-independent pathways (e.g., NOS, COX-2, TGF-β, and MAPK), or that such toxicity may be more closely associated with the local CNI exposure [58].

Based on the initial clinical findings among long-term stable renal transplant patients treated with CsA, an optimal level of RGE has been suggested to be 20–30% [4]. However, the proposed range for CsA may not be applicable in other patient populations and tacrolimus-based immunosuppressive regimens. The clinical studies of NFAT-regulated gene expression involve different patient populations with various diagnoses, types of transplantation, immune status, immunosuppressive regimens, and comedication. Moreover, the time between the gene expression measurement and the observed clinical events varies. In some reports, the gene expression analysis was performed at single time points at the inclusion or end of the study, whereas other studies involved repeated gene expression measurements (Tables 11.2 and 11.3). The observed changes in gene expression response with time indicate that single gene expression measurements may not be sufficient to predict the pharmacodynamic response [57,76]. Furthermore, immunological complications may be more closely related to the overall immunosuppression than to CNI effects alone. Currently, there is only limited knowledge of the impact of concomitant immunosuppressive drugs on NFAT-regulated gene expression. Altogether, this emphasizes the need for further investigations of NFAT-regulated gene expression in different patient populations, including relevant immunosuppressive regimens and time periods after transplantation.

The efficacy and safety of tacrolimus dose adjustments based on NFAT-regulated gene expression are currently being investigated in a randomized controlled trial. The planned enrollment is 40 renal transplant patients divided into a standard of care group and an experimental group in which tacrolimus doses are adjusted if RGE is less than 15% or greater than 80% (ClinicalTrials.gov identifier NCT01771705; https://clinicaltrials.gov/ct2/show/NCT01771705). The results of the ongoing study may provide valuable knowledge considering the clinical potential of pharmacodynamic monitoring based on NFAT-regulated gene expression.

11.7 PERSPECTIVES

The investigations so far indicate that NFAT-regulated gene expression holds promise as an assay for pharmacodynamic monitoring of the CNIs. To take this further as a tool for individualized dosing, prospective clinical studies are needed that provide evidence for the correlation between CNI dosing based on NFAT-regulated gene expression and clinical outcome. Such studies will require inclusion of a large number of patients and should be performed in several transplantation centers. In this context, the following subjects should be addressed:

- Reported results must be harmonized between laboratories. Assays should be established with sufficient standardization and robustness for comparison or pooling of results. The principle of calculating the RGE at a time point within the dosing interval, relative to the pre-dose value, will eliminate much of the potential variability between assays. However, considerations about standardization should particularly focus on sample timing and materials, ex vivo stimulation of cells, and selection of reference genes.

- Adjustments for practicability of the assay will be requested. Although hands-on time for the assay may be acceptable, the collection of a sample within the dosing interval and the need for mitogen stimulation for several hours implies that it will be difficult to report the results within the same day. One may ask whether this is crucial or not, and in a setting in which occasional pharmacodynamic assessments are combined with more frequent measurements of drug concentrations, a response lag of 1 day might be fully acceptable.

- The NFAT-regulated gene expression differs between transplant populations. Therefore, therapeutic ranges of the RGE should be investigated and documented according to the kind of transplantation, comorbidity, immunogenic risk profile, immunosuppressive drug regimen and exposure, and time since transplantation.

- How to adjust the CNI dose based on the RGE? It should be noted that the development of RGE as a pharmacodynamic biomarker relies on simultaneous pharmacokinetic monitoring that ensures trough values within rather narrow ranges. Thus, the interpretation of the RGE and also adjustment of the CNI dosing has to be performed in relation to the drug exposure, keeping in mind the nonlinear nature of the pharmacodynamic response. A change in CNI dose will influence both C_0 and $C_{1.5/2}$, and the influence on the RGE has to be carefully assessed in order to make recommendations for dosing strategies.

- Could other target genes be of relevance to the CNI efficacy and toxicity? The combined gene expression of *IL2*, *IFNG*, and *CSF2* has been selected and extensively investigated as a response marker for CNIs. However, the possibility for other genes should not be ruled out. When performing studies on the NFAT-regulated gene expression in CNI-treated patients, it would be advantageous to include parallel investigations of other genes, NFAT-regulated or not, that may be identified as supplementary markers of the CNI response.

- What kind of outcome parameters could be improved by the introduction of pharmacodynamic monitoring such as the NFAT-regulated gene expression? Although the incidence of acute rejection episodes has decreased in recent years, chronic allograft damage is still a limiting factor for long-term graft survival. Lifelong immunosuppression is still the only option for most transplant recipients, and even with the currently lower doses, adverse effects and long-term risks and complications are significant to the degree that the quality of life and life expectancy are reduced. This applies to general effects of immunosuppression, such as infections and malignancies, as well as drug-specific effects such as diabetes (new-onset diabetes after transplantation), lipidemia, nephrotoxicity, and other risks affecting life expectancy. Hence, for the transplanted patient, the most interesting achievement of improved individualization would be that the immunosuppressant doses could safely be reduced. In this respect, the required prospective studies become even more challenging because they will need to assess such long-term parameters.

11.8 CONCLUSIONS

NFAT-regulated gene expression holds promise as a potential useful pharmacodynamic marker for CNIs. Such an assay could be applied together with pharmacokinetic monitoring in order to further individualize the dosing of immunosuppressive drugs, reducing doses to a level that minimizes the long-term adverse effects and complications of such therapy. In order to obtain this, harmonization of the assays is required, and the impact on outcome must be documented, ideally in prospective controlled intervention studies.

REFERENCES

[1] Kapturczak MH, Meier-Kriesche HU, Kaplan B. Pharmacology of calcineurin antagonists. Transplant Proc 2004;36:25S–32S.

[2] Ekberg H, Tedesco-Silva H, Demirbas A, Vitko S, et al. Reduced exposure to calcineurin inhibitors in renal transplantation. N Engl J Med 2007;357:2562–75.

[3] de Jonge H, Naesens M, Kuypers DR. New insights into the pharmacokinetics and pharmacodynamics of the calcineurin inhibitors and mycophenolic acid: possible consequences for therapeutic drug monitoring in solid organ transplantation. Ther Drug Monit 2009;31:416–35.

[4] Sommerer C, Meuer S, Zeier M, Giese T. Calcineurin inhibitors and NFAT-regulated gene expression. Clin Chim Acta 2012;413:1379–86.

[5] Macian F, Lopez-Rodriguez C, Rao A. Partners in transcription: NFAT and AP-1. Oncogene 2001;20:2476–89.

[6] Palkowitsch L, Marienfeld U, Brunner C, Eitelhuber A, et al. The Ca^{2+}-dependent phosphatase calcineurin controls the formation of the Carma1-Bcl10-Malt1 complex during T cell receptor-induced NF-kappaB activation. J Biol Chem 2011;286:7522–34.

[7] Vafadari R, Kraaijeveld R, Weimar W, Baan CC. Tacrolimus inhibits NF-kappaB activation in peripheral human T cells. PLoS One 2013;8:e60784.

[8] Matsuda S, Shibasaki F, Takehana K, Mori H, et al. Two distinct action mechanisms of immunophilin-ligand complexes for the blockade of T-cell activation. EMBO Rep 2000;1:428–34.

[9] Vafadari R, Hesselink DA, Cadogan MM, Weimar W, et al. Inhibitory effect of tacrolimus on p38 mitogen-activated protein kinase signaling in kidney transplant recipients measured by whole-blood phosphospecific flow cytometry. Transplantation 2012;93:1245–51.

[10] Karin M. The regulation of AP-1 activity by mitogen-activated protein kinases. J Biol Chem 1995;270:16483–6.

[11] Shin GT, Khanna A, Ding R, Sharma VK, et al. *In vivo* expression of transforming growth factor-beta1 in humans: stimulation by cyclosporine. Transplantation 1998;65:313–8.

[12] Khanna A, Cairns V, Hosenpud JD. Tacrolimus induces increased expression of transforming growth factor-beta1 in mammalian lymphoid as well as nonlymphoid cells. Transplantation 1999;67:614–9.

[13] Goppelt-Struebe M, Esslinger B, Kunzendorf U. Failure of cyclosporin A to induce transforming growth factor beta (TGF-beta) synthesis in activated peripheral blood lymphocytes. Clin Transplant 2003;17:20–5.

[14] van Rossum HH, Romijn FP, Sellar KJ, Smit NP, et al. Variation in leukocyte subset concentrations affects calcineurin activity measurement: implications for pharmacodynamic monitoring strategies. Clin Chem 2008;54:517–24.

[15] Heidt S, Roelen DL, Eijsink C, Eikmans M, et al. Calcineurin inhibitors affect B cell antibody responses indirectly by interfering with T cell help. Clin Exp Immunol 2010;159:199–207.

[16] Morteau O, Blundell S, Chakera A, Bennett S, et al. Renal transplant immunosuppression impairs natural killer cell function *in vitro* and *in vivo*. PLoS One 2010;5:e13294.

[17] Harrison CA, Bastan R, Peirce MJ, Munday MR, et al. Role of calcineurin in the regulation of human lung mast cell and basophil function by cyclosporine and FK506. Br J Pharmacol 2007;150:509–18.

[18] Vandewalle A, Tourneur E, Bens M, Chassin C, et al. Calcineurin/NFAT signaling and innate host defence: a role for NOD1-mediated phagocytic functions. Cell Commun Signal 2014;12:8.

[19] Hamalainen M, Lahti A, Moilanen E. Calcineurin inhibitors, cyclosporin A and tacrolimus inhibit expression of inducible nitric oxide synthase in colon epithelial and macrophage cell lines. Eur J Pharmacol 2002;448:239–44.

[20] Hocherl K, Dreher F, Vitzthum H, Kohler J, et al. Cyclosporine A suppresses cyclooxygenase-2 expression in the rat kidney. J Am Soc Nephrol 2002;13:2427–36.

[21] Hocherl K, Kees F, Kramer BK, Kurtz A. Cyclosporine A attenuates the natriuretic action of loop diuretics by inhibition of renal COX-2 expression. Kidney Int 2004;65: 2071–80.

[22] White M, Cantin B, Haddad H, Kobashigawa JA, et al. Cardiac signaling molecules and plasma biomarkers after cardiac transplantation: impact of tacrolimus versus cyclosporine. J Heart Lung Transplant 2013;32:1222–32.

[23] Kino T, Hatanaka H, Miyata S, Inamura N, et al. FK-506, a novel immunosuppressant isolated from a *Streptomyces*. II. Immunosuppressive effect of FK-506 *in vitro*. J Antibiot (Tokyo) 1987;40:1256–65.

[24] Fukudo M, Yano I, Masuda S, Fukatsu S, et al. Pharmacodynamic analysis of tacrolimus and cyclosporine in living-donor liver transplant patients. Clin Pharmacol Ther 2005;78:168–81.

[25] Fukudo M, Yano I, Masuda S, Okuda M, et al. Distinct inhibitory effects of tacrolimus and cyclosporin a on calcineurin phosphatase activity. J Pharmacol Exp Ther 2005;312:816–25.

[26] Sommerer C, Zeier M, Meuer S, Giese T. Individualized monitoring of nuclear factor of activated T cells-regulated gene expression in FK506-treated kidney transplant recipients. Transplantation 2010;89:1417–23.

[27] Jiang H, Wynn C, Pan F, Ebbs A, et al. Tacrolimus and cyclosporine differ in their capacity to overcome ongoing allograft rejection as a result of their differential abilities to inhibit interleukin-10 production. Transplantation 2002;73:1808–17.

[28] Jordan ML, Naraghi R, Shapiro R, Smith D, et al. Tacrolimus rescue therapy for renal allograft rejection—five-year experience. Transplantation 1997;63:223–8.

[29] Jiang H, Kobayashi M. Differences between cyclosporin A and tacrolimus in organ transplantation. Transplant Proc 1999;31:1978–80.

[30] Almawi WY, Melemedjian OK. Clinical and mechanistic differences between FK506 (tacrolimus) and cyclosporin A. Nephrol Dial Transplant 2000;15:1916–8.

[31] Jiang H, Yang XF, Soriano R, Fujitsu T, et al. Inhibition of IL-10 by FK 506 may be responsible for overcoming ongoing allograft rejection in the rat. Transplant Proc 1999;31:1203–5.

[32] Kung L, Halloran PF. Immunophilins may limit calcineurin inhibition by cyclosporine and tacrolimus at high drug concentrations. Transplantation 2000;70:327–35.

[33] Barraclough KA, Staatz CE, Isbel NM, McTaggart SJ. Review: pharmacodynamic monitoring of immunosuppression in kidney transplantation. Nephrology (Carlton) 2010;15:522–32.

[34] Sanquer S, Amrein C, Grenet D, Guillemain R, et al. Expression of calcineurin activity after lung transplantation: a 2-year follow-up. PLoS One 2013;8:e59634.

[35] Maguire O, Tornatore KM, O'Loughlin KL, Venuto RC, et al. Nuclear translocation of nuclear factor of activated T cells (NFAT) as a quantitative pharmacodynamic parameter for tacrolimus. Cytometry A 2013;83:1096–104.

[36] Giese T, Zeier M, Schemmer P, Uhl W, et al. Monitoring of NFAT-regulated gene expression in the peripheral blood of allograft recipients: a novel perspective toward individually optimized drug doses of cyclosporine A. Transplantation 2004;77:339–44.

[37] Pena JA, Titus L, Jackson J, Kirk AD, et al. Differential regulation of calcineurin isoforms in transplant patients: a new look at an old problem. Transplantation 2013;96:239–44.

[38] Perrino BA, Wilson AJ, Ellison P, Clapp LH. Substrate selectivity and sensitivity to inhibition by FK506 and cyclosporin A of calcineurin heterodimers composed of the alpha or beta catalytic subunit. Eur J Biochem 2002;269:3540–8.

[39] Macian F. NFAT proteins: key regulators of T-cell development and function. Nat Rev Immunol 2005;5:472–84.

[40] Millan O, Brunet M, Campistol JM, Faura A, et al. Pharmacodynamic approach to immunosuppressive therapies using calcineurin inhibitors and mycophenolate mofetil. Clin Chem 2003;49:1891–9.

[41] Paliogianni F, Raptis A, Ahuja SS, Najjar SM, et al. Negative transcriptional regulation of human interleukin 2 (IL-2) gene by glucocorticoids through interference with nuclear transcription factors AP-1 and NF-AT. J Clin Invest 1993;91:1481–9.

[42] Stein CM, Murray JJ, Wood AJ. Inhibition of stimulated interleukin-2 production in whole blood: a practical measure of cyclosporine effect. Clin Chem 1999;45:1477–84.

[43] Sindhi R, LaVia MF, Paulling E, McMichael J, et al. Stimulated response of peripheral lymphocytes may distinguish cyclosporine effect in renal transplant recipients receiving a cyclosporine + rapamycin regimen. Transplantation 2000;69:432–6.

[44] Grinyo JM, Cruzado JM, Millan O, Caldes A, et al. Low-dose cyclosporine with mycophenolate mofetil induces similar calcineurin activity and cytokine inhibition as does standard-dose cyclosporine in stable renal allografts. Transplantation 2004;78:1400–3.

[45] Ahmed M, Venkataraman R, Logar AJ, Rao AS, et al. Quantitation of immunosuppression by tacrolimus using flow cytometric analysis of interleukin-2 and interferon-gamma inhibition in CD8(−) and CD8(+) peripheral blood T cells. Ther Drug Monit 2001;23:354–62.

[46] Hodge G, Hodge S, Reynolds P, Holmes M. Intracellular cytokines in blood T cells in lung transplant patients—a more relevant indicator of immunosuppression than drug levels. Clin Exp Immunol 2005;139:159–64.

[47] Stalder M, Birsan T, Holm B, Haririfar M, et al. Quantification of immunosuppression by flow cytometry in stable renal transplant recipients. Ther Drug Monit 2003;25:22–7.

[48] Boleslawski E, Conti F, Sanquer S, Podevin P, et al. Defective inhibition of peripheral CD8+ T cell IL-2 production by anti-calcineurin drugs during acute liver allograft rejection. Transplantation 2004;77:1815–20.

[49] Akoglu B, Kriener S, Martens S, Herrmann E, et al. Interleukin-2 in CD8+ T cells correlates with Banff score during organ rejection in liver transplant recipients. Clin Exp Med 2009;9:259–62.

[50] Millan O, Rafael-Valdivia L, Torrademe E, Lopez A, et al. Intracellular IFN-gamma and IL-2 expression monitoring as surrogate markers of the risk of acute rejection and personal drug response in *de novo* liver transplant recipients. Cytokine 2013;61:556–64.

[51] Tary-Lehmann M, Hricik DE, Justice AC, Potter NS, et al. Enzyme-linked immunosorbent assay spot detection of interferon-gamma and interleukin 5-producing cells as a predictive marker for renal allograft failure. Transplantation 1998;66:219–24.

[52] Zucker C, Zucker K, Asthana D, Carreno M, et al. Longitudinal induced IL-2 mRNA monitoring in renal transplant patients immunosuppressed with cyclosporine and in unmodified canine renal transplant rejection. Hum Immunol 1996;45:1–12.

[53] Hartel C, Fricke L, Schumacher N, Kirchner H, et al. Delayed cytokine mRNA expression kinetics after T-lymphocyte costimulation: a quantitative measure of the efficacy of cyclosporin A-based immunosuppression. Clin Chem 2002;48:2225–31.

[54] Giese T, Zeier M, Meuer S. Analysis of NFAT-regulated gene expression *in vivo*: a novel perspective for optimal individualized doses of calcineurin inhibitors. Nephrol Dial Transplant 2004;19(Suppl. 4) iv55–60.

[55] Halloran PF, Helms LM, Kung L, Noujaim J. The temporal profile of calcineurin inhibition by cyclosporine *in vivo*. Transplantation 1999;68:1356–61.

[56] Sommerer C, Zeier M, Czock D, Schnitzler P, et al. Pharmacodynamic disparities in tacrolimus-treated patients developing cytomegalus virus viremia. Ther Drug Monit 2011;33:373–9.

[57] Steinebrunner N, Sandig C, Sommerer C, Hinz U, et al. Pharmacodynamic monitoring of nuclear factor of activated T cell-regulated gene expression in liver allograft recipients on immunosuppressive therapy with calcineurin inhibitors in the course of time and correlation with acute rejection episodes—a prospective study. Ann Transplant 2014;19:32–40.

[58] Sommerer C, Konstandin M, Dengler T, Schmidt J, et al. Pharmacodynamic monitoring of cyclosporine A in renal allograft recipients shows a quantitative relationship between immunosuppression and the occurrence of recurrent infections and malignancies. Transplantation 2006;82:1280–5.

[59] Mallone R, Mannering SI, Brooks-Worrell BM, Durinovic-Bello I, et al. Isolation and preservation of peripheral blood mononuclear cells for analysis of islet antigen-reactive T cell responses: position statement of the T-Cell Workshop Committee of the Immunology of Diabetes Society. Clin Exp Immunol 2011;163:33–49.

[60] Hartel C, Schumacher N, Fricke L, Ebel B, et al. Sensitivity of whole-blood T lymphocytes in individual patients to tacrolimus (FK 506): impact of interleukin-2 mRNA expression as surrogate measure of immunosuppressive effect. Clin Chem 2004;50:141–51.

[61] El-Safa EA, Fredericks S, MacPhee I, Holt DW, et al. Paradoxical response to tacrolimus assessed by interleukin-2 gene expression. Transplant Proc 2006;38:3327–30.

[62] Fan J, Nishanian P, Breen EC, McDonald M, et al. Cytokine gene expression in normal human lymphocytes in response to stimulation. Clin Diagn Lab Immunol 1998;5:335–40.

[63] Barreau C, Paillard L, Osborne HB. AU-rich elements and associated factors: are there unifying principles? Nucleic Acids Res 2005;33:7138–50.

[64] Bustin SA, Nolan T. Pitfalls of quantitative real-time reverse-transcription polymerase chain reaction. J Biomol Tech 2004;15:155–66.

[65] Bustin SA, Benes V, Garson JA, Hellemans J, et al. The MIQE guidelines: minimum information for publication of quantitative real-time PCR experiments. Clin Chem 2009;55:611–22.

[66] Bai X, Fischer S, Keshavjee S, Liu M. Heparin interference with reverse transcriptase polymerase chain reaction of RNA extracted from lungs after ischemia-reperfusion. Transpl Int 2000;13:146–50.

[67] Schrader C, Schielke A, Ellerbroek L, Johne R. PCR inhibitors—occurrence, properties and removal. J Appl Microbiol 2012;113:1014–26.

[68] Jacob F, Guertler R, Naim S, Nixdorf S, et al. Careful selection of reference genes is required for reliable performance of RT-qPCR in human normal and cancer cell lines. PLoS One 2013;8:e59180.

[69] Bengtsson M, Stahlberg A, Rorsman P, Kubista M. Gene expression profiling in single cells from the pancreatic islets of Langerhans reveals lognormal distribution of mRNA levels. Genome Res 2005;15:1388–92.

[70] Dundas J, Ling M. Reference genes for measuring mRNA expression. Theory Biosci 2012;131:215–23.

[71] Herden U, Kromminga A, Hagel C, Hartleb J, et al. Monitoring of nuclear factor of activated T-cell-regulated gene expression in de novo and long-term liver transplant recipients treated with cyclosporine A. Ther Drug Monit 2011;33:185–91.

[72] Billing H, Giese T, Sommerer C, Zeier M, et al. Pharmacodynamic monitoring of cyclosporine A by NFAT-regulated gene expression and the relationship with infectious complications in pediatric renal transplant recipients. Pediatr Transplant 2010;14:844–51.

[73] Andreucci M, Faga T, Lucisano G, Uccello F, et al. Mycophenolic acid inhibits the phosphorylation of NF-kappaB and JNKs and causes a decrease in IL-8 release in H_2O_2-treated human renal proximal tubular cells. Chem Biol Interact 2010;185:253–62.

[74] Riesbeck K, Gullberg M, Forsgren A. Evidence that the antibiotic ciprofloxacin counteracts cyclosporine-dependent suppression of cytokine production. Transplantation 1994;57:267–72.

[75] Sommerer C, Schnitzler P, Meuer S, Zeier M, et al. Pharmacodynamic monitoring of cyclosporin A reveals risk of opportunistic infections and malignancies in renal transplant recipients 65 years and older. Ther Drug Monit 2011;33:694–8.

[76] Zahn A, Schott N, Hinz U, Stremmel W, et al. Immunomonitoring of nuclear factor of activated T cells-regulated gene expression: the first clinical trial in liver allograft recipients. Liver Transpl 2011;17:466–73.

[77] Billing H, Breil T, Schmidt J, Tonshoff B, et al. Pharmacodynamic monitoring by residual NFAT-regulated gene expression in stable pediatric liver transplant recipients. Pediatr Transplant 2012;16:187–94.

[78] Konstandin MH, Sommerer C, Doesch A, Zeier M, et al. Pharmacodynamic cyclosporine A-monitoring: relation of gene expression in lymphocytes to cyclosporine blood levels in cardiac allograft recipients. Transpl Int 2007;20:1036–43.

[79] Koefoed-Nielsen PB, Karamperis N, Hojskov C, Poulsen JH, et al. The calcineurin activity profiles of cyclosporin and tacrolimus are different in stable renal transplant patients. Transpl Int 2006;19:821–7.

[80] Barraclough KA, Isbel NM, Johnson DW, Campbell SB, et al. Once- versus twice-daily tacrolimus: are the formulations truly equivalent? Drugs 2011;71:1561–77.

[81] Capron A, Mourad M, De Meyer M, De Pauw L, et al. CYP3A5 and ABCB1 polymorphisms influence tacrolimus concentrations in peripheral blood mononuclear cells after renal transplantation. Pharmacogenomics 2010;11:703–14.

[82] Sommerer C, Giese T, Schmidt J, Meuer S, et al. Ciclosporin A tapering monitored by NFAT-regulated gene expression: a new concept of individual immunosuppression. Transplantation 2008;85:15–21.

[83] Tumlin JA, Roberts BR, Kokko KE, El Minshawy O, et al. T-cell receptor-stimulated calcineurin activity is inhibited in isolated T cells from transplant patients. J Pharmacol Exp Ther 2009;330:602–7.

[84] Mortensen DM, Koefoed-Nielsen PB, Jorgensen KA. Calcineurin activity in tacrolimus-treated renal transplant patients early after and 5 years after transplantation. Transplant Proc 2006;38:2651–3.

[85] Buchler M, Chadban S, Cole E, Midtvedt K, et al. Evolution of the absorption profile of cyclosporine A in renal transplant recipients: a longitudinal study of the *de novo* and maintenance phases. Nephrol Dial Transplant 2006;21:197–202.

[86] Kuypers DR, Claes K, Evenepoel P, Maes B, et al. Time-related clinical determinants of long-term tacrolimus pharmacokinetics in combination therapy with mycophenolic acid and corticosteroids: a prospective study in one hundred *de novo* renal transplant recipients. Clin Pharmacokinet 2004;43:741–62.

[87] Zidek Z, Anzenbacher P, Kmonickova E. Current status and challenges of cytokine pharmacology. Br J Pharmacol 2009;157:342–61.

[88] Steinebrunner N, Sandig C, Sommerer C, Hinz U, et al. Reduced residual gene expression of nuclear factor of activated T cells-regulated genes correlates with the risk of cytomegalovirus infection after liver transplantation. Transpl Infect Dis 2014;16:379–86.

[89] Sommerer C, Hartschuh W, Enk A, Meuer S, et al. Pharmacodynamic immune monitoring of NFAT-regulated genes predicts skin cancer in elderly long-term renal transplant recipients. Clin Transplant 2008;22:549–54.

[90] Giese T, Sommerer C, Zeier M, Meuer S. Monitoring immunosuppression with measures of NFAT decreases cancer incidence. Clin Immunol 2009;132:305–11.

Index

Note: Page numbers followed by "*b*," "*f*," and "*t*" refer to boxes, figures, and tables, respectively.

291

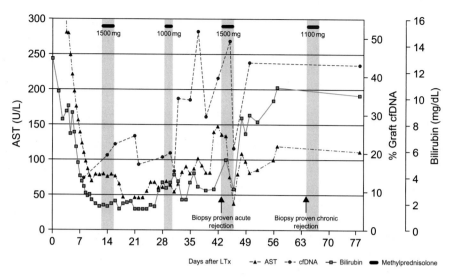

FIGURE 7.2

LTx patient with several rejection episodes. GcfDNA, AST, and bilirubin values are shown over time (days) post LTx. Methylprednisolone doses and tacrolimus target concentrations (shaded area) are also indicated. Results show that during rejection episodes, there was an increase in GcfDNA days before increases were seen in AST or bilirubin.

With permission from Beck et al. [50].

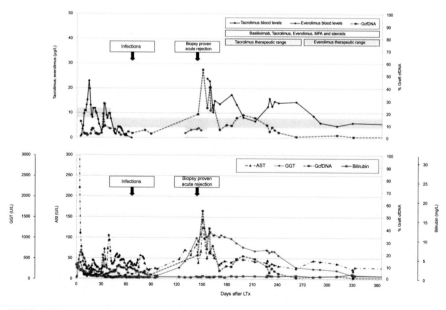

FIGURE 7.3

GcfDNA, LFTs, and ISD concentrations are shown for a patient who had an infection that resulted in decreases in ISD dosing, which led to an acute rejection episode that responded to increased ISD exposure.

Adapted from Kanzow [51].

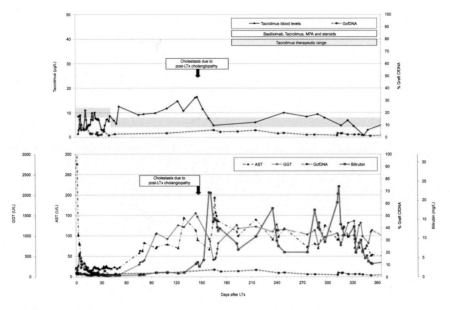

FIGURE 7.4

GcfDNA, LFTs, and ISD concentrations in a HCV+ patient who had an episode of cholestasis post-LTx. The therapeutic (target) ranges used to adjust ISD dosing are shown as shaded areas.

Adapted from Kanzow [51].

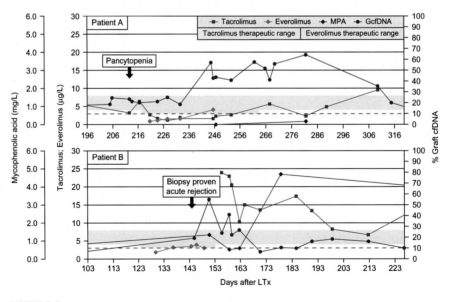

FIGURE 7.8

GcfDNA, LFTs, and ISD in patients whose IS therapies were switched.

Adapted from Kanzow [51].